Musculoskeletal Systems: Injuries and Disorders

Musculoskeletal Systems: Injuries and Disorders

Edited by Benjamin West

hayle medical

New York

Hayle Medical,
750 Third Avenue, 9th Floor,
New York, NY 10017, USA

Visit us on the World Wide Web at:
www.haylemedical.com

ISBN: 978-1-63241-539-4

Cataloging-in-Publication Data

Musculoskeletal systems : injuries and disorders / edited by Benjamin West.
p. cm.
Includes bibliographical references and index.
ISBN 978-1-63241-539-4
1. Musculoskeletal system--Wounds and injuries. 2. Musculoskeletal system--Diseases.
I. West, Benjamin.
RC925.5 .M87 2019
617.47--dc23

Table of Contents

Preface

It is often said that books are a boon to mankind. They document every progress and pass on the knowledge from one generation to the other. They play a crucial role in our lives. Thus I was both excited and nervous while editing this book. I was pleased by the thought of being able to make a mark but I was also nervous to do it right because the future of students depends upon it. Hence, I took a few months to research further into the discipline, revise my knowledge and also explore some more aspects. Post this process, I begun with the editing of this book.

The musculoskeletal system refers to the muscular and skeletal systems of humans that facilitate the support, stability and movement of the body. It also provides protection to the vital organs of the body. The musculoskeletal system comprises of muscles, bones of the skeleton, tendons, joints, ligaments and other connective tissue that binds tissues and organs together. Many diseases and disorders affect the system. Musculoskeletal disorders can arise due to sudden exertion, repetitive strain or awkward posture. Some examples are carpal tunnel syndrome, tendinitis, tension neck syndrome, epicondylitis, etc. Musculoskeletal injury refers to the damage to the musculoskeletal system, and can include arthritis, rheumatic diseases, etc. This book is a valuable compilation of topics, ranging from the basic to the most complex advancements in the treatment of musculoskeletal injuries and disorders. It includes contributions of experts and scientists, which will provide innovative insights in this domain. It is an essential guide for both academicians, orthopedic surgeons, physical therapists, physiatrists and students who wish to pursue this discipline further.

I thank my publisher with all my heart for considering me worthy of this unparalleled opportunity and for showing unwavering faith in my skills. I would also like to thank the editorial team who worked closely with me at every step and contributed immensely towards the successful completion of this book. Last but not the least, I wish to thank my friends and colleagues for their support.

Editor

1

Development of the "Treatment beliefs in knee and hip OsteoArthritis (TOA)" questionnaire

Ellen M. H. Selten[1*], Johanna E. Vriezekolk[1], Henk J. Schers[2], Marc W. Nijhof[3], Willemijn H. van der Laan[4], Roelien G. van der Meulen-Dilling[5], Rinie Geenen[6] and Cornelia H. M. van den Ende[1]

Abstract

Background: Use of conservative treatment modalities in osteoarthritis (OA) is suboptimal, which appears to be partly due to patients' beliefs about treatments. The aim of this study was to develop a research instrument assessing patients' beliefs about various treatment modalities of hip and knee OA: the 'Treatment beliefs in OA (TOA) questionnaire'.

Methods: The item pool that was retrieved from interviews with patients and healthcare providers comprised beliefs regarding five treatment modalities: physical activity, pain medication, physiotherapy, injections and arthroplasty. After an extensive selection procedure, a draft questionnaire with 200 items was constructed. Descriptive analyses and exploratory factor analyses with oblique rotation were conducted for each treatment modality separately to decide upon the final questionnaire. Internal consistency and test-retest reliability were determined.

Results: The final questionnaire comprised 60 items. It was completed by 351 patients with knee or hip OA. Each of the five treatment modalities yielded a two factor solution with 37% to 51% explained variance and high face validity. Factor I included 'positive treatment beliefs' and factor II 'negative treatment beliefs'. Internal consistency (Cronbach α's from 0.72 to 0.87) and test-retest reliability (i.e. intraclass correlation coefficient from 0.66–0.88; standard error of measurement from 0.06–0.11) were satisfactory to good.

Conclusions: The TOA questionnaire is the first questionnaire assessing positive and negative treatment beliefs regarding five treatment modalities for knee and hip OA. The instrument will help to understand whether and to what extent treatment beliefs influence treatment choices.

Keywords: Osteoarthritis, Knee, Hip, Treatment beliefs, Measurement instrument

Background

Osteoarthritis (OA) of the knee and hip causes pain, stiffness and decreased physical functioning [1]. Because OA cannot be cured, treatment is directed towards the reduction of symptoms, improvement of quality of life, and prevention of progression. Treatment options can be classified into conservative treatment modalities, such as lifestyle education, pain medication and physiotherapy, and surgical treatment modalities, such as an arthroplasty and osteotomy [1].

Several national and international recommendations and guidelines for the management of hip and knee OA recommend that patients first are provided with conservative treatment options, and that they are referred to surgical treatment only when conservative treatment does not lead to adequate pain relief and functional improvement [2–4]. However, in clinical practice, health care utilisation is suboptimal in terms of underutilisation of conservative treatment modalities [5–7] and an increased use of surgical treatment modalities [8]. This is undesirable because surgery does not always result in

* Correspondence: e.selten@maartenskliniek.nl
[1]Department of Rheumatology, Sint Maartenskliniek, Sint Maartenskliniek, P.O. Box 9011, 6500, GM, Nijmegen, The Netherlands
Full list of author information is available at the end of the article

good outcomes and pain reduction [9, 10] and may lead to higher health care costs.

Amongst others, a possible pathway to optimise the imbalanced use of treatment options is through understanding patients' beliefs about treatment modalities of knee and hip OA [11, 12]. Patients' beliefs influence health-related behaviour as postulated by health beliefs models, such as the Theory of Planned Behaviour [13]. Previous research found that patients' beliefs about the efficacy and safety of medication influence both their decision to take medication and their preference for the type of medication [14]. Moreover, it has been suggested that treatment choices can be better predicted when beliefs about multiple treatment options are assessed, instead of assessing beliefs about a single treatment option [15]. Therefore, identifying patients' beliefs about various treatment modalities of OA may help to increase the understanding of treatment decisions.

At present, little is known about how and to what extent patients' beliefs about treatment modalities of knee and hip OA influence patients' treatment choices. Previous qualitative studies indicate that many considerations such as patients' beliefs about the effectiveness and side-effects of the treatment may play a role in their treatment choice [16–18]. While qualitative studies are ideal to get an encompassing overview of all possible determinants of treatment choices, a measurement instrument based on self-reports is needed to get insight into the relative importance of treatment beliefs in the one patient as compared to the other. Therefore, guided by the results of these qualitative studies, a self-report instrument is needed in order to be able to systematically assess patients' beliefs about treatment modalities for knee and hip OA. This instrument can be used in research to examine to what extent patients' treatment beliefs contribute to the patients' decision making process, and ultimately help to understand why conservative treatment modalities are underused in the management of knee and hip OA.

In the context of knee and hip OA, no questionnaire is available that comprehensively assesses patients' beliefs about both surgical and conservative treatment modalities. Existing questionnaires assess fears and beliefs related to the consequences of knee OA [19] and expectations about the role of their physician in the management of knee OA [20]. Existing self-report instruments about treatment beliefs refer to low back pain [21], medicines [22] and surgery [15]. Therefore, the aim of the current study was to develop a questionnaire to assess patients' beliefs about treatment modalities of knee and hip OA: the TOA (Treatment beliefs in OsteoArthritis) questionnaire, and to examine its factorial structure, internal consistency and test-retest reliability.

Methods

Development of item pool

For the development of a first draft of the TOA questionnaire an elaborated process was undertaken to generate and select items based on the findings of three previous studies among patients with knee and hip OA in the Netherlands. These were two qualitative studies [17, 23] on treatment beliefs in patients and healthcare providers and a concept mapping study [24] to define the most important themes. A total of 2207 statements reflecting beliefs about treatment modalities of knee or hip OA (which could be potentially included as items in the TOA questionnaire) were extracted from the interviews. Items were selected from 4 major themes originated from the concept mapping study: 'contextual barriers' (e.g. the healthcare system), disadvantages (e.g. risks), treatment outcomes (e.g. physical functioning) and 'outcomes for personal life' (e.g. activities of daily living) [24].

The draft TOA questionnaire consisted of five modules, based on five treatment options recommended in the 'stepped care strategy' for knee and hip OA in the Netherlands [3]: physical activities, pain medication, physiotherapy, injections and arthroplasty. We aimed for a feasible set of approximately 50 items to include in each module in the draft version of the TOA questionnaire. In a careful and thorough consensus process, as described previously [24], all 2207 statements about specific treatment modalities derived from the interviews were reduced by a project group comprising researchers and health professionals including medical specialists. The selection procedure comprised several steps. For each step, cut-off points were developed to reach a representative set of 51 general items (Additional file 1). Two patient partners assessed this set of 51 items for its representativeness and comprehensiveness. In the next step, all 51 items were assessed for its applicability to each of the 5 treatment modalities. For instance, the item 'the treatment may cause an infection' was applicable for the treatment modality injections and arthroplasty, but not for physical activity, pain medication and physiotherapy. If applicable, the item was included in the module. The final draft version of the TOA questionnaire comprised 200 items, distributed over 5 modules: physical activities (41 items), pain medication (37 items), physiotherapy (42 items), injections (41 items) and arthroplasty (39 items). A 5-point Likert scale with scoring options ranging from 1 to 5 was chosen, labelled from 'disagree' to 'agree' in order to avoid end-aversion bias (i.e. avoiding absolute statements as 'completely disagree' and 'completely agree' to overcome the reluctance of some people to use extreme categories of a scale) [25]. The TOA questionnaire was developed in Dutch. An English translation of the items can be found in Additional file 2.

Pilot testing

The draft TOA questionnaire was pilot tested in a stepwise way. The first draft of the questionnaire was tested by five researchers and health professionals. Subsequently, ten patients were recruited via a primary care physiotherapy practice in the Northern part of the Netherlands. Besides the clinical diagnosis of knee or hip OA, no other inclusion criteria were required. Patients were asked to fill out the questionnaire at home and to make notes if they thought a question was difficult to understand. Hereafter, the researcher contacted the patient for a telephone interview. All items of the questionnaire were discussed, using the probing method for pilot-testing whether the patient understood the items, whether items were interpreted according to their intended meaning, and whether the length of the questionnaire was considered acceptable [26, 27]. Including patients for the pilot test was stopped after 10 interviews because no new information emerged from interviewing the last two patients (data saturation). Based on the results of the pilot test, minor alterations were made in the instructions and lay-out.

Patients and measures

Two different samples were recruited for this study. The first sample was recruited to examine the factor structure and internal consistency of the TOA questionnaire; the second sample was recruited to examine the test-retest reliability of the TOA questionnaire.

Sample 1: Factor structure and internal consistency

Eligible patients who visited the department of Rheumatology of the Sint Maartenskliniek in 2013–2014 (n = 600, randomly selected from the electronic patient record system) or the department of Orthopaedics in June–August 2015 (n = 240, consecutively), who were clinically diagnosed with knee or hip OA, and were aged ≥18 received an information letter and informed consent form. Assuming a number of 4–10 participants per item and 51 unique items, a sample size of at least 204 patients was needed to perform the factor analysis [26]. These patients filled out the TOA questionnaire once. In addition, demographic and clinical characteristics were collected: body mass index (BMI), duration of OA symptoms, affected joint(s), comorbidities (question 70 from the DUTCH-AIMS2 [28]), treatment use, and the Dutch version of the Western Ontario and McMaster Universities Arthritis LK3.1 Index (WOMAC). The WOMAC is a health status measure assessing the dimensions of pain, stiffness and function in patients with OA of the hip/knee [29].

Sample 2: Test-retest reliability analysis

Patients were consecutively selected from a larger study sample with similar eligibility criteria as sample 1. To determine test-retest reliability by calculating an ICC of 0.8 with a 95% confidence interval ± 0.1 using 2 repeated measurements, 50 respondents are required [26]. Eligible patients of the department of Rheumatology of the Sint Maartenskliniek in 2015–2016 (n = 39) or the department of Orthopaedics in September 2015–September 2016 (n = 41) were randomly selected from the electronic patient record system. Patients were invited to fill out the final TOA questionnaire twice, with a 2 weeks interval. The first 50 respondents who sent the questionnaire back were included in the analysis, to keep the time between the first and second measurement close to the aimed interval of 2 weeks.

The medical ethical board of the Radboud University Medical Center, Nijmegen concluded that the Dutch Medical Research Involving Human Subjects Act did not apply to this study (protocol number: 2015–1772 for sample 1 and protocol number 2016–2605 for sample 2).

Statistical analyses

Because the TOA questionnaire comprises five treatment modalities, we aimed for a brief set of items per treatment module. Therefore, rigorous item reduction and exploratory factor analysis were used to design the final TOA questionnaire. This was conducted per module in three consecutive steps: initial item reduction, factor analysis and further refinement. Furthermore, internal consistency (Cronbach's alpha) and the test-retest reliability of the final TOA questionnaire were examined per module.

Step 1: Initial item reduction

Items were considered to be deleted if: a) missing values were >15%; b) >50% of patients scored 1 (disagree) or 5 (agree) on an item (floor or ceiling effect); c) skewness of the item was >1; d) inter-item correlations were >.80 (in this case one of the redundant paired items was considered for deletion) [25].

Step 2: Factor analysis and internal consistency

Exploratory factor analyses were conducted for each modality separately to examine the dimensionality of the TOA questionnaire. First, exploratory factor analysis without rotation was used to determine the initial numbers of factors. This was determined by two researchers (JV and ES) by visual inspection of the scree plot, percentages of explained variance (>5%) and eigenvalues >1 [30]. Thereafter, for each module exploratory factor analysis with oblique (direct oblimin) rotation was conducted for 2-factor to 4-factor solutions. Oblique rotation was chosen because it allowed the extracted factors to be correlated. To select the most salient items two criteria were used: only items with factor loadings ≥0.45 were retained, and items with cross loadings on more than one factor within 0.3 of the primary loading were dropped because of inadequate discrimination [31]. The final number of factors per module was determined by the project group based on factor interpretability and revealed a 2-factor solution for each module.

Step 3: Further refinement

Guided by the results of a previous concept mapping study [24], items were further considered for deletion. Briefly, in this concept mapping study, 36 patients sorted the 51 items (each item printed on a card) from the TOA questionnaire into piles with a similar meaning; subsequently hierarchical cluster analysis yielded a 15-cluster solution that was grouped in 4 higher-order categories and 2 overarching categories. The following additional rules (set by the project group) were applied for further item reduction per module:

1. Each factor should contain preferably a maximum of 1 item per cluster
2. If more than 1 item per cluster loaded on the factor, the item with the highest factor loading was retained
3. If internal consistency of a factor, as assessed with Cronbach's alpha, dropped below .70, the item with the next highest factor loading was retained.
4. If internal consistency of the factor, as assessed with Cronbach's alpha, was still < .70, an item with the next highest factor loading from another cluster was added.

Lastly, a final two-factor factor analysis with the remaining items per module was conducted. Cronbach's alpha was calculated for each factor, and Pearson's correlation coefficients were calculated between factor I and factor II per module.

Test-retest reliability

Because each method to assess test-retest reliability of a questionnaire has its advantages and disadvantages and is difficult to interpret without other methods [32], multiple methods were used to assess the test-retest reliability of the TOA questionnaire. Test-retest reliability was determined by 1) Intraclass correlation coefficients (ICCs) (two-way mixed effects model, measuring consistency of individual differences) [33]; 2) Limits of agreement (LoA); and 3) Standard errors of measurement (SEMs) of the whole model including systematic differences between repeated measures. Scale scores of the TOA questionnaire were calculated by summation of the items for each factor. When a respondent had ≤25% missing items on a subscale, these missing items were substituted by the respondent's mean sum score on the subscale. When a respondent had >25% missing items on a subscale, these were taken into account as missing values in the analysis. Unstandardised scores for each subscale per module were used for calculating ICCs and the LoA. For calculating the SEM, standardised scores were calculated (raw total score of subscale / total items on subscale). Thus, total scores on each subscale were comparable on a scale from 1 to 5. ICCs range from 0 to 1, whereby 1 reflects perfect reliability. In general, ICCs ≥0.70 are considered acceptable [34]. LoA were calculated with the following formula: mean difference ± 1.96 x $SD_{difference}$. SEM of the whole model including systematic variation of repeated measures was calculated for each subscale with: $\sqrt{(\sigma^2_m + \sigma^2_{residual})}$. Where σ^2_m = variance between the two repeated measures; and $\sigma^2_{residual}$ = variance of the residual ("error"). A smaller SEM reflects better test-retest reliability [26].

All analyses were performed using STATA 13.1.

Results

Participants

Sample 1

Of 840 invited patients, 351 filled out the TOA questionnaire and provided informed consent (response rate: 41.8%). Eighty-two patients indicated they did not want to participate in the study. Some patients provided a reason for non-participation, e.g.: no knee or hip OA (n = 25), not wanting to (n = 5), comorbidities (n = 4), not satisfied about care provided by the hospital (n = 3). Ten patients who did fill out the questionnaire were excluded because they did not provide informed consent. Three patients did not fill out the additional questionnaire assessing demographic and clinical characteristics but were included in the factor analysis. Table 1 shows the demographic and clinical characteristics of the study sample.

Sample 2

Of the 80 patients who were invited to fill out the final TOA questionnaire twice, 67 patients returned the questionnaire (response rate: 83.8%). The first 50 respondents who sent the questionnaire back were included in the analysis, to keep the time between the first and second measurement close to the aimed interval of 2 weeks (Mean time interval = 13 days, SD = 2.5, range = 6–18). The mean age of sample 2 was 63.8 years (SD = 10.5), and 56% was female.

Step 1: Initial item reduction

Item reduction resulted in dropping 9, 8, 8, 2, and 4 items respectively in modules 1 to 5. Two pairs of items in module 4 had a correlation of 0.81 and 0.82, but because the items reflected different contents, none of the items were deleted.

Step 2: Factor structure and internal consistency

Based on exploratory factor analyses and interpretability, a two-factor solution for each module was obtained.

Table 1 Characteristics of the study sample (*N*=348[a])

Demographic characteristics	
Age (years), mean (SD)	62.8 (12.3)
Gender (female), *n* (%)	217 (63.1)
Married or cohabiting, *n* (%)	273 (79.4)
Currently employed, *n* (%)[b]	145 (44.1)
Education level, *n* (%)[c]	
Low	62 (18.0)
Middle	175 (50.9)
High	107 (31.1)
Clinical characteristics	
Body Mass Index (BMI) (kg/m^2), n(%)	
Normal weight (BMI <25)	106 (31.0)
Overweight (BMI 25–30)	146 (42.7)
Obese (BMI > 30)	90 (26.3)
Duration of OA symptoms (years), mean (SD)[b]	11.1 (9.8)
Affected joint(s), *n* (%)	
Hip	82 (24)
Knee	169 (49.5)
Hip and knee	91 (26.5)
Comorbidities, n(%)[d]	
No comorbidities	141 (40.8)
High blood pressure	97 (28.0)
Heart disease	39 (11.2)
Diabetes	27 (7.8)
Lung disease	28 (8)
Other	42 (12)
Previous or current treatments for OA, *n* (%)[d]	
Pain medication	291 (85.3)
Physiotherapy	234 (68.6)
Injections	133 (39.0)
Surgery	112 (32.8)
WOMAC[e] (Likert scale 0–4), unstandardized mean (SD), theoretical range	
Pain[b]	10.0 (4.5), 0–20
Stiffness	4.5 (2.0), 0–8
Functioning	32.4 (14.8), 0–68
Total (sum score)[b]	46.7 (20.0), 0–96

[a] *3 respondents did not fill out these questions*
[b]Missing values > 5%: Currently employed = 6%; Duration of OA symptoms = 7%; WOMAC subscale pain = 5%, WOMAC total (sum score) = 8%
[c]Low = no education, primary school, lower vocational education; Middle = secondary school, middle vocational education; High = higher vocational education, university
[d]More than 1 answer possible
[e]Western Ontario and McMaster Universities Arthritis Index. Higher scores reflect worse pain, stiffness and functioning

Respectively 8, 12, 16, 18, 14 items were dropped because of factor loadings ≥0.45 or cross loadings <0.3 in module 1 to 5 (Additional file 2).

Step 3: Further refinement

After the previous steps of item reduction, a total of 24, 17, 18, 22 and 21 items remained for module 1 to 5 respectively). After the third step of refinement, 13 items remained for module 1 (physical activities), 12 items for module 2 (pain medication), 9 items for module 3 (physiotherapy), 12 items for module 4 (injections), and 14 items for module 5 (arthroplasty). After this last round of item reduction, a final 2-factor factor analysis with oblique (direct oblimin) rotation was performed for all modules. The explained percentage of variance per module ranged from 37% to 51%, Cronbach's alpha's of the final TOA questionnaire ranged from .72 to .87, and correlations between factors ranged from −.03 to −.51 (Table 2).

Factor interpretation

For each module, the first factor reflected positive beliefs about the treatment, such as health benefits and perceived advantages (e.g. "I learn to deal with my symptoms better by the treatment"). The second factor reflected negative beliefs about the treatment, such as treatment risks and disadvantages (e.g. "I think that the treatment involves risks"). Therefore, for each module, Factor I was labelled 'positive treatment beliefs' and Factor II was labelled 'negative treatment beliefs'. For each subscale in each module of the TOA questionnaire, a sum score can be calculated whereby a higher sum score on subscale I reflects more positive treatment beliefs and a higher sum score on subscale II reflects more negative treatment beliefs. Scorings on the questions M5Q4 and M5Q9 should be reversed. Missing item scores on a subscale are replaced with the mean of the other items; when more than 25% of the items are missing, the subscale score is not valid.

Table 2 presents the factor loadings, eigenvalues, percentages of explained variance, Cronbach's alpha for each factor per treatment module, and the correlations between factors per treatment module.

Test-retest reliability

Table 3 shows 3 different measures of test-retest reliability for each subscale of the TOA questionnaire. Considering the moderate to high ICCs (0.66–0.88) and small SEM (0.06–0.11) obtained for all subscales, test-retest reliability of the TOA questionnaire was satisfactory.

Discussion

The TOA questionnaire is the first questionnaire assessing treatment beliefs regarding surgical and conservative (physical activities, pain medication, physiotherapy, injections) modalities for knee and hip OA. The TOA questionnaire comprises five treatment modalities with each a positive and negative subscale. Each part of the

Table 2 Factor loadings, eigenvalues, percentage of explained variance and Cronbach's alpha for the final TOA questionnaire

Module 1: Physical activities		
Items	*Factor loadings*	
M1 = Module 1, Q = Question number (see Additional file 1*)*	*Factor I*	*Factor II*
M1Q32: I learn to deal with my symptoms better by doing physical activities	.77	
M1Q19: I can do household chores better by doing physical activities	.72	
M1Q22: Doing physical activities produces good results at my age	.71	
M1Q33: I can do my job better by doing physical activities	.70	
M1Q39: I can tailor doing physical activities to my goals	.63	
M1Q10: I can postpone surgery by doing physical activities	.53	
M1Q14: I can do physical activities together with others	.48	
M1Q8: The only way to reduce my OA symptoms is by doing physical activities	.47	
M1Q20: I enjoy doing physical activities	.45	
M1Q24: By doing physical activities I will overload my knee/hip		.72
M1Q23: I think that doing physical activities causes pain		.66
M1Q7: I think that doing physical activities involves risks		.65
M1Q28: I am scared to do physical activities		.55
Eigenvalue	4.03	1.06
Percentage of variance	31%	8%
Cronbach's Alpha	.84	.79
Correlation between factors	−.51	
Module 2: Pain medication		
Items	*Factor loadings*	
M2 = Module 2, Q = Question number (see Additional file 1*)*	*Factor I*	*Factor II*
M2Q10: I can move more freely by using painkillers	.80	
M2Q18: I can do household chores better by using painkillers	.76	
M2Q2: My quality of life increases by using painkillers	.74	
M2Q20: Using painkillers produces good results at my age	.73	
M2Q9: I can postpone surgery by using painkillers	.50	
M2Q15: Using painkillers is harmful to my health		.70
M2Q6: I think that using painkillers involves risks		.67
M2Q11: I think that painkillers have side-effects		.64
M2Q28: I think that using painkillers is invasive		.52

Table 2 Factor loadings, eigenvalues, percentage of explained variance and Cronbach's alpha for the final TOA questionnaire *(Continued)*

M2Q25: I am scared to use painkillers		.47
M2Q19: I think that using painkillers leads to habituation		.38
M2Q22: By using painkillers I will overload my knee/hip		.35
Eigenvalue	2.74	2.00
Percentage of variance	23%	17%
Cronbach's Alpha	.82	.72
Correlation between factors	−.14	
Module 3: Physiotherapy		
Items	*Factor loadings*	
M3 = Module 3, Q = Question number (see Additional file 1*)*	*Factor I*	*Factor II*
M3Q23: Doing physiotherapy produces good results at my age	.86	
M3Q20: I can do household chores better by physiotherapy	.85	
M3Q34: I can do my job better by physiotherapy	.76	
M3Q3: My quality of life increases by physiotherapy	.71	
M3Q22: I need to actively get going with physiotherapy myself	.60	
M3Q10: I can postpone surgery by physiotherapy	.52	
M3Q25: By physiotherapy I will overload my knee/hip		.71
M3Q24: I think that physiotherapy causes pain		.70
M3Q7: I think that physiotherapy involves risks		.62
Eigenvalue	3.49	1.09
Percentage of variance	39%	12%
Cronbach's Alpha	.86	.74
Correlation between factors	−.36	
Module 4: Injections		
Items	*Factor loadings*	
M4 = Module 4, Q = Question number (see Additional file 1*)*	*Factor I*	*Factor II*
M4Q33: I can do my job better by an injection	.89	
M4Q20: I can do household chores better by an injection	.88	
M4Q3: My quality of life increases by an injection	.76	
M4Q30: An injection gives quick results	.76	
M4Q10: I can postpone surgery by an injection	.62	
M4Q31: I think that an injection can be repeated	.47	

Table 2 Factor loadings, eigenvalues, percentage of explained variance and Cronbach's alpha for the final TOA questionnaire *(Continued)*

M4Q24: By an injection I will overload my knee/hip		.62
M4Q15: I am becoming dependent on an injection		.61
M4Q34: An injection damages my knee/hip		.60
M4Q32: I think that an injection is invasive		.54
M4Q7: I think that an injection involves risks		.48
M4Q40: An injection takes a lot of my time		.38
Eigenvalue	3.54	1.78
Percentage of variance	30%	15%
Cronbach's Alpha	.87	.72
Correlation between factors	–.11	
Module 5: Arthroplasty		
Items	*Factor loadings*	
M5 = Module 5, Q = Question number (see Additional file 1*)*	*Factor I*	*Factor II*
M5Q4: My pain increases by a joint replacement	–.61	
M5Q9: My knee/hip deteriorates faster by a joint replacement	–.51	
M5Q10: I can move more freely after a joint replacement	.78	
M5Q17: I can do household chores better after a joint replacement	.77	
M5Q18: A joint replacement produces good results at my age	.81	
M5Q21: More people with OA choose to do a joint replacement	.43	
M5Q29: I think that a joint replacement can be repeated	.45	
M5Q38: I think that an artificial joint lasts a long time	.44	
M5Q1: I think a joint replacement is painful		.51
M5Q23: I think an artificial joint carries the chance of an infection		.57
M5Q24: I think a joint replacement carries the chance of an infection		.67
M5Q27: A joint replacement takes up my energy		.53
M5Q30: I think that a joint replacement is invasive		.62
M5Q37: A joint replacement takes a lot of my time		.60
Eigenvalue	3.13	2.14
Percentage of variance	22%	15%
Cronbach's Alpha	.81	.75
Correlation between factors	–.03	

Table 3 Intraclass correlation coefficient (ICC), mean difference between repeated measures, limits of agreement (LoA), and standard error of measurement (SEM) including systematic differences between repeated measures and error variance

Module	Subscale	ICC	Mean difference	LoA	SEM
Physical activity	positive *9 items*	.88	–.44	–7.65; 6.78	.06
	negative *4 items*	.74	.81	–4.60; 6.23	.10
Pain medication	positive *5 items*	.80	.19	–6.44; 6.82	.09
	negative *7 items*	.83	.59	–6.82; 8.00	.08
Physiotherapy	positive *6 items*	.88	.16	–6.35; 6.67	.08
	negative *3 items*	.72	–0.40	–4.81; 4.01	.11
Injections	positive *6 items*	.88	0.05	–5.85; 5.96	.07
	negative *6 items*	.83	.45	–5.06; 5.96	.07
Arthroplasty	positive *8 items*	.66	–.20	–9.14; 8.75	.08
	negative *6 items*	.77	.45	–5.52; 6.41	.07

questionnaire can be used independently, so beliefs regarding either one or multiple treatment modalities can be measured. A main strength of this study was the design used to generate the items. For the selection of items, we used two previous in-depth interview studies in which both patients and healthcare providers were asked about their beliefs and views regarding treatment modalities for knee and hip OA [17, 23]. The item pool was generated very carefully in several consensus rounds by the project team, and selected items were assessed by patients. As a result, based on the perspective of patients and professionals, we developed a questionnaire to comprehensively assess both positive and negative treatment beliefs in knee and hip OA. The qualitative approach will have contributed to the face validity. The internal consistency and test-retest reliability of the TOA questionnaire were satisfactory to good. Confirmatory factor analysis and replication of clinimetric properties in other samples as well as validation studies such as studies examining the association with actual treatment choices are needed in order to fully establish the validity and reliability of the TOA questionnaire.

The 2-factor structure reflected individual differences in positive and negative beliefs about treatment modalities. Similarly to existing generic questionnaires about medication (Beliefs about Medicines Questionnaire (BMQ) [22]) and surgery (Beliefs about Surgery Questionnaire (BSQ) [15]), the TOA questionnaire assesses negative treatment beliefs as a distinct dimension. In contrast to the BMQ and BSQ, the TOA questionnaire also assesses positive beliefs about treatment modalities. The small correlations between the factors – especially for the modules pain medication, injections and arthroplasty – show that positive and negative beliefs are not the opposite poles of a single dimension. This indicates the importance of measuring both patients' negative and positive treatment beliefs in order to fully understand patients' treatment preferences.

The TOA questionnaire can primarily be used as a research tool to assess individual differences in treatment beliefs and to examine to what extent treatment beliefs influence treatment choices in OA. Previous research showed that patients with knee or hip OA differ in their willingness to undergo surgery, and that this difference might be due to individual differences in sex, ethnicity, socioeconomic status [35], severity, age and income [36]. In interaction with, and in addition to these sociodemographic characteristics, treatment beliefs will likely play a role in treatment choices, specifically in suboptimal use of conservative treatment modalities. Previous studies have demonstrated the practice variation in primary care settings with regard to diagnostic procedures and referrals [37, 38], and that referrals by the GP to other disciplines are associated with patients' preferences [39]. This suggests that besides organisational and healthcare provider-related factors, patients' treatment beliefs should be taken into account, in order to choose a treatment that fits best to the patient's individual situation and preferences. In clinical practice, individual scores at the TOA questionnaire could be used as an input for shared decision making. However, users should be aware that the item pool reflects a restricted number of items that predominantly reflect individual differences. To get an encompassing overview of treatment beliefs that may be important for an individual patient, it is better to use all statements from a previous concept mapping study [24] which represent a wide range of potential benefits and barriers.

Some limitations of the study need to be addressed. Firstly, our findings in a secondary care sample cannot be generalised to other samples or settings without empirical replication. With respect to external validity, cross-cultural validation studies are needed to examine whether the TOA questionnaire is valid to use in other languages and cultures than Dutch. Also other aspects of validity need to be more extensively evaluated, such as construct validity and criterion validity. In new samples, the structural validity of the TOA questionnaire could be further evaluated by using confirmatory factor analyses to verify whether the factor structure is replicated and Item-Response Theory to improve the precision of the measurement instrument [26]. On average, our sample reported moderate OA complaints in terms of pain, stiffness and functioning [29, 40]. Future research needs to examine the robustness of the factor structure of the TOA in other samples. Secondly, the response rate for sample 1 in this study was 42%, which could indicate a response bias. The questionnaire was quite long, which might have been burdensome for patients. The response rate, however, is comparable to other studies in knee or hip OA [41]. Moreover, 351 respondents filled in the questionnaire, which is sufficient for a factor analysis [26]. Thirdly, patients' involvement in the item reduction process for the TOA questionnaire was limited to an assessment of the comprehensiveness and completeness of the items by two patients and an extensive pilot-test in 10 primary care patients. However, items for the TOA questionnaire were selected in a careful and thorough process to enhance the validity of the questionnaire.

Conclusions

The TOA questionnaire assesses positive and negative treatment beliefs of patients with knee or hip OA about 5 treatment modalities: physical activities, pain medication, physiotherapy, injections and arthroplasty. Initial analyses of the clinimetric properties of the TOA questionnaire are promising. The questionnaire can be used in research to clarify treatment choices. Future research should assess the validity and reliability of the TOA questionnaire in other OA samples, and should verify whether treatment beliefs in interaction with other variables influence intended and actual treatment choices.

Additional files

Additional file 1: Procedure that was used for selecting a representative set of items from statements resulting from interviews. Description: Procedure that was used for selecting a representative set of items from statements resulting from interviews. (DOCX 22 kb)

Additional file 2: Initial factor loadings for items in the Treatment beliefs in OsteoArthritis Questionnaire in patients with knee and hip osteoarthritis ($N = 351$). Description: Initial factor loadings for items in the Treatment beliefs in OsteoArthritis Questionnaire. (DOCX 42 kb)

Abbreviations

BMI: Body mass index; ICC: Intraclass correlation coefficient; LoA: Limits of agreement; OA: Osteoarthritis; SD: Standard deviation; SEM: Standard error of measurement; TOA: Treatment beliefs in osteoarthritis; WOMAC: Western ontario and McMaster universities arthritis index

Acknowledgements

Not applicable.

Funding

Not applicable.

Authors' contributions

Study conception and design: ES, JV, CE. Acquisition of data: ES. Contributions to the analysis and interpretation of data: ES; JV; HS; MW; WL; RM; RG; CE. Drafting the article and revising it critically for important intellectual content: ES; JV; HS; MW; WL; RM; RG; CE. Approval of the final version to be submitted for publication: ES; JV; HS; MW; WL; RM; RG; CE. Accountable for all aspects of the work: ES; JV; HS; MW; WL; RM; RG; CE.

Competing interests

All authors declare that they have no competing interests.

Author details

[1]Department of Rheumatology, Sint Maartenskliniek, Sint Maartenskliniek, P.O. Box 9011, 6500, GM, Nijmegen, The Netherlands. [2]Department of Primary and Community Care, Radboud University Nijmegen Medical Center, Nijmegen, The Netherlands. [3]Department of Orthopedics, Sint Maartenskliniek, Nijmegen, The Netherlands. [4]Department of Rheumatology, Sint Maartenskliniek, Woerden, The Netherlands. [5]Physical Therapy and Manual Therapy Velperweg Partnership, Arnhem, The Netherlands. [6]Department of Psychology, Utrecht University, Utrecht, The Netherlands.

References

1. Bijlsma JW, Berenbaum F, Lafeber FP. Osteoarthritis: an update with relevance for clinical practice. Lancet. 2011;377:2115–26.
2. McAlindon TE, Bannuru RR, Sullivan MC, Arden NK, Berenbaum F, Bierma-Zeinstra SM, et al. OARSI guidelines for the non-surgical management of knee osteoarthritis. Osteoarthr Cartil. 2014;22:363–88.
3. Smink AJ, van den Ende CH, Vliet Vlieland TP, Swierstra BA, Kortland JH, Bijlsma JW, et al. "Beating osteoARThritis": development of a stepped care strategy to optimize utilization and timing of non-surgical treatment modalities for patients with hip or knee osteoarthritis. Clin Rheumatol. 2011;30:1623–9.
4. Zhang W, Moskowitz RW, Nuki G, Abramson S, Altman RD, Arden N, et al. OARSI recommendations for the management of hip and knee osteoarthritis, Part II: OARSI evidence-based, expert consensus guidelines. Osteoarthr Cartil. 2008;16:137–62.
5. McHugh GA, Luker KA, Campbell M, Kay PR, Silman AJ. A longitudinal study exploring pain control, treatment and service provision for individuals with end-stage lower limb osteoarthritis. Rheumatology (Oxford). 2007;46:631–7.
6. Shrier I, Feldman DE, Gaudet MC, Rossignol M, Zukor D, Tanzer M, et al. Conservative non-pharmacological treatment options are not frequently used in the management of hip osteoarthritis. J Sci Med Sport. 2006;9:81–6.
7. Snijders GF, den Broeder AA, van Riel PL, Straten VH, de Man FH, van den Hoogen FH, et al. Evidence-based tailored conservative treatment of knee and hip osteoarthritis: between knowing and doing. Scand J Rheumatol. 2011;40:225–31.
8. Otten R, van Roermund PM. Picavet HS: [Trends in the number of knee and hip arthroplasties: considerably more knee and hip prostheses due to osteoarthritis in 2030]. Ned Tijdschr Geneeskd. 2010;154:A1534.
9. Beswick AD, Wylde V, Gooberman-Hill R, Blom A, Dieppe P. What proportion of patients report long-term pain after total hip or knee replacement for osteoarthritis? A systematic review of prospective studies in unselected patients. BMJ Open. 2012;2:e000435.
10. Nilsdotter AK, Toksvig-Larsen S, Roos EM. Knee arthroplasty: are patients' expectations fulfilled? A prospective study of pain and function in 102 patients with 5-year follow-up. Acta Orthop. 2009;80:55–61.
11. Hofstede SN, Marang-van de Mheen PJ, Vliet Vlieland TP, van den Ende CH, Nelissen RG, van Bodegom-Vos L. Barriers and Facilitators Associated with Non-Surgical Treatment Use for Osteoarthritis Patients in Orthopaedic Practice. PLoS One. 2016;11:e0147406.
12. Tariman JD, Doorenbos A, Schepp KG, Becker PS, Berry DL. Patient, Physician and Contextual Factors Are Influential in the Treatment Decision Making of Older Adults Newly Diagnosed with Symptomatic Myeloma. Cancer Treat Commun. 2014;2:34–47.
13. Ajzen I. The Theory of Planned Behavior. Organ Behav Hum Decis Process. 1991;50:179–211.
14. Uebelacker LA, Bailey G, Herman D, Anderson B, Stein M. Patients' Beliefs About Medications are Associated with Stated Preference for Methadone, Buprenorphine, Naltrexone, or no Medication-Assisted Therapy Following Inpatient Opioid Detoxification. J Subst Abus Treat. 2016;66:48–53.
15. Francis JJ, Wileman SM, Bekker H, Barton GR, Ramsay CR. Beliefs about surgery: Development and validation of an instrument to assess cognitive representations about surgery, in the context of a chronic illness. Psychol Health. 2009;24:1125–37.
16. O'Neill T, Jinks C, Ong BN. Decision-making regarding total knee replacement surgery: a qualitative meta-synthesis. BMC Health Serv Res. 2007;7:52.
17. Selten EM, Vriezekolk JE, Geenen R, van der Laan WH, van der Meulen-Dilling RG, Nijhof MW, et al. Reasons for Treatment Choices in Knee and Hip Osteoarthritis: A Qualitative Study. Arthritis Care Res (Hoboken). 2016;68:1260–7.
18. Smith TO, Purdy R, Lister S, Salter C, Fleetcroft R, Conaghan PG. Attitudes of people with osteoarthritis towards their conservative management: a systematic review and meta-ethnography. Rheumatol Int. 2014;34:299–313.
19. Benhamou M, Baron G, Dalichampt M, Boutron I, Alami S, Rannou F, et al. Development and validation of a questionnaire assessing fears and beliefs of patients with knee osteoarthritis: the Knee Osteoarthritis Fears and Beliefs Questionnaire (KOFBeQ). PLoS One. 2013;8:e53886.
20. Benhamou M, Boutron I, Dalichampt M, Baron G, Alami S, Rannou F, et al. Elaboration and validation of a questionnaire assessing patient expectations about management of knee osteoarthritis by their physicians: the Knee Osteoarthritis Expectations Questionnaire. Ann Rheum Dis. 2013;72:552–9.
21. Dima A, Lewith GT, Little P, Moss-Morris R, Foster NE, Hankins M, et al. Patients' treatment beliefs in low back pain: development and validation of a questionnaire in primary care. Pain. 2015;156:1489–500.
22. Horne R, Weinman J, Hankins M. The Beliefs about Medicines Questionnaire: the development and evaluation of a new method for assessing the cognitive representation of medication. Psychol Health. 1999;4:1–24.
23. Selten EMH, Vriezekolk JE, Nijhof MW, Schers HJ, Van der Meulen-Dilling RG, van der Laan WH et al. Barriers impeding the use of non-pharmacological, non-surgical care in hip and knee osteoarthritis: the views of general practitioners, physiotherapists and medical specialists. Journal of Clinical Rheumatology. 2017; in press.
24. Selten EM, Geenen R, van der Laan WH, van der Meulen-Dilling RG, Schers HJ, Nijhof MW, et al. Hierarchical structure and importance of patients' reasons for treatment choices in knee and hip osteoarthritis: a concept mapping study. Rheumatology (Oxford). 2017;56:271–8.
25. Streiner DL, Norman GR. Health Measurement Scales, a practical guide to their development and use. 4th ed. New York: Oxford University Press; 2008.
26. De Vet HCW, Terwee CB, Mokkink LB, Knol DL. Measurement in Medicine. 1st ed. New York: Cambridge University Press; 2011.
27. Willis GB, Artino AR Jr. What Do Our Respondents Think We're Asking? Using Cognitive Interviewing to Improve Medical Education Surveys. J Grad Med Educ. 2013;5:353–6.
28. Riemsma RP, Taal E, Rasker JJ, Houtman PM, VAn Paassen HC, Wiegman O. Evaluation of a Dutch version of the AIMS2 for patients with rheumatoid arthritis. Br J Rheumatol. 1996;35:755–60.
29. Bellamy N. The WOMAC Knee and Hip Osteoarthritis Indices: development, validation, globalization and influence on the development of the AUSCAN Hand Osteoarthritis Indices. Clin Exp Rheumatol. 2005;23:S148–53.
30. Costello AB, Osborne JW. Best Practices in Exploratory Factor Analysis: Four Recommendations for Getting the Most From Your Analysis. Pract Assess Res Eval. 2005;10
31. Tabachnick BG, Fidell LS. Using Multivariate Statistics. 5th ed. Boston: Allyn and Bacon; 2007.
32. Rankin G, Stokes M. Reliability of assessment tools in rehabilitation: an illustration of appropriate statistical analyses. Clin Rehabil. 1998;12:187–99.
33. Shrout PE, Fleiss JL. Intraclass correlations: uses in assessing rater reliability. Psychol Bull. 1979;86:420–8.
34. Terwee CB, Mokkink LB, Steultjens MP, Dekker J. Performance-based methods for measuring the physical function of patients with osteoarthritis of the hip or knee: a systematic review of measurement properties. Rheumatology (Oxford). 2006;45:890–902.
35. Hawker GA. Who, when, and why total joint replacement surgery? The patient's perspective. Curr Opin Rheumatol. 2006;18:526–30.
36. Ratcliffe J, Buxton M, McGarry T, Sheldon R, Chancellor J. Patients' preferences for characteristics associated with treatments for osteoarthritis. Rheumatology (Oxford). 2004;43:337–45.
37. Allen KD, Bosworth HB, Chatterjee R, Coffman CJ, Corsino L, Jeffreys AS, et al. Clinic variation in recruitment metrics, patient characteristics and treatment use in a randomized clinical trial of osteoarthritis management. BMC Musculoskelet Disord. 2014;15:413.
38. Jordan KP, Tan V, Edwards JJ, Chen Y, Englund M, Hubertsson J, et al. Influences on the decision to use an osteoarthritis diagnosis in primary care: a cohort study with linked survey and electronic health record data. Osteoarthr Cartil. 2016;24:786–93.
39. Musila N, Underwood M, McCaskie AW, Black N, Clarke A, van der Meulen JH. Referral recommendations for osteoarthritis of the knee incorporating patients' preferences. Fam Pract. 2011;28:68–74.

2

Efficacy of nerve growth factor antibody in a knee osteoarthritis pain model in mice

Masayuki Miyagi[1*], Tetsuhiro Ishikawa[2], Hiroto Kamoda[2], Miyako Suzuki[2], Gen Inoue[1], Yoshihiro Sakuma[2], Yasuhiro Oikawa[2], Sumihisa Orita[2], Kentaro Uchida[1], Kazuhisa Takahashi[2], Masashi Takaso[1] and Seiji Ohtori[2]

Abstract

Background: Nerve growth factor (NGF) is not only an important factor in nerve growth but also a major contributor to the production of inflammation. It has been reported that inhibiting NGF could reduce several types of pain in several animal models. Here, we aimed to clarify the efficacy of NGF antibody in a knee osteoarthritis (OA) pain model in mice.

Method: Six-week-old male C57BR/J mice were used (n = 30). Ten mice comprised the control group, which received saline injection into the right knee joints; the other 20 mice comprised the experimental group, which received monoiodoacetate (MIA) injection into the right knee joints. Three weeks after surgery, the 20 experimental mice were randomly placed into treatment groups which received either sterile saline (non-treat group: 10 mg/kg, i.p.) or an anti-NGF antibody (anti-NGF group: 10 mg/kg, i.p.). Simultaneously, all mice received fluorogold (FG) retrograde neurotracer injection into their right joints. In a behavioral study, we evaluated gait using the CatWalk quantitative gait analysis system before surgery, 3 weeks after surgery (before treatment), 4 weeks after surgery (one week after surgery), and 5 weeks after surgery (2 weeks after surgery). In immunohistochemical analysis, the right dorsal root ganglia (DRGs) from the L4–L6 levels were resected 5 weeks after surgery (2 weeks after surgery). They were immunostained for calcitonin gene-related peptide (CGRP), and the number of FG-labeled or CGRP-immunoreactive (IR) DRG neurons was counted.

Results: On gait analysis using the CatWalk system, duty cycle, swing speed, and print area were decreased in non-treat group compared with those in control group and improved in the anti-NGF group compared with those in non-treat group. CGRP expression in DRGs was up-regulated in non-treat group compared with that in control group and suppressed in the anti-NGF group compared with that in non-treat group (both $p < 0.05$).

Conclusions: MIA injection into the knee joint induced gait impairment and the up-regulation of CGRP in DRG neurons in a knee OA pain model in mice. Intraperitoneal injection of anti-NGF antibody suppressed this impairment of gait and up-regulation of CGRP in DRG neurons. These finding suggest that anti-NGF therapy might be valuable in the treatment of OA pain in the knee.

Keywords: Nerve growth factor, Anti-nerve growth factor therapy, Knee osteoarthritis, Monoiodoacetate, CatWalk, Calcitonin gene-related peptide, Dorsal root ganglia

* Correspondence: masayuki008@aol.com
[1]Department of Orthopaedic Surgery, Kitasato University, School of Medicine, 1-15-1, Kitasato, Minami-ku, Sagamihara city, Kanagawa 252-0374, Japan
Full list of author information is available at the end of the article

Background

Knee osteoarthritis (OA) is a common chronic degenerative disease characterized by degeneration of articular cartilage components, synovitis, remodeling of subchondral bone and atrophy of joint muscles. Knee OA patients usually suffer from knee pain and are treated with several treatment modes, including medication, intraarticular injection of hyaluronic acid, and surgery [1]. Understanding of the mechanism of knee OA pain is incomplete, and medication for knee OA pain were sometimes insufficient.

As part of studies into new targets of knee OA pain, we have focused on pain-related molecules, including nerve growth factor (NGF) [2]. NGF not only plays an important role in the maintenance and development of the sensory nervous system [3] but is also a major contributor to inflammation and nociception [4]. Lewin et al. reported that the systemic injection of NGF induced thermal and mechanical hyperalgesia [5]. In addition, systemic injection of anti-NGF antibody reduced allodynia and hyperalgesia in animal models of neuropathic pain, including nerve trunk or spinal nerve ligation [6–8].

Basic research into knee OA has been aided by the development of several animal models, including the anterior cruciate ligament transection model [9], destabilization of the medial meniscus model [10], the rat medical meniscal tear model [11], GDF5 deficiency mice [12], and monoiodoacetate (MIA) injection model [13–16]. The MIA injection model has been reported to result in progressive joint damage, with some features that may be considered similar to OA [14–16] and significant pain-related behavior [13, 16]. The MIA injection model is superior for evaluating knee pain; although it seems animal models including the medical meniscus model better approximate the anatomic pathology found in OA in humans. Some of these previous reports evaluated pain-related behavior using the von Frey test, which is for evaluation of mechanical allodynia. Clinically, however, knee OA patients suffer from knee pain that includes gait impairment but not mechanical allodynia. Several authors have evaluated knee pain behavior using weight bearing assays [17–20]. For instance, the CatWalk gait analysis system can provide quantitative assessment of gait and motor function in rats and mice. This system has recently been used to assay impaired gait function in knee OA pain models [17–19]. Regarding the pathological mechanism of knee OA pain, our previous immunohistochemical analysis showed that the expression of pain-related molecules in the sensory nervous system was increased in a knee OA pain model [16]. Thus, this finding demonstrated the upregulation of pain-related molecules in the sensory nervous system in the pain state.

We therefore hypothesized that anti-NGF therapy was effective for knee pain in a mouse model of knee OA. The aim of the current study is to evaluate the efficacy of NGF antibody in a knee OA pain model using the CatWalk gait analysis system and immunohistochemical analysis of the sensory nervous system in mice.

Method

Knee osteoarthritis pain model

Thirty 8-week-old male C57 BL/6 mice were used. (Control group: n = 10, Monoiodeacete (MIA) without treatment (non-treat) group: n = 10, and MIA + anti-NGF therapy (anti-NGF) group: n = 10) Animals were anesthetized with sodium pentobarbital (40 mg/kg, intraperitoneal) and treated aseptically throughout the experiments. In the non-treatment group and anti-NGF group, the right knees were treated with a single intraarticular injection of 0.2 mg of MIA (Sigma-Aldrich, St. Louis, MO) in 10 μl of sterile saline. The solution was injected through the patellar ligament by using a 27G needle with the leg flexed at a 90 degrees angle at the knee as described previously [16]. Three weeks after surgery, mice were randomly assigned to treatment groups receiving either sterile saline (10 mg/kg, i.p.) (non-treat group) or an anti-NGF antibody (L148 M; Exalpha Biological Inc., Shirley, MA) (10 mg/kg, i.p.) (anti-NGF group). We have previously confirmed this medication's efficacy for treating neuropathic pain [2]. Simultaneously, to detect dorsal root ganglia (DRG) neurons innervating the right knee joint, the right knees of all 20 animals were treated with intraarticular injection of 2% retrograde neurotracer FG (Fluorochrome, Denver, CO) as we have previously described [16]. The control group was treated with a single intraarticular injection of 10 μl of sterile saline to the right knee, followed three weeks later by intraarticular injection of 2% retrograde neurotracer FG.

Behavioral evaluation (gait analysis)

Gait was analysed in detail using the CatWalk system (Noldus Information Technology, Wageningen, The Netherlands). This system has been described in detail elsewhere [19]. Briefly, mice are placed on a glass plate located in a darkened room and allowed to walk freely. A light beam from a fluorescent lamp is aimed through the glass plate. The light beams are completely reflected internally. However, when a paw touches the glass plate, the light beams are reflected downwards. This results in a sharp bright image of the paw print. The entire run is recorded with a video camera. The data are acquired, compressed, and analyzed using CatWalk software as described previously [21].

Before surgery and 3 (before treatment; pre-treat) 4, or 5 weeks (1 or 2 weeks after treatment, respectively; treat-1w or treat-2w) after surgery, all mice were walked on the glass plate three times. The gait of all mice was recorded three times and analyzed using the CatWalk system. We compared the ratio of movement of the ipsi and contralateral hind paws with regard to three variables, namely duty cycle (standing as a percentage of the step cycle: stand/(stand time + swing time) × 100%); swing speed (speed of the paw during swing: stride length/swing time); and print area (surface area of the complete print) among the three groups.

Immunohistochemical analysis

All procedure, including anesthetization, perfusion, sectioning, immunostaining and the observation and evaluation of immunoreactive neurons, were used the same manner as discribed previously [21, 22].

In all three groups, four (n = 5, each) or five (n = 5, each) weeks after surgery (one or two weeks after treatment), mice were anesthetized with sodium pentobarbital (40 mg/kg, intraperitoneal) and perfused transcardially with 0.9% saline, followed by 30 mL of 4% paraformaldehyde in phosphate buffer (0.1 M, pH 7.4). Next, the right DRGs from the L3 to L5 levels were resected and the specimens were immersed in the same fixative solution overnight at 4 °C, and then stored in 0.01 M phosphate-buffered saline (PBS) containing 20% sucrose for 20 h at 4 °C.

For DRGs, each ganglion was sectioned at a 10 μm thickness on a cryostat and mounted on POLY-L-LYSINE-coated slides. Endogenous tissue peroxidase activity was quenched by soaking sections in 0.3% hydrogen peroxide solution in 0.01 M PBS for 30 min. Specimens were then treated for 90 min at room temperature in blocking solution consisting of 0.01 M PBS containing 0.3% Triton X-100 and 3% skim milk. To evaluate the expression of neuropeptides in DRGs, the sections were processed for CGRP immunohistochemistry using a rabbit antibody to CGRP (1:1000; Chemicon, Temecula, CA) diluted in blocking solution, and incubated for 20 h at 4 °C. To detect CGRP in the DRGs, sections were incubated for 3 h with goat antirabbit Alexa 488 fluorescent antibody conjugate (1:400; Molecular Probes, Eugene, OR).

Thirty sections in each group (two sections per each DRG (L3, L4, L5) in 5 animals) were examined using a fluorescence microscope. For each DRG section, we counted the number of all Fluoro-Gold-labeled neurons and the number of Fluoro-Gold-labeled and CGRP-immunoreactive (IR) neurons per 0.45 mm^2 in 10 randomly-selected fields among 30 sections in each group at ×400 magnification using a counting grid, as we have previously reported [16]. The proportion of FG-labeled and CGRP-IR DRG neurons among all FG-labeled neurons was then calculated. All FG-labeled neurons indicated neurons innervating the right knee joint, while FG-labeled and CGRP-IR neurons indicated pain-related neurons innervating the right knee joint.

Statistical analysis

Using the ratio of ipsi and contralateral hind paw values for the three CatWalk variables of duty cycle, swing speed, and print area, the proportion of FG-labeled and CGRP-IR DRG neurons among all FG-labeled DRG neurons was compared among the three groups using a non-repeated measures ANOVA with Bonferroni's correction. A p-value less than 0.05 was considered statistically significant.

Results

Behavioral analysis

In the non-treatment group, the ratio of ipsi to contralateral hind paw values for duty cycle was significantly decreased at pre-treat, treat-1w, and treat-2w compared with that in control group. ($p < 0.05$) In contrast, in the anti-NGF group, the ratio of ipsi to contralateral hind paws values for duty cycle were significantly decreased only at pre-treat ($p < 0.05$) compared with that in control group, and not at treat-1w and treat-2w ($p > 0.05$). In addition, the ratio in the anti-NGF group was significantly improved at treat-1w compared with that in the non-treat group. ($p < 0.05$) (Fig. 1).

In the non-treated group, the ratio of ipsi to contralateral hind paw values for swing speed were significantly decreased at pre-treat, treat-1w, and treat-2w compared with that in the control group. ($p < 0.05$) In contrast, in the anti-NGF group, this ratio was significantly decreased only at pre-treat ($p < 0.05$) compared with that

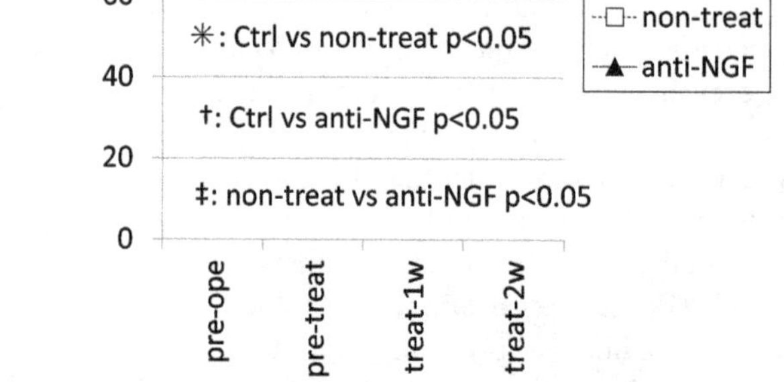

Fig. 1 Ratio of ipsi and contralateral hind paw values of the duty cycle from the CatWalk system. ($p < 0.05$, compared among 3 groups using with a non-repeated measures ANOVA with Bonferroni's *post-hoc* correction.). MIA injection of the knee joint induced a significant small duty cycle within 5 weeks after injection. In contrast, systemic injection of anti-NGF antibody induced significant improvement after only one week of treatment

in control group, and not at treat-1w and treat-2w ($p > 0.05$). In addition, this ratio in the anti-NGF group was significantly improved at treat-1w compared with that in the non-treat group. ($p < 0.05$) (Fig. 2).

In the non-treated group, the ratio of ipsi and contralateral hind paw values for print area were significantly decreased at pre-treat, treat-1w, and treat-2w compared with that in control group. ($p < 0.05$) In contrast, in the anti-NGF group, this ratio was significantly decreased only at pre-treat ($p < 0.05$) compared with that in control group, and not at treat-1w and treat-2w ($p > 0.05$). In addition, the ratio in the anti-NGF group was significantly improved at treat-1w and treat-2w compared with that in the non-treat group. ($p < 0.05$) (Fig. 3).

Immunohistochemical analysis

FG-labeled DRG neurons, which indicated where FG was transported from the right knee, were present in the right L3 to L5 DRGs in all 3 groups (Fig. 4).

The proportion of FG-labeled/CGRP-IR neurons among all FG-labeled neurons was significantly increased in the non-treated group at treat-1w and treat-2w compared with that in control group. ($p < 0.05$) Conversely, the expression of CGRP was significantly decreased in the anti-NGF group at treat-1w and treat-2w compared with the non-treated group ($p < 0.05$). (Figs. 4 and 5).

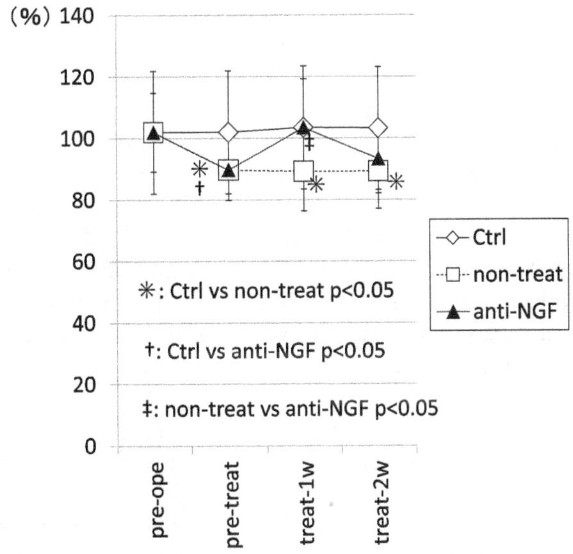

Fig. 2 The ratio of ipsi and contralateral hind paw values for swing speed from the CatWalk system. ($p < 0.05$, compared among 3 groups using with a non-repeated measures ANOVA with Bonferroni's *post-hoc* correction.). MIA injection of the knee joint induced a significant small swing speed within 5 weeks after injection. In contrast, systemic injection of anti-NGF antibody induced significant improvement after only one week of treatment

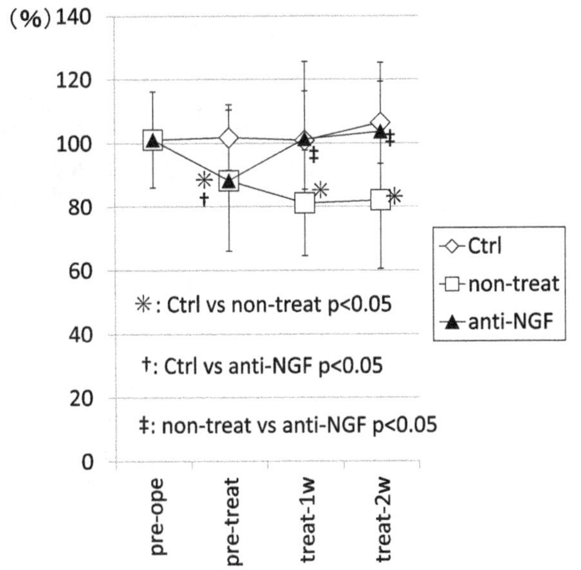

Fig. 3 The ratio of ipsi and contralateral hind paw values of print area from the CatWalk system. ($p < 0.05$, compared among 3 groups using with a non-repeated measures ANOVA with Bonferroni's *post-hoc* correction.). MIA injection of the knee joint induced a significant small print area within 5 weeks after injection. In contrast, systemic injection of anti-NGF antibody induced significant improvement after only 2 weeks of treatment

Discussion

In this study, intraarticular injection of MIA to the knee joints induced gait disturbances, including a small duty cycle, small swing speed, and small print area, and the up-regulation of neuropeptides in DRG neurons innervating the knee joints. Systemic injection of anti-NGF antibody improved these gait disturbances and the expression of neuropeptides in DRG neurons in this model.

Regarding the Knee OA model, multiple authors have reported various surgery-induced animal models. Myers et al. reported that anterior cruciate ligament transection induced changes in the articular cartilage of the unstable knee that are consistent with OA [23]. In addition, Marijnissen et al. reported the usability of the "Groove" model, in which knee articular cartilage is damaged as a knee OA model [24]. Further, Bendele AM report that medial meniscal tear in rats results in rapidly progressive degenerative changes to the cartilage with similarities to OA [11]. These surgically induced knee OA models are suitable for basic research, to the extent that they simulate clinical situations. Nevertheless, the MIA injection model which results in severe joint damage seems superior for evaluating knee pain. MIA injection to the knee joints has been reported to cause joint pathology via the inhibition of glycolysis, and thereby targets avascular cartilage and causes chondrocyte death [25]. We also previously reported that MIA-treated knees exhibited behavioral disturbances within four days and osteoarthritic histological

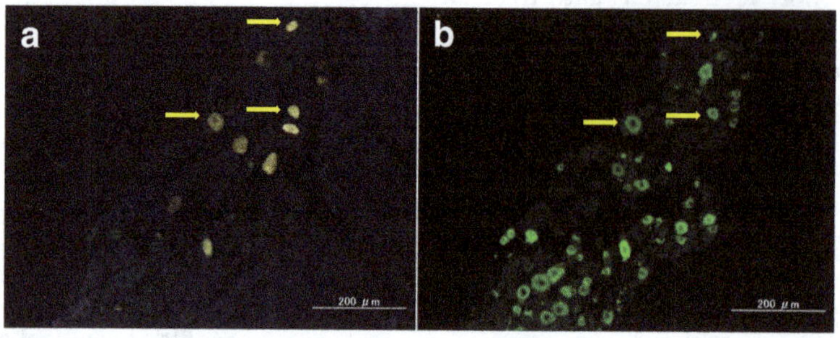

Fig. 4 Representative FG-labeled (**a**) and CGRP-IR (**b**) DRG neurons. **a** and **b** are the same section. The arrow indicates FG- and CGRP-double labeled DRG neurons

changes within four weeks [16]. We therefore used the MIA injection model as a knee OA model in this study.

Regarding knee pain behavior, several authors reported that knee pain models exhibited mechanical allodynia using the von Frey test [13, 16]. In addition, Shelton DL et al. report NGF induced mechanical allodynia in autoimmune arthritis [26]. Therefore, evaluating knee pain using the von Frey test seems to be appropriate for basic research using animal models. However, there is doubt about whether these models of knee pain simulate clinical situations, because knee OA patients do not typically complain of mechanical allodynia in their foot. Recently, gait analysis studies have focused on behavioral studies to evaluate pain behavior. The CatWalk system was initially developed to evaluate motor function, such as that modified in a spinal cord injury model, a Parkinson's disease model, or an olivocerebellar degeneration model [19, 27–29]. Recently, this system has been applied to various models to evaluate behavior associated with pain, such as mechanical allodynia models [30]. We also previously evaluated low back pain behavior using the CatWalk system, and concluded that rat models of low back pain exhibit changes in rat gait, including a long standing time and short strides [21, 31]. Recently several authors applied the CatWalk system to evaluate behavior associated with knee pain. Ferland et al. reported that the MIA-induced knee pain model shows gait changes, including a short Duty cycle and a small Swing Speed. In our previous preliminary study, the MIA-induced knee pain model exhibited a small duty cycle, small swing speed, and small print area. (un-published date) Therefore, in this study, we compared the ratio of ipsi and contralateral hind paw values for the three variables, namely duty cycle, swing speed, and print area among the three groups to evaluate the effect of anti-NGF therapy.

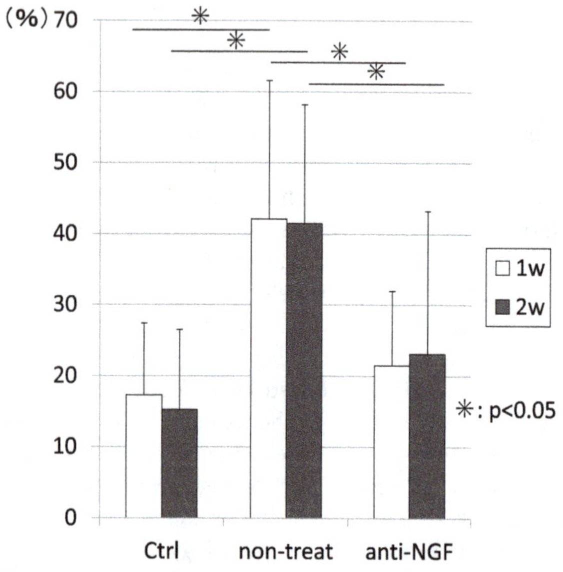

Fig. 5 Percentages of FG and CGRP double labeling of DRGneurons among all FG labeled DRG neurons. (*$p < 0.05$, compared among the three groups using a non-repeated measures ANOVA with Bonferroni's *post-hoc* correction)

Regarding the up-regulation of CGRP in the sensory nervous system, we previously evaluated potential pain-like states by evaluating the up-regulation of pain-related neuropeptides such as CGRP and substance P in the sensory nervous system using a combination of immunohistochemistry and retrograde tracing instead of evaluating pain behavior [22]. CGRP-IR DRG neurons have been reported to be NGF-dependent DRG neurons involved in pain perception related to inflammation [32], suggesting that CGRP is a marker of inflammatory pain. We previously reported that MIA injection to the knee joint induced the up-regulation of CGRP in DRGs [16]. These results suggest that the animals in the group receiving MIA injection to their knee joints were in a state of knee pain.

We focused on NGF as target for the treatment for knee OA pain based on our previous report that MIA injection induced the up-regulation not only inflammatory cytokines but also NGF in the knee joints [16]. Regarding the efficacy of anti-NGF therapy for knee OA pain, NGF is generally involved in chronic inflammatory or neuropathic pain states [33]. Several basic and clinical research had been reported the efficacy of anti-NGF therapy for knee OA pain [34, 35]. However, the pathological mechanism of knee OA pain was not fully understood. NGF is physically produced in articular structures and expressed in both normal and OA synovial tissues, but is increased in synovial inflammation, especially upon synovial tissue exposure to inflammatory cytokines including TNF-alpha [36, 37]. Thus, the up-regulation of inflammatory cytokines in OA knee joints promoted NGF production, which induced the up-regulation of CGRP in the sensory nervous system and chronic inflammatory or neuropathic pain states. Ashraf S et al. report that NGF injection into knee OA joints results in gait disturbance as compared to NGF injection into non-OA joints. This group used two models of knee OA, including an MIA injection model and a meniscal transection model [38]. Further, McNamee KE et al. report NGF expression is correlated with knee pain but that TNF alpha is not up-regulated in the late stages of OA [39]. These findings indicate inflammatory cytokines including TNF might only develop during the pain state, but that NGF might play a role in maintaining as well as in development of the pain state in knee OA patients. Therefore, NGF represents a possible important therapeutic target in the treatment of knee OA pain. In preclinical studies, newly developed tanezumab and its murine precursor muMab-911 have effectively targeted the NGF pathway in various chronic and inflammatory pain models [40]. In addition, phase I and II clinical trials for osteoarthritic pain and chronic lower back pain have demonstrated efficacy for the compound, as well as a good safety and tolerability profile [41]. In the present study, anti-NGF therapy suppressed the impairment gait and up-regulation of CGRP in DRG neurons. These findings may explain the pathological mechanism of knee OA pain.

There were some limitations in this study. First, we should have used tanezumab and its murine precursor muMab-911 for this study. We also did not evaluate differences in efficacy between muMab-911 and anti-NGF antibody, which we used in this study. Second, we did not evaluate the efficacy of positive control including non-steroid anti-inflammatory drugs for knee OA pain. Third, we also evaluated the efficacy of only a one-time injection of anti-NGF antibody. In the future, it will be necessary to evaluate the effect of repeated injections for knee pain. Fourth, we did not evaluate the histopathology of the knee joint. In clinical trials of the monoclonal NGF antibody tanezumab for knee and hip OA pain, osteonecrosis was reported as a side effect [42]. Therefore, further study focusing on side effects of anti-NGF therapy is necessary. Fifth, we did not include a power calculation to justify the group sizes. Further, due to ethical concerns related to using the animals, we combined our behavioral and immunohistochemical evaluations. Therefore, with regard to behavioral evaluation, some experiments ended after 4 weeks and others ended after 5 weeks.

Conclusions

MIA injection into the knee joint induced gait impairment and the up-regulation of CGRP in DRG neurons in a knee OA pain model in mice. Further, intraperitoneal injection of anti-NGF antibody suppressed gait impairment and the up-regulation of CGRP in DRG neurons. These finding indicate that anti-NGF therapy might be valuable in the treatment of OA pain in the knee.

Abbreviations

CGRP: Calcitonin gene related peptide; DRG: dorsal root ganglion; FG: FluoroGold; IR: immunoreactive; MIA: monoiodeacetate; NGF: nerve growth factor; OA: osteoarthritis

Acknowledgments

Not applicable.

Funding

MM was supported by Mitsui Sumitomo Insurance Welfare Foundation.

Authors' contributions

MM conceived this study and carried out the behavioral studies and immunohistochemical studies, participated in its design and coordination and drafted the manuscript, TI carried out behavioral studies and immunohistochemical studies and drafted the manuscript, HK MS and GI made animal models and helped to revise the manuscript, YS, YO, SO carried out behavioral studies and participated in the design of the study, KU carried out statistical analysis and revised the manuscript, KT and MT participated in the design of the study and SO conceived the study and participated in its design and coordination. All authors have read and approved the final manuscript.

Competing interests

This work was supported by Mitsui Sumitomo Insurance Welfare Foundation. The authors declare that they have no competing interests.

Author details

[1]Department of Orthopaedic Surgery, Kitasato University, School of Medicine, 1-15-1, Kitasato, Minami-ku, Sagamihara city, Kanagawa 252-0374, Japan. [2]Department of Orthopaedic Surgery, Graduate School of Medicine, Chiba University, Chiba, Japan.

References

1. Vaishya R, Pariyo GB, Agarwal AK, Vijay V. Non-operative management of osteoarthritis of the knee joint. J Clin. Orthop Trauma. 2016;7(3):170–6.
2. Miyagi M, Ishikawa T, Kamoda H, Suzuki M, Inoue G, Sakuma Y, Oikawa Y, Uchida K, Suzuki T, Takahashi K, Takaso M, Ohtori S. The efficacy of nerve growth factor antibody in a mouse model of neuropathic cancer pain. Exp. Anim 2016; 65 (4):337–343.
3. Mendell LM. Neurotrophins and sensory neurons: role in development, maintenance and injury. A thematic summary. Philos.Trans.R.Soc.Lond B Biol. Sci. 1996;351(1338):463–7.
4. Lewin GR, Mendell LM. Nerve growth factor and nociception. Trends Neurosci. 1993;16(9):353–9.

5. Lewin GR, Rueff A, Mendell LM. Peripheral and central mechanisms of NGF-induced hyperalgesia. EurJ Neurosci. 1994;6(12):1903–12.
6. Ramer MS, Bisby MA. Adrenergic innervation of rat sensory ganglia following proximal or distal painful sciatic neuropathy: distinct mechanisms revealed by anti-NGF treatment. Eur. J Neurosci. 1999;11(3):837–46.
7. Ro LS, Chen ST, Tang LM, Jacobs JM. Effect of NGF and anti-NGF on neuropathic pain in rats following chronic constriction injury of the sciatic nerve. Pain. 1999;79(2–3):265–74.
8. Wild KD, Bian D, Zhu D, Davis J, Bannon AW, Zhang TJ, Louis JC. Antibodies to nerve growth factor reverse established tactile allodynia in rodent models of neuropathic pain without tolerance. J Pharmacol.Exp.Ther. 2007; 322(1):282–7.
9. Ochiai N, Ohtori S, Sasho T, Nakagawa K, Takahashi K, Takahashi N, Murata R, Takahashi K, Moriya H, Wada Y, Saisu T. Extracorporeal shock wave therapy improves motor dysfunction and pain originating from knee osteoarthritis in rats. Osteoarthritis. Cartilage. 2007;15(9):1093–6.
10. Muramatsu Y, Sasho T, Saito M, Yamaguchi S, Akagi R, Mukoyama S, Akatsu Y, Katsuragi J, Fukawa T, Endo J, Hoshi H, Yamamoto Y, Takahashi K. Preventive effects of hyaluronan from deterioration of gait parameters in surgically induced mice osteoarthritic knee model. Osteoarthritis. Cartilage. 2014;22(6):831–5.
11. Bendele AM. Animal models of osteoarthritis. J Musculoskelet. Neuronal. Interact. 2001;1(4):363–76.
12. Daans M, Luyten FP, Lories RJ. GDF5 deficiency in mice is associated with instability-driven joint damage, gait and subchondral bone changes. Ann. Rheum.Dis. 2011;70(1):208–13.
13. Combe R, Bramwell S, Field MJ. The monosodium iodoacetate model of osteoarthritis: a model of chronic nociceptive pain in rats? Neurosci.Lett. 2004;370(2–3):236–40.
14. Guingamp C, Gegout-Pottie P, Philippe L, Terlain B, Netter P, Gillet P. Mono-iodoacetate-induced experimental osteoarthritis: a dose-response study of loss of mobility, morphology, and biochemistry. Arthritis Rheum. 1997;40(9): 1670–9.
15. Guzman RE, Evans MG, Bove S, Morenko B, Kilgore K. Mono-iodoacetate-induced histologic changes in subchondral bone and articular cartilage of rat femorotibial joints: an animal model of osteoarthritis. Toxicol.Pathol. 2003;31(6):619–24.
16. Orita S, Ishikawa T, Miyagi M, Ochiai N, Inoue G, Eguchi Y, Kamoda H, Arai G, Toyone T, Aoki Y, Kubo T, Takahashi K, Ohtori S. Pain-related sensory innervation in monoiodoacetate-induced osteoarthritis in rat knees that gradually develops neuronal injury in addition to inflammatory pain. BMCMusculoskeletDisord. 2011;12:134.
17. Ferland CE, Laverty S, Beaudry F, Vachon P. Gait analysis and pain response of two rodent models of osteoarthritis. Pharmacol.Biochem.Behav. 2011; 97(3):603–10.
18. Ferreira-Gomes J, Adaes S, Castro-Lopes JM. Assessment of movement-evoked pain in osteoarthritis by the knee-bend and CatWalk tests: a clinically relevant study. J Pain. 2008;9(10):945–54.
19. Hamers FP, Lankhorst AJ, van Laar TJ, Veldhuis WB, Gispen WH. Automated quantitative gait analysis during overground locomotion in the rat: its application to spinal cord contusion and transection injuries. J Neurotrauma. 2001;18(2):187–201.
20. Nwosu LN, Mapp PI, Chapman V, Walsh DA. Relationship between structural pathology and pain behaviour in a model of osteoarthritis (OA). Osteoarthritis. Cartilage. 2016;24(11):1910–7.
21. Miyagi M, Ishikawa T, Kamoda H, Orita S, Kuniyoshi K, Ochiai N, Kishida S, Nakamura J, Eguchi Y, Arai G, Suzuki M, Aoki Y, Toyone T, Takahashi K, Inoue G, Ohtori S. Assessment of gait in a rat model of myofascial inflammation using the CatWalk system. Spine (Phila Pa 1976). 2011;36(21):1760–4.
22. Miyagi M, Ishikawa T, Orita S, Eguchi Y, Kamoda H, Arai G, Suzuki M, Inoue G, Aoki Y, Toyone T, Takahashi K, Ohtori S. Disk injury in rats produces persistent increases in pain-related neuropeptides in dorsal root ganglia and spinal cord glia but only transient increases in inflammatory mediators: pathomechanism of chronic diskogenic low back pain. Spine (Phila Pa 1976). 2011;36(26):2260–6.
23. Myers SL, Brandt KD, O'Connor BL, Visco DM, Albrecht ME. Synovitis and osteoarthritic changes in canine articular cartilage after anterior cruciate ligament transection. Effect of surgical hemostasis. Arthritis Rheum. 1990; 33(9):1406–15.
24. Marijnissen AC, van Roermund PM, TeKoppele JM, Bijlsma JW, Lafeber FP. The canine 'groove' model, compared with the ACLT model of osteoarthritis. Osteoarthritis. Cartilage. 2002;10(2):145–55.
25. Janusz MJ, Bendele AM, Brown KK, Taiwo YO, Hsieh L, Heitmeyer SA. Induction of osteoarthritis in the rat by surgical tear of the meniscus: inhibition of joint damage by a matrix metalloproteinase inhibitor. Osteoarthritis. Cartilage. 2002;10(10):785–91.
26. Shelton DL, Zeller J, Ho WH, Pons J, Rosenthal A. Nerve growth factor mediates hyperalgesia and cachexia in auto-immune arthritis. Pain. 2005; 116(1–2):8–16.
27. Cendelin J, Voller J, Vozeh F. Ataxic gait analysis in a mouse model of the olivocerebellar degeneration. Behav. Brain Res. 2010;210(1):8–15.
28. Chuang CS, Su HL, Cheng FC, Hsu SH, Chuang CF, Liu CS. Quantitative evaluation of motor function before and after engraftment of dopaminergic neurons in a rat model of Parkinson's disease. J Biomed.Sci. 2010;17:9.
29. Koopmans GC, Deumens R, Honig WM, Hamers FP, Steinbusch HW, Joosten EA. The assessment of locomotor function in spinal cord injured rats: the importance of objective analysis of coordination. J Neurotrauma. 2005;22(2): 214–25.
30. Vrinten DH, Hamers FF. CatWalk' automated quantitative gait analysis as a novel method to assess mechanical allodynia in the rat; a comparison with von Frey testing. Pain. 2003;102(1–2):203–9.
31. Miyagi M, Ishikawa T, Kamoda H, Suzuki M, Sakuma Y, Orita S, Oikawa Y, Aoki Y, Toyone T, Takahashi K, Inoue G, Ohtori S. Assessment of pain behavior in a rat model of intervertebral disc injury using the CatWalk gait analysis system. Spine (Phila Pa 1976). 2013;38(17):1459–65.
32. Averill S, McMahon SB, Clary DO, Reichardt LF, Priestley JV. Immunocytochemical localization of trkA receptors in chemically identified subgroups of adult rat sensory neurons. Eur. J Neurosci. 1995;7(7):1484–94.
33. Pezet S, McMahon SB. Neurotrophins: mediators and modulators of pain. Annu.Rev.Neurosci. 2006;29:507–38.
34. Ishikawa G, Koya Y, Tanaka H, Nagakura Y. Long-term analgesic effect of a single dose of anti-NGF antibody on pain during motion without notable suppression of joint edema and lesion in a rat model of osteoarthritis. Osteoarthritis. Cartilage. 2015;23(6):925–32.
35. Schnitzer TJ, Marks JAA. Systematic review of the efficacy and general safety of antibodies to NGF in the treatment of OA of the hip or knee. Osteoarthritis. Cartilage. 2015;23(Suppl 1):S8–17.
36. Manni L, Lundeberg T, Fiorito S, Bonini S, Vigneti E, Aloe L. Nerve growth factor release by human synovial fibroblasts prior to and following exposure to tumor necrosis factor-alpha, interleukin-1 beta and cholecystokinin-8: the possible role of NGF in the inflammatory response. Clin.Exp.Rheumatol. 2003;21(5):617–24.
37. Takano S, Uchida K, Miyagi M, Inoue G, Fujimaki H, Aikawa J, Iwase D, Minatani A, Iwabuchi K, Takaso M. Nerve growth factor regulation by TNF-alpha and IL-1beta in synovial macrophages and fibroblasts in osteoarthritic mice. J Immunol Res. 2016;2016:5706359.
38. Ashraf S, Mapp PI, Burston J, Bennett AJ, Chapman V, Walsh DA. Augmented pain behavioural responses to intra-articular injection of nerve growth factor in two animal models of osteoarthritis. Ann.Rheum.Dis. 2014; 73(9):1710–8.
39. McNamee KE, Burleigh A, Gompels LL, Feldmann M, Allen SJ, Williams RO, Dawbarn D, Vincent TL, Inglis JJ. Treatment of murine osteoarthritis with TrkAd5 reveals a pivotal role for nerve growth factor in non-inflammatory joint pain. Pain. 2010;149(2):386–92.
40. Xu L, Nwosu LN, Burston JJ, Millns PJ, Sagar DR, Mapp PI, Meesawatsom P, Li L, Bennett AJ, Walsh DA, Chapman V. The anti-NGF antibody muMab 911 both prevents and reverses pain behaviour and subchondral osteoclast numbers in a rat model of osteoarthritis pain. Osteoarthritis. Cartilage. 2016; 24(9):1587–95.
41. Cattaneo A. Tanezumab, a recombinant humanized mAb against nerve growth factor for the treatment of acute and chronic pain. Curr.Opin.Mol. Ther. 2010;12(1):94–106.
42. Balanescu AR, Feist E, Wolfram G, Davignon I, Smith MD, Brown MT, West CR. Efficacy and safety of tanezumab added on to diclofenac sustained release in patients with knee or hip osteoarthritis: a double-blind, placebo-controlled, parallel-group, multicentre phase III randomised clinical trial. Ann.Rheum.Dis. 2014;73(9):1665–72.

3

Analysis of medical service use of knee osteoarthritis and knee meniscal and ligament injuries in Korea: a cross-sectional study of national patient sample data

Chang Yong Suh[1†], Yoon Jae Lee[1†], Joon-Shik Shin[1], Jinho Lee[1], Me-riong Kim[2], Wonil Koh[1], Yun-Yeop Cha[3], Byung-Cheul Shin[4,5], Eui-Hyoung Hwang[4,5], Kristin Suhr[6], Mia Kim[7] and In-Hyuk Ha[1*]

Abstract

Background: Osteoarthritis (OA) and meniscal and ligament injuries of the knee are the two most common knee disorders in Korea. The aim of this study was to analyze the demographic characteristics, medical service use and related costs for these disorders, and the results are expected to help inform practitioners, researchers, and policy-makers.

Methods: The present study aimed to evaluate incidence and patient characteristics, and to assess current medical service use, usual care, and medical expenses of knee disorders by analyzing 2014 national patient sample data from the Korean Health Insurance Review and Assessment Service. Data was extracted using 3% stratified sampling from all Korea national health insurance claims submitted in 2014, and analyzed. Usual care for M17 knee osteoarthritis and S83 knee meniscal and ligament injury codes of the International Classification of Diseases, 10th revision (ICD-10) were determined by investigating total number of patients, sociodemographic characteristics, days in care, number of visits, and expenses.

Results: Knee OA showed the highest incidence in females aged ≥60 years, whereas meniscal and ligament injuries of the knee were most prevalent among patients aged <20 years and young adults. Total inpatient care expenses exceeded the cost of ambulatory care for both disorders. Ambulatory care was mainly provided at primary care clinics, with 90% of these visits made to orthopedic specialists. Medical expenses for knee OA and meniscal and ligament injuries were largely due to procedures/surgeries and injections, and procedures/surgeries and hospitalizations, respectively. Total replacement arthroplasty was the most commonly performed surgery for knee OA, while meniscectomy and cruciate ligament reconstruction were the most often performed surgeries for meniscal and ligament injuries. Intra-articular injection rates were 55% in knee OA patients and 3% in meniscal and ligament injury patients. Aceclofenac, diclofenac, and tramadol were the most frequently prescribed analgesics.

Conclusions: The current findings may be used as basic data for establishing medical policies and can benefit researchers and clinicians in recognizing trends and patterns of treatment for knee disorders.

Keywords: Knee osteoarthritis, Knee meniscal and ligament injury, Medical service use, Usual care, Korean Health Insurance Review and Assessment Service-National Patient Sample (HIRA-NPS) data

* Correspondence: hanihata@gmail.com
†Equal contributors
[1]Jaseng Spine and Joint Research Institute, Jaseng Medical Foundation, 858 Eonju-ro, Gangnam-gu, Seoul, Republic of Korea
Full list of author information is available at the end of the article

Background

Knee osteoarthritis (OA) is one of the most common disorders in the U.S., and symptomatic OA prevalence was found to be as high as 10% in men and 13% in women aged ≥60 [1]. Similarly, symptomatic knee OA was shown to affect 9.3% and 28.5% of Korean men and women aged ≥50, respectively, with a steep increase in prevalence in older populations [2]. Meanwhile, knee meniscal injury patients tend to be younger than knee OA patients, and incidence was reported as 3–5% in the U.S. [3] and 10.6% in Korean populations [4]. According to the U.S. Medical Expenditure Panel Survey, insurance coverage and out-of-pocket expenses for knee OA amounted to 185 billion U.S. dollars, denoting its significant socioeconomic impact [5]. In addition, arthroscopic partial meniscectomy is one of the most frequently performed orthopedic surgeries in the U.S., with 700,000 new cases performed each year, and estimates for direct annual medical costs were put at 4 billion U.S. dollars [6].

The epidemiology and pathology of knee OA and meniscal injury differ substantially regarding their onset, age, and etiology. Population-wide studies have purported that incidence estimates of knee meniscal injury are highest in adolescent and young men [7], stating that these populations are at higher risk of injury as they are more likely to engage in competitive sports such as ball games, while older adults are at lower risk of injury as they are more likely to participate in non-competitive sports such as walking, jogging and swimming [8]. On the other hand, knee OA prevalence increases rapidly after the age of 50, which is especially pronounced in post-menopausal women due to the effect of hormonal imbalance on cartilaginous tissue [9]. Although the epidemiology of knee osteoarthritis and injury varies considerably, their etiology is often viewed to share certain traits; injury of the anterior cruciate ligament (ACL) or the meniscus may incur joint instability and damage the cartilage surface, leading to chronic disability and potential knee OA [10, 11].

The National Health Insurance Service (NHIS) in Korea covers 47 million out of 51 million South Korean residents. Claims data are generated when a medical institution provides medical services to a patient and applies for reimbursement from the NHIS, and therefore contain information on the patient and medical institution, a complete list of insured medical services that were provided (e.g., treatment, examinations, and prescriptions), and their related costs. The two highest frequency knee disorders, knee OA and knee meniscal and ligament injuries, were comprehensively analyzed for patient characteristics and expenditure (i.e., surgery, hospitalization, physical therapy and medication costs) to the aim of providing basic information to policymakers and practitioners in Korea. Moreover, given that standard care based on evidence and the usual care provided in real world settings frequently digress and that by country and culture, the implications of current reports on high-frequency medical service use (i.e., pharmacological, nonpharmacological, and surgical interventions) hold relevance at an international level also through illustration of concurrent clinical practice in knee disorders.

The aim of this study was to provide preliminary data towards establishing a basic guideline for general medical care based on the prevalence, current use of medical services, and costs of knee OA and meniscal and ligament injuries from the 2014 claims data submitted to the Korea Health Insurance Review and Assessment Service (HIRA). This analysis may be used to assist policymakers, practitioners, and researchers by providing a window into the most common treatments for knee conditions.

Methods

Data and subjects

The 2014 Health Insurance Review and Assessment Service-National Patient Sample (HIRA-NPS) data were analyzed. Claims data are generated when medical institutions apply for reimbursement of medical costs partially covered by Korea National Health Insurance. The data include medical record details (e.g., treatments, procedures, examinations, and prescriptions), diagnosis codes, co-payment paid by the patient and the insurance benefit paid by Korea National Health Insurance, patient demographics (e.g., age and sex), and information on the service provider (medical institution).

Provided yearly for research purposes, the HIRA-NPS datasets are extracted from the raw claims database using random sampling, stratified according to age groups and sex, with removal of identifying personal and institutional information. Each dataset consists of claims records for the corresponding year. Regardless of inpatient/outpatient status, 3% of the total patient population for each year was sampled and extracted, which approximates to 1.4 million patients. As each individual patient is coded with a unique identifier which is randomly generated and not privacy-sensitive, multiple visits of individual patients are easily traceable [12]. The current study chose to analyze the total number of patients by treatment type as opposed to total number of visits to the aim of illustrating individual medical service use in this patient population. Upon analysis, the results were presented both as inpatient and outpatient groups separately, and in total. The number of in- and outpatients indicate the number of patients who were hospitalized and those who visited the outpatient department one or more times for knee disorder-related diagnosis codes during the corresponding year, respectively. Multiple hospitalizations or outpatient visits of individual patients were viewed as duplicates and disregarded. Total counts for medical services were similarly tallied as the number of patients who used each respective service and not the number of treatment sessions. The actual parameters of the South Korean population may therefore be estimated from the current sample data statistics by multiplying the weighting value of 33.3 as the database is generated from 3% stratified sampling of total patients. In the present study, the statistical weight was not applied as the weighting was identical across all data and therefore did not affect the interpretation of results.

Knee OA and knee meniscal and ligament injuries

Knee disorders were classified as M17 (arthrosis of the knee), S83 (dislocation, sprain, and strain of joints and ligaments of the knee), M22 (disorders of the patella) and M23 (internal derangement of the knee), according to the International Statistical Classification of Diseases and Related Health Problems, 10th revision (ICD-10). The number of individuals with knee disorder codes and radiological imaging of the knee were 48,321 with M17, 3087 with M22, 7103 with M23, and 19,136 with S83 in the 2014 dataset (Additional file 1: Table S1). Only those coded as M17 and S83 were included in this study as relatively few individuals were diagnosed with M22 and M23. A total of 48,000 outpatients and 3084 inpatients were diagnosed and treated under M17, and 18,540 outpatients and 2434 inpatients were diagnosed and treated under S83. Duplicate cases existed when a patient received both ambulatory and hospital care under the same code; thus, the total number of patients was smaller than the numerical sum of inpatients and outpatients. Through literature review and author discussion, M17 was diagnosed as knee OA [13–15] and S83 as knee meniscal and ligament injury [16].

Analysis

The demographic characteristics of knee disorder patients as classified using ICD-10 diagnostic codes were examined. Age groups were divided into 10-year intervals: less than 20 years, 20–29 years, 30–39 years, and so on. Each patient was also classified by type of insurance as being eligible for either National Health Insurance or Medicaid. Medical institutions were categorized as primary care clinics, hospitals, general hospitals, tertiary hospitals, long-term care hospitals, or public health centers. The specialty of the attending physician was also assessed. The total treatment expenses were divided and analyzed according to the medical service codes designated by the Korean Ministry of Health and Welfare (i.e., costs per visit (consultation), hospitalization, medication, injection, anesthesia, physiotherapy, psychotherapy, procedure/surgery, examination, and radiographic evaluation/intervention). Total expense was defined as the total costs incurred for healthcare of the insured patient at medical institutions, which equaled the sum of benefit paid by the National Health Insurance Service and co-payment expenses paid by patients, of which the reimbursement amount was reviewed and determined by HIRA.

Details on the use of surgeries, injections, physiotherapy, and analgesics were investigated according to the corresponding code count; the relevant codes for these services are summarized in Additional file 2: Table S2. When assessing surgical patterns, the procedure codes were excluded from the procedure/surgery analysis because surgery codes were always accompanied by collateral procedure codes. Surgery codes that are not limited to the knee such as joint excision, osteochondral autograft transplantation, osteotomy and internal fixation, and subcutaneous tenotomy were also excluded.

Injection use was investigated according to the administration route, with intra-articular, subcutaneous, and intramuscular injections being of particular interest. Although intravenous, continuous intravenous, and perineural injections were often administered for knee disorders in clinical settings, the authors concluded that these injection types were generally not directly related to knee disorder treatment or for anti-nociceptive purposes, and these codes were accordingly excluded.

The most frequently applied physiotherapies are arranged in order of their prescription frequencies. Analgesics prescribed for inpatient and outpatient use were classified in order of prescription frequency, according to the 5th Anatomical Therapeutic Chemical (ATC) Classification System levels. Narcotic and non-narcotic substances were categorized as previously reported by the Korean National Evidence-based Health Care Collaborating Agency [17]. ATC codes were developed by the WHO Collaborating Centre for Drug Statistics Methodology in 1976 [18]. The 1st, 2nd, 3rd, 4th, and 5th ATC code levels indicate the anatomical target groups, therapeutic groups, therapeutic/pharmacologic subgroups, chemical/therapeutic/pharmacologic subgroups, and chemical substances, respectively, for the systematic classification of drug substances [19].

Most 5th ATC level drug substances have corresponding chemical names, with a few exceptions such as acetaminophen and paracetamol. Although this study used 5th ATC level terms to standardize nomenclature, four analgesics (7 in Additional file 3: Table S3) did not have corresponding 5th level codes, and in those instances, chemical names were used instead. Drug prescriptions were identified using the relevant claims data, regardless of dose.

Statistical analysis

The demographic characteristics and medical details regarding surgeries, injections, physiotherapy, and drug prescriptions of patients with knee OA and meniscal and ligament injury are presented as frequencies and percentages (%) following frequency analyses. Patient percentages were determined using the total number of patients in each relevant diagnosis group as the denominator, and medical expense percentages were similarly calculated for total expenses, per-patient expenses, and costs per service using the total treatment expense for knee OA and knee meniscal and ligament injury as the denominator, respectively. Statistical analyses were performed using SAS, ver. 9.3 package (SAS Institute Inc., Cary, NC, USA).

Results

Current use of medical treatment for knee OA and knee meniscal and ligament injuries

The total number of patients, total expenses, per-patient expenses, average days of care, and average number of visits were higher for patients with knee OA than for those with knee meniscal and ligament injuries, regardless of whether the patients were treated as inpatients or outpatients. Although the total number of inpatients was smaller than the total number of outpatients, the total expenses for inpatients were higher in both types of knee disorders. The per-patient expense for inpatients was approximately 20 times higher than that for outpatients, irrespective of the type of knee disorder. However, the average number of days of care and number of visits were more than three times higher for hospitalized patients than for those receiving ambulatory care (Table 1).

Sociodemographic characteristics of knee OA and knee meniscal and ligament injury patients

The majority of patients with OA of the knee and knee meniscal and ligament injury received ambulatory care with approximately 6% of knee OA patients and 12% of meniscal and ligament injury patients hospitalized. The incidence of knee OA was positively correlated with age, showing a steep increase after the age of 50 years. However, the number of knee meniscal and ligament injury patients was highest in age < 20 years, with the numbers remaining constant from age 20 to 60 years, and declining thereafter. The age distribution was similar for both inpatients and outpatients with knee OA. On the other hand, the percentage of knee meniscal and ligament injury in patients aged <20 years who were hospitalized was approximately half the number of those receiving outpatient care. Knee OA was found to be more prevalent in women than in men, as was clearly evidenced by the fact that 82% percent of inpatients were women. On the contrary, the incidence of knee meniscal and ligament injuries was slightly higher in men than in women.

Almost all knee disorder patients were covered by National Health Insurance, and the treatment patterns did not differ substantially between inpatients and outpatients. About 70% of all patients visited primary care clinics, while the rest visited hospitals, general hospitals, and tertiary hospitals (listed in order of decreasing frequency of use). Notably, more than half of all knee OA and meniscal and ligament injury inpatients received medical care in hospitals instead of more accessible primary care clinics, which differed from the pattern seen in outpatients, and the percentage of general, tertiary, and long-term care hospitals increased substantially in inpatients. However, overall usage of medical institutions did not differ greatly between knee OA and meniscal and ligament injury patients. Approximately 90% of all patients, regardless of the type of disorder or whether they were receiving inpatient or outpatient care, sought medical care from an orthopedics department. Apart from orthopedics, knee OA patients were treated in anesthesiology, general surgery, and neurosurgery departments, and knee meniscal and ligament injury patients were treated in general surgery, neurosurgery, and emergency medicine (EM) departments. Other than orthopedics, inpatients were often treated in specialty departments such as rehabilitative medicine and general surgery, whereas radiology, EM, and general practice departments were utilized for outpatients (Table 2).

Distribution of medical expenses in knee OA and knee meniscal and ligament injuries

Medical expenses for knee OA and knee meniscal and ligament injury cases were classified into 10 categories:

Table 1 General medical service use and expenses for knee osteoarthritis and knee meniscal and ligament injury in Korea

Visit type	Diagnostic groups	Number of patients	Total expense[a]	Expense-per-patient[a]	Days of treatment[b]	Number of visits[c]
Total	Knee OA	48,321	24,526,738,820	507,579.3	11.0	9.1
	Knee meniscal and ligament injury	19,136	5,800,760,680	303,133.4	5.8	4.7
Outpatients	Knee OA	48,000	10,758,908,490	224,143.9	8.7	7.8
	Knee meniscal and ligament injury	18,540	1,660,439,710	89,559.9	3.4	3.2
Inpatients	Knee OA	3084	13,767,830,330	4,464,277.0	36.4	22.2
	Knee meniscal and ligament injury	2434	4,140,320,970	1,701,035.7	20.1	12.3

OA Osteoarthritis
[a]Displayed in KRW; 1 USD = 1104 KRW (as of September 30th, 2016)
[b]The total days of treatment indicated in the claims statement including drug prescription days without medical treatment
[c]The number of outpatient visits or the number of inpatient care days of the patient indicated in the claims statement

Table 2 Sociodemographic characteristics of knee osteoarthritis and knee meniscal and ligament injury patients

Characteristics		Total				Inpatient				Outpatient			
		Knee OA		Knee meniscal and ligament injury		Knee OA		Knee meniscal and ligament injury		Knee OA		Knee meniscal and ligament injury	
		N = 48,321	%	*N* = 19,136	%	*N* = 3084	%	*N* = 2434	%	*N* = 48,000	%	*N* = 18,540	%
Age (years)	< 20	243	0.50	4290	22.42	1	0.03	272	11.18	242	0.50	4252	22.93
	20~29	457	0.95	2665	13.93	11	0.36	411	16.89	450	0.94	2592	13.98
	30~39	890	1.84	2488	13.00	38	1.23	359	14.75	877	1.83	2415	13.03
	40~49	3812	7.89	3131	16.36	199	6.45	470	19.31	3758	7.83	3032	16.35
	50~59	12,856	26.61	3542	18.51	772	25.03	539	22.14	12,736	26.53	3387	18.27
	60~69	14,790	30.61	1865	9.75	960	31.13	251	10.31	14,729	30.69	1777	9.58
	≥ 70	15,273	31.61	1155	6.04	1103	35.77	132	5.42	15,208	31.68	1085	5.85
Sex	Male	13,141	27.20	10,445	54.58	546	17.70	1438	59.08	13,054	27.20	10,171	54.86
	Female	35,180	72.80	8691	45.42	2538	82.30	996	40.92	34,946	72.80	8369	45.14
Insurance type[a]	NHI	45,183	93.51	18,483	96.59	2853	92.51	2356	96.80	44,879	93.50	17,912	96.61
	MD	3234	6.69	651	3.40	230	7.46	74	3.04	3215	6.70	625	3.37
	VH	135	0.28	21	0.11	11	0.36	6	0.25	133	0.28	19	0.10
Medical institution type[b]	Clinic	36,731	76.01	13,343	69.73	592	19.20	590	24.24	36,570	76.19	13,115	70.74
	Hospital	12,925	26.75	4814	25.16	1816	58.88	1263	51.89	12,616	26.28	4452	24.01
	GH	5371	11.12	2053	10.73	646	20.95	569	23.38	5251	10.94	1872	10.10
	TH	1801	3.73	437	2.28	243	7.88	129	5.30	1774	3.70	408	2.20
	LCH	621	1.29	85	0.44	176	5.71	25	1.03	457	0.95	65	0.35
	PHC	407	0.84	21	0.11	2	0.06	–	–	407	0.85	21	0.11
	KMH	126	0.26	59	0.31	80	2.59	34	1.40	50	0.10	26	0.14
Medical specialty[c]	OS	43,654	90.34	17,056	89.13	2852	92.48	2304	94.66	43,379	90.37	16,486	88.92
	AN	3108	6.43	300	1.57	32	1.04	11	0.45	3083	6.42	293	1.58
	GS	2350	4.86	588	3.07	91	2.95	56	2.30	2281	4.75	554	2.99
	NS	1957	4.05	493	2.58	76	2.46	27	1.11	1899	3.96	470	2.54
	IM	1888	3.91	428	2.24	50	1.62	23	0.94	1846	3.85	410	2.21
	RM	1532	3.17	354	1.85	166	5.38	53	2.18	1408	2.93	323	1.74
	FM	1656	3.43	220	1.15	110	3.57	26	1.07	1563	3.26	195	1.05
	RD	258	0.53	295	1.54	1	0.03	1	0.04				
	ER	101	0.21	451	2.36	1	0.03	4	0.16				
	GP	326	0.67	19	0.10	1	0.03	1	0.04				
	Other[d]	470	0.97	93	0.49								

OA Osteoarthritis
[a]NHI, National Health Insurance; MD, Medicaid; VH, Veteran Healthcare
[b]GH, General Hospital; TH, Tertiary Hospital; LCH, Long-term Care Hospital; PHC, Public Health Center; KMH, Korean Medicine Hospital
[c]OS, Orthopedic surgery; AN, Anesthesiology; GS, General Surgery; NS, Neurosurgery; IM, Internal Medicine; RM, Rehabilitation Medicine; FM, Family Medicine; RD, Radiology; EM, Emergency Medicine; GP, General Physician
[d]Including Neurology, Thoracic and Cardiovascular Surgery, Pediatrics, Obstetrics and Gynecology, Urology, and Neuropsychiatry

costs of visits (consultations), hospitalizations, medications, injections, anesthesia, physiotherapy, psychotherapy, procedures/surgeries, examinations, and radiologic evaluations/interventions. The categories reflecting the bulk of total expenses for each diagnostic group were, in decreasing order, procedures/surgeries, injections, visits (consultations), and hospitalizations for knee OA patients, and procedures/surgeries, hospitalizations, visits (consultations), and injections for knee meniscal and ligament injury cases. Procedures/surgeries constituted ≥30% of total expenses in both knee disorder categories, and injection costs comprised nearly 20% of the total expenses for knee OA patients, ranking 2nd in total costs, but only 6% of the total expenses for meniscal and ligament injury patients. More than 99% of all patients, irrespective of specific knee disorder, paid for cost of visits (consultations), and this category represented the third highest percentage of total costs for patients with either disorder. In addition, hospitalization costs also comprised a considerable portion of total medical expenses. In particular, hospitalization costs represented almost 20% (second highest percentage) of the total expenses for knee meniscal and ligament injury patients. Although more than 13% of all patients were prescribed medications, total medication costs were <2% of the total expenses for patients with either knee disorder. Similarly, ≥53% of all patients underwent physiotherapy, but this treatment cost represented only 6% of total expenses. The other subcategories (i.e., radiographic evaluations/interventions, examinations, and anesthesia) took up <6% of all expenses, and psychotherapy was rarely performed. Despite its relatively low proportion out of total costs, radiographic evaluations/interventions were widely applied to 98% of knee OA patients and 94% of meniscal and ligament injury patients (Table 3).

Usual care of knee OA and knee meniscal and ligament injuries, excluding medications

Frequently used surgeries, injections, and physiotherapies were investigated to determine usual practice patterns. Replacement arthroplasty was the most frequently performed surgery for knee OA patients, and cruciate ligament or meniscus surgery was the most common for knee meniscal and ligament injuries. Specifically, replacement arthroplasty usually involved total arthroplasty, and menisectomy was performed as either unilateral medial or unilateral lateral menisectomy. Patients who received surgical care were generally hospitalized.

Subcutaneous and intramuscular injections were performed in 19,722 knee OA cases and in 7390 meniscal and ligament injury cases, taking up approximately 40% of the cases of each disorder. In contrast, intra-articular injections were performed in 26,883 (55%) knee OA cases and in 549 (3%) meniscal and ligament injury cases. Upon hospitalization, subcutaneous and intramuscular injection rates increased to 83% and 65% for knee OA and meniscal and ligament injury patients, respectively, representing rates that were approximately twice those observed in outpatients. Intra-articular injections were administered to 55% of knee OA outpatients, but to only 14% of inpatients.

Of various physiotherapy modalities, superficial heat therapy, deep heat therapy, transcutaneous electrical nerve stimulation, and interferential current therapy were prescribed to about 25% of patients of either knee disorder; other physiotherapies were seldom used. Physiotherapy use was slightly more common for knee OA than meniscal and ligament injury patients. However, in hospitalized patients, exercise therapy was prescribed to 59% of knee OA and 27% of meniscal and ligament injury patients, which is significantly higher than the rates observed in ambulatory settings (Table 4).

Medication use in usual care of knee OA and knee meniscal and ligament injuries

The medications, including both narcotics and non-narcotics, frequently used for knee disorders were organized according to 5th ATC levels. The most frequently used medication, for both knee OA and meniscal and ligament injury patients, was aceclofenac, which was administered to 20–30% of all knee disorder patients. Tramadol and diclofenac were also commonly prescribed, but their use was more pronounced in inpatients than in outpatients. In contrast, paracetamol was more frequently used among outpatients than among

Table 3 Distribution of medical expenditure in knee osteoarthritis and knee meniscal and ligament injury

Classification	Knee OA					Knee meniscal and ligament injury				
	Case (n)		Cost[a]		Per-case cost[a]	Case (n)		Cost[a]		Per-case cost[a]
	N = 48,321	%	Total	%		*N* = 19,136	%	Total	%	
Procedure/surgery	5403	11.18	7,593,254,872	31.41	1,405,377.5	4555	23.80	1,887,655,557	34.31	414,414.0
Injection	37,050	76.67	4,732,291,088	19.58	127,727.2	8315	43.45	365,245,211	6.64	43,926.1
Outpatient visit (consultation)	48,283	99.92	4,021,230,425	16.64	83,284.6	19,084	99.73	715,896,835	13.01	37,512.9
Hospitalization	3033	6.28	2,757,254,594	11.41	909,084.9	2403	12.56	1,186,629,123	21.57	493,811.5
Physiotherapy	25,667	53.12	1,337,965,293	5.54	52,127.8	11,048	57.73	334,564,005	6.08	30,282.8
Radiographic evaluation/ intervention	47,232	97.75	1,277,960,897	5.29	27,057.1	17,919	93.64	323,895,267	5.89	18,075.5
Examination	10,310	21.34	1,144,231,241	4.73	110,982.7	3351	17.51	357,995,050	6.51	106,832.3
Anesthesia	8576	17.75	907,924,433	3.76	105,868.1	1829	9.56	224,006,652	4.07	122,474.9
Medication	6327	13.09	399,489,786	1.65	63,140.5	3043	15.90	105,707,519	1.92	34,737.9
Psychotherapy	21	0.04	674,087	0.00	32,099.4	1	0.01	12,579	0.00	12,579.0

OA Osteoarthritis
[a]Displayed in KRW; 1 USD = 1104 KRW (as of September 30th, 2016)

Table 4 Usual care of knee osteoarthritis and knee meniscal and ligament injury, excluding prescription medication use

	Subtypes	Total				Inpatient				Outpatient			
		Knee OA		Knee meniscal and ligament injury		Knee OA		Knee meniscal and ligament injury		Knee OA		Knee meniscal and ligament injury	
		N = 48,321	%	N = 19,136	%	N = 3084	%	N = 2434	%	N = 48,000	%	N = 18,540	%
Surgery	Replacement Arthroplasty, Total Arthroplasty, knee	1466	3.03	1	0.01	1466	47.54	1	0.04	–	–	–	–
	Replacement Arthroplasty, Hemiarthroplasty, knee	89	0.18	–	–	89	2.89	–	–	–	–	–	–
	Revision of Replacement Arthroplasty, Total Arthroplasty, knee	26	0.05	–	–	26	0.84	–	–	–	–	–	–
	Revision of Replacement Arthroplasty, Hemiarthroplasty, knee	8	0.02	–	–	8	0.26	–	–	–	–	–	–
	Menisectomy, Medial or Lateral	182	0.38	586	3.06	182	5.90	584	23.99	–	–	2	0.01
	Menisectomy, Medial and Lateral	44	0.09	151	0.79	44	1.43	151	6.20	–	–	–	–
	Repair of Meniscus, Medial or Lateral	18	0.04	222	1.16	18	0.58	222	9.12	–	–	–	–
	Repair of Meniscus, Medial and Lateral	2	0.00	35	0.18	2	0.06	35	1.44	–	–	–	–
	Reconstruction of Cruciate Ligament	–	–	446	2.33	–	–	446	18.32	–	–	–	–
	Repair of Cruciate Ligament	1	0.00	11	0.06	1	0.03	11	0.45	–	–	–	–
Injection	Intraarticular Injection	26,883	55.63	334	1.75	427	13.85	107	4.40	26,695	55.61	296	1.60
	Subcutaneous or Intramuscular Injection	19,722	40.81	6457	33.74	2572	83.40	1775	72.93	18,265	38.05	5279	28.47
Physiotherapy	Superficial Heat Therapy	24,261	50.21	8774	45.85	1486	48.18	952	39.11	23,575	49.11	8319	44.87
	Deep Heat Therapy	22,128	45.79	8032	41.97	1285	41.67	863	35.46	21,511	44.81	7603	41.01
	Transcutaneous Electrical Nerve Stimulation	14,281	29.55	4804	25.10	969	31.42	572	23.50	13,736	28.62	4467	24.09
	Interferential Current Therapy	12,306	25.47	4195	21.92	980	31.78	563	23.13	11,698	24.37	3853	20.78
	Laser Therapy[a]	3423	7.08	1705	8.91	327	10.60	216	8.87	3172	6.61	1557	8.40
	Therapeutic Exercise[a]	2016	4.17	811	4.24	1806	58.56	652	26.79	612	1.28	381	2.06
	Simple Therapeutic Exercise	1712	3.54	673	3.52	434	14.07	174	7.15	1358	2.83	537	2.90
	Cold Therapy, Cold Pack	1119	2.32	785	4.10	423	13.72	195	8.01	774	1.61	647	3.49
	Myofascial Trigger Point Injection Therapy[b]	609	1.26	58	0.30	37	1.20	7	0.29	576	1.20	51	0.28

OA Osteoarthritis

[a]Simple rehabilitation treatments, which can be prescribed by specialists of rehabilitation medicine, orthopedic surgery, neurosurgery, neurology, general surgery, cardiovascular surgery, and anesthesiology

[b]Complex rehabilitation treatment, which can only be prescribed by specialists of rehabilitation medicine

inpatients. Meloxicam and celecoxib were also largely used for knee OA patients, but their use was not evident in knee meniscal and ligament injury patients. Pethidine was the most commonly used narcotic analgesic, with 25% of knee OA inpatients receiving pethidine, although the overall prescription rate was low (Table 5).

Discussion

The total expenses, per-patient expenses, average days of care, and average number of visits were higher for inpatients than for outpatients, regardless of the specific type of knee disorder diagnosis (knee OA or meniscal and ligament injury). These results may be partly attributed to differences in disease and symptom severity as patients with more severe disease and/or symptoms may be more likely to undergo hospitalized care. Another possible explanation is that surgical interventions are more often performed in inpatient settings (Table 4). The current results support the view that surgical interventions take up a substantial portion of knee disorder-related costs. The incidence of knee OA was highest among females aged ≥50 years, which is consistent with a previous report by Arden et al. [20]. Conversely, knee meniscal and ligament injuries occurred more often among those aged <60 years. Although the incidence of these injuries was highest among children and adolescents, hospitalized patients amounted to only half of the outpatient sector in this age group, suggesting that physically active younger individuals may be more prone to injury but injuries may be milder.

The costs for procedures/surgeries, injections, visits (consultations), and hospitalizations comprised ≥75% of the total expenses for patients with either type of knee disorder. Although the large number of injection treatments is mainly responsible for this finding, it is worth note that the number of surgery and hospitalization cases was relatively small compared to the total costs. It can be carefully inferred that performing surgical operations in inpatient settings is likely to drastically increase per-patient expenses. Injection treatments constituted the second largest expense in knee OA patients, and hospitalization was the 2nd largest expense for knee meniscal and ligament injury patients. To ease the socioeconomic burden of these disorders (i.e., total expenses and per-patient expenses), studies should be conducted, from the policymakers' perspective, on appropriate practice guidelines and adequate compensation costs, especially regarding surgical interventions, injection treatments, and hospitalization.

The types of surgical interventions performed in the two diagnostic groups were highly disparate, with

Table 5 Medication prescribed for knee osteoarthritis and knee meniscal and ligament injury as assessed at the 5th Anatomical Therapeutic Chemical Classification System level

5th ATC level	Total				Inpatient				Outpatient			
	Knee OA		Knee meniscal and ligament injury		Knee OA		Knee meniscal and ligament injury		Knee OA		Knee meniscal and ligament injury	
	N = 48,321	%	*N* = 19,136	%	*N* = 3084	%	*N* = 2434	%	*N* = 48,000	%	*N* = 18,540	%
Aceclofenac	15,810	32.72	4961	25.92	840	27.24	858	35.25	15,357	31.99	4499	24.27
Tramadol	10,651	22.04	2982	15.58	1743	56.52	837	34.39	9364	19.51	2291	12.36
Diclofenac	9068	18.77	3688	19.27	1764	57.20	1132	46.51	7734	16.11	2832	15.28
Meloxicam	10,785	22.32	597	3.12	524	16.99	178	7.31	10,544	21.97	486	2.62
Loxoprofen sodium hydrate[a]	5598	11.59	3295	17.22	291	9.44	358	14.71	5375	11.20	3043	16.41
Tramadol, combinations	7082	14.66	1588	8.30	582	18.87	248	10.19	6741	14.04	1423	7.68
Talniflumate[a]	5273	10.91	3127	16.34	432	14.01	519	21.32	4944	10.30	2747	14.82
Paracetamol	4988	10.32	1435	7.50	843	27.33	364	14.95	4299	8.96	1133	6.11
Celecoxib	4791	9.91	134	0.70	634	20.56	43	1.77	4490	9.35	106	0.57
Piroxicam	2085	4.31	307	1.60	220	7.13	116	4.77	1908	3.98	200	1.08
Zaltoprofen[a]	1531	3.17	753	3.93	138	4.47	113	4.64	1432	2.98	666	3.59
Chlorphenesin carbamate[a]	1597	3.30	599	3.13	69	2.24	46	1.89	1565	3.26	568	3.06
Dexibuprofen	1105	2.29	509	2.66	36	1.17	23	0.94	1072	2.23	488	2.63
Ketorolac	777	1.61	279	1.46	633	20.53	230	9.45	152	0.32	49	0.26
Nabumetone	904	1.87	114	0.60	46	1.49	37	1.52	873	1.82	83	0.45
Pethidine[b]	858	1.78	151	0.79	843	27.33	145	5.96	18	0.04	7	0.04

ATC Anatomical Therapeutic Chemical, *OA* Osteoarthritis
[a]Chemical name of medicine with no corresponding 5th level ATC codes
[b]Narcotics; otherwise, non-narcotics

replacement arthroplasty being performed most frequently in cases of knee OA, and meniscal and ligament operations (i.e., injured menisci or ligaments) being most common in cases of knee meniscal and ligament injury. Subcutaneous and intramuscular injection treatments were conducted in 19,722 knee OA cases and in 7390 knee meniscal and ligament injury cases, each comprising about 40% of all cases. However, the percentages of patients receiving subcutaneous and intramuscular injections rose to 83% in knee OA inpatients and to 65% in meniscal and ligament injury inpatients. Although intra-articular injections were frequently employed for knee OA outpatients, they were seldom used in patients with knee meniscal and ligament injury.

Heat therapy and electrostimulation are two types of physiotherapy that may be considered typical care for knee OA and meniscal and ligament injuries. More than 58% of hospitalized knee OA patients were prescribed therapeutic exercise, which was more common than superficial heat therapy. Therapeutic exercise is speculated to be mainly used as a means of post-surgical rehabilitation. Laser therapy and therapeutic exercise were considered simple rehabilitation treatment methods; myofascial trigger point injection, a complex rehabilitation method; and the other subtypes to be basic physiotherapies. Basic physiotherapy can be prescribed by all physicians without restriction as opposed to simple and complex rehabilitation therapies which can only be prescribed by relevant specialists. Therefore, limitations in the ability to prescribe laser therapy, therapeutic exercise, and myofascial trigger point injection treatments should be considered when interpreting these results.

Diclofenac is a non-steroidal anti-inflammatory drug (NSAID) that is widely used as first-line therapy for chronic inflammatory states including OA. However, prolonged use of diclofenac has been associated with gastrointestinal adverse events such as bleeding, ulcers, and perforations in severe cases. Aceclofenac, which has a similar chemical structure, was developed to address such complications and has been proven to be a safer alternative [21]. Aceclofenac was shown to be used more frequently than diclofenac in this study, possibly because it exhibits fewer side effects. Diclofenac tended to be more frequently administered in inpatient settings where adverse event monitoring is easier.

Tramadol is an opioid-like analgesic that affects the central nervous system (CNS) [22]. Tramadol, a μ-opioid receptor agonist, exerts nociceptive effects by increasing serotonin and noradrenaline levels in the CNS [23]. As the mechanisms of action differ between tramadol and NSAIDs, tramadol can be effectively used in patients with pain not responding adequately to NSAID treatment [24]. The present study results revealed that tramadol was the second most commonly prescribed drug. Moreover, tramadol combinations were the sixth most common prescription, under a separate ATC code, and taken together, the number of tramadol prescriptions was nearly as high as those for aceclofenac.

Paracetamol, also known as acetaminophen, is recommended as a first-line analgesic for knee OA patients by the European League against Rheumatism, American College of Rheumatology (ACR), and Osteoarthritis Research Society International. Long-term use of paracetamol is also preferred over other medications [25]. Although the analgesic effect of paracetamol is relatively weak compared to that of NSAIDs or COX-2 selective inhibitors, it is widely used as it is better tolerated [26]. However, paracetamol is often implicated in drug-induced liver injuries with approximately 30,000 patients being hospitalized annually for paracetamol-related liver injuries in the United States [27]. Nevertheless, paracetamol hepatotoxicity has been reported to be minimized by avoiding overdosing [28, 29].

One strength of classifying drugs according to 5th ATC levels is that complete identification of specific chemicals is possible, while limitations include the fact that identification and recognition of prescription patterns is not easy. The most frequently prescribed drug substances are listed in Table 5. Complete listings of prescribed drugs are organized by non-narcotics and narcotics in Additional file 3: Table S3 and Additional file 4: Table S4. At the 4th ATC level, the non-narcotic and narcotic drugs consisted of 18 and 4 subgroups, respectively (Additional file 5: Table S5). In order of prescription frequency, acetic acid derivatives and related substances, other opioids, propionic acid derivatives, oxicams, other anti-inflammatory and anti-rheumatic agents, and non-steroids were the most frequently used drugs in the non-narcotic analgesic subgroups, and phenylpiperidine derivatives, natural opium alkaloids, opioid anesthetics, and opium alkaloids and their derivatives were the most frequently prescribed drugs from the narcotic analgesic subgroups.

Investigations of medical service use at a national level hold heightened significance in that various disparities exist between evidence-based medicine and the actual practice selected for knee disorders in real world settings. For example, while use of meniscectomy is similarly high in Korea as in the U.S., a recent high-quality RCT reported that its effects did not surpass that of sham controls [30]. Similarly, although total knee replacement (TKR) is the most common surgical intervention for knee OA in Korea and is performed in 670,000 new cases in the U.S. annually, comparison of TKR and 12 weeks of conservative treatment found that while TKR resulted in significant differences in pain reduction, it also entailed serious complications, and most of the conservative treatment group exhibited meaningful improvement without surgery [31]. Moreover, intra-articular triamcinolone injections, which are commonly used in knee OA patients, failed to provide pain relief over saline, and were associated with a significantly larger decrease in joint cartilage [32].

Study limitations include the following: While the study analyses were based on codes filed in the national claims database, the level of accuracy of the diagnosing process itself could not be verified and is beyond the scope of this study. For example, a physician may have reached a diagnosis not conforming to such well-established diagnostic standards as proposed by the ACR [33]. In addition, outpatient medication intake could only be assessed from database prescription records rather than actual medication intake records. Regarding terminology, although the term incidence was used throughout the manuscript to indicate new cases within the index period, readers should take into account that the incidence was limited to new symptomatic cases that received diagnosis and treatment through visits to medical institutions for medical service use. Moreover, the current database does not contain information regarding treatments and medications not covered by National Health Insurance or over-the-counter medication. While other studies using claims data carry similar limitations, these uncertainties need to be given due consideration when interpreting these results.

Records of medical services, including surgeries, injections, physiotherapy, and analgesic use, could not be solely attributed to knee disorders if the patient had coexisting conditions and was coded with different subsets of disease codes. Although codes that were clearly non-knee-associated were excluded, such consolidations may be an additional limitation of this study, as it may have introduced unintentional selection bias. Also of note is that both conventional and traditional Korean medicine (TKM) are recognized by Korean medical and legal regulatory bodies in a dual medical system and are covered by National Health Insurance. Many patients seek acupuncture and pharmacopuncture for treatment of musculoskeletal disorders. In a previous report on TKM care and low back pain in Korea using 2011 HIRA-NPS data, TKM use was highest (28.8%) in patients with low back pain [34]. Unfortunately, the 2014 dataset currently available to the public does not include records on TKM use, limiting the present study results to conventional medicine services, and precluding a more comprehensive and complete assessment of knee disorder treatments in Korea.

Conclusions

This study analyzed HIRA-NPS data to investigate the current incidence of knee disorders and clinical practice patterns for knee OA and knee meniscal and ligament injuries. The medical expense analysis (i.e., amounts and distribution) may provide further information to policy-makers. Further, the detailed description of injection, physiotherapy, and analgesic use may prove valuable for researchers and practitioners seeking to understand the constituents of usual care in actual clinical practice. Additional research is warranted, particularly regarding treatment codes (e.g., M22 and M23) not covered in the present study. Also, the HIRA-NPS dataset only contains billing records for a single calendar year, rendering longitudinal studies with time series analyses of natural history and causal relationships impossible; national cohort data extracted from national health insurance claims data [35] may be analyzed for such purposes in future studies.

Additional files

Additional file 1: Table S1. Diagnostic codes of knee disorders following the Korean Standard Classification of Diseases, 6th revision (KCD-6) adapted from the International Classification of Diseases, 10th revision. (ICD-10) (DOCX 20 kb)

Additional file 2: Table S2. Definition of medical care for knee disorders from given codes. (DOCX 18 kb)

Additional file 3: Table S3. Non-narcotic medications in knee osteoarthritis and knee meniscal and ligament injury as assessed at the 5th Anatomical Therapeutic Chemical Classification System level. (DOCX 30 kb)

Additional file 4: Table S4. Narcotic medications in knee osteoarthritis and knee meniscal and ligament injury as assessed at the 5th Anatomical Therapeutic Chemical Classification System level. (DOCX 19 kb)

Additional file 5: Table S5. Total medications in knee osteoarthritis and knee meniscal and ligament injury as assessed at the 4th Anatomical Therapeutic Chemical Classification System level. (DOCX 23 kb)

Abbreviations

ACL: Anterior cruciate ligament; ACR: American College of Rheumatology; ATC: Anatomical Therapeutic Chemical; CNS: Central nervous system; COX-2: Cyclooxygenase-2; EM: Emergency medicine; HIRA: Korean Health Insurance Review and Assessment Service; ICD: International Classification of Diseases; NHIS: National Health Insurance Service; NPS: National Patient Sample; NSAID: Non-steroidal anti-inflammatory drug; OA: Osteoarthritis; TKM: Traditional Korean medicine; TKR: Total knee replacement

Acknowledgements

Not applicable.

Funding

This research was supported by the Traditional Korean Medicine R&D program funded by the Ministry of Health & Welfare through the Korea Health Industry Development Institute (KHIDI) (HI17C0761).

Authors' contributions

CYS, YJL, MRK, and IHH conceptualized and designed the study. JSS and JL acquired the data. CYS, WK, YYC, BCS, EHH, KS and MK analyzed and interpreted the data. CYS, JSS, MRK, and WK drafted the manuscript. JL, YJL, YYC, BCS, EHH, KS, MK, and IHH revised the manuscript critically for important intellectual content. YJL acquired funding. All authors have read and approved the final manuscript.

Competing interests
The authors declare that they have no competing interests.

Author details
[1]Jaseng Spine and Joint Research Institute, Jaseng Medical Foundation, 858 Eonju-ro, Gangnam-gu, Seoul, Republic of Korea. [2]Department of Applied Korean Medicine, College of Korean Medicine, Graduate School, Kyung Hee University, Dongdaemun-gu, Seoul, Republic of Korea. [3]Department of Rehabilitation Medicine of Korean Medicine, College of Korean Medicine, Sangji University, Wonju-si, Gangwon-do, Republic of Korea. [4]Spine & Joint Center, Pusan National University Korean Medicine Hospital, Yangsan-si, Gyeongsangnam-do, Republic of Korea. [5]Department of Korean Rehabilitation Medicine, School of Korean Medicine, Pusan National University, Yangsan-si, Gyeongsangnam-do, Republic of Korea. [6]Prevention Sciences, Rollins School of Public Health, Emory University, Atlanta, GA, USA. [7]Department of Cardiovascular and Neurological Diseases (Stroke Center), College of Korean Medicine, Kyung Hee University, Seoul, Republic of Korea.

References

1. Zhang Y, Jordan JM. Epidemiology of osteoarthritis. Clin Geriatr Med. 2010; 26(3):355–69.
2. Park J-H, Hong J-Y, Han K, Suh S-W, Park S-Y, Yang J-H, et al. Prevalence of symptomatic hip, knee, and spine osteoarthritis nationwide health survey analysis of an elderly Korean population. Medicine. 2017;96(12)
3. Jordan MR. Lateral meniscal variants: evaluation and treatment. J Am Acad Orthop Surg. 1996;4(4):191–200.
4. Kim S-J, Lee Y-T, Kim D-W. Intraarticular anatomic variants associated with discoid meniscus in Koreans. Clin Orthop Relat Res. 1998;356:202–7.
5. Kotlarz H, Gunnarsson CL, Fang H, Rizzo JA. Osteoarthritis and absenteeism costs: evidence from US National Survey Data. J Occup Environ Med. 2010; 52(3):263–8.
6. Cullen KA, Hall MJ, Golosinskiy A. Ambulatory surgery in the United States, 2006. Natl Health Stat Report. 2009;(11):1-25.
7. Peat G, Bergknut C, Frobell R, Jöud A, Englund M. Population-wide incidence estimates for soft tissue knee injuries presenting to healthcare in southern Sweden: data from the Skåne healthcare register. Arthritis research & therapy. 2014;16(4):R162.
8. Kujala UM, Taimela S, Viljanen T. Leisure physical activity and various pain symptoms among adolescents. Br J Sports Med. 1999;33(5):325–8.
9. Ding C, Cicuttini F, Jones G. Tibial subchondral bone size and knee cartilage defects: relevance to knee osteoarthritis. Osteoarthr Cartil. 2007;15(5):479–86.
10. Yelin E, Callahan LF. Special article the economic cost and social and psychological impact of musculoskeletal conditions. Arthritis. Rheumatology. 1995;38(10):1351–62.
11. Muthuri S, McWilliams D, Doherty M, Zhang W. History of knee injuries and knee osteoarthritis: a meta-analysis of observational studies. Osteoarthr Cartil. 2011;19(11):1286–93.
12. Kim L, Kim J-A, Kim SA. Guide for the utilization of health insurance review and assessment service national patient samples. Epidemiology and health. 2014;36
13. Bergkvist D, Dahlberg LE, Neuman P, Englund M. Knee arthroscopies: who gets them, what does the radiologist report, and what does the surgeon find? An evaluation from southern Sweden. Acta Orthop. 2016;87(1):12–6.
14. Prieto-Alhambra D, Judge A, Javaid MK, Cooper C, Diez-Perez A, Arden NK. Incidence and risk factors for clinically diagnosed knee, hip and hand osteoarthritis: influences of age, gender and osteoarthritis affecting other joints. Ann Rheum Dis. 2014;73(9):1659–64.
15. Hubertsson J, Petersson IF, Thorstensson CA, Englund M. Risk of sick leave and disability pension in working-age women and men with knee osteoarthritis. Ann Rheum Dis. 2013;72(3):401–5.
16. Peat G, Bergknut C, Frobell R, Joud A, Englund M. Population-wide incidence estimates for soft tissue knee injuries presenting to healthcare in southern Sweden: data from the Skane healthcare register. Arthritis Res Ther. 2014;16(4):R162.
17. Lee SM, Han SK, Kim JH, Jang BH, Cheong CL, Son HJ, et al. Clinical effectiveness of injection therapy for chronic low back pain. In: Korean national evidence-based health care collaborating agency; 2010. p. 1–232.
18. ATC/DDD Methodology: History [http://www.whocc.no/atc_ddd_methodology/history].
19. ATC: Structure and principles [http://www.whocc.no/atc/structure_and_principles].
20. Arden N, Nevitt MC. Osteoarthritis: epidemiology. Best Pract Res Clin Rheumatol. 2006;20(1):3–25.
21. Sharma G, Singh J, Anand D, Kumar M, Raza K, Pareek A, et al. Aceclofenac: species-dependent metabolism and newer paradigm shift from oral to non-oral delivery. Curr Top Med Chem. 2016;
22. Merashly M, Uthman I. Management of knee osteoarthritis: an evidence-based review of treatment options. J Med Liban. 2012;60(4):237–42.
23. Desmeules JA. The tramadol option. Eur J Pain. 2000; 4 Suppl A:15–21.
24. Inage K, Orita S, Yamauchi K, Suzuki T, Suzuki M, Sakuma Y, et al. Low-dose tramadol and non-steroidal anti-inflammatory drug combination therapy prevents the transition to chronic low back pain. Asian. Spine J. 2016;10(4):685–9.
25. American Geriatrics Society Panel on the Pharmacological Management of Persistent Pain in Older. P. Pharmacological management of persistent pain in older persons. Pain Med. 2009;10(6):1062–83.
26. Graham GG, Davies MJ, Day RO, Mohamudally A, Scott KF. The modern pharmacology of paracetamol: therapeutic actions, mechanism of action, metabolism, toxicity and recent pharmacological findings. Inflammopharmacology. 2013;21(3):201–32.
27. Blieden M, Paramore LC, Shah D, Ben-Joseph RA. Perspective on the epidemiology of acetaminophen exposure and toxicity in the United States. Expert Rev Clin Pharmacol. 2014;7(3):341–8.
28. Sinatra RS, Jahr JS, Reynolds LW, Viscusi ER, Groudine SB, Payen-Champenois C. Efficacy and safety of single and repeated administration of 1 gram intravenous acetaminophen injection (paracetamol) for pain management after major orthopedic surgery. Anesthesiology. 2005;102(4):822–31.
29. Clark R, Fisher JE, Sketris IS, Johnston GM. Population prevalence of high dose paracetamol in dispensed paracetamol/opioid prescription combinations: an observational study. BMC Clin Pharmacol. 2012;12:11.
30. Sihvonen R, Paavola M, Malmivaara A, Itälä A, Joukainen A, Nurmi H, et al. Arthroscopic partial meniscectomy versus sham surgery for a degenerative meniscal tear. N Engl J Med. 2013;369(26):2515–24.
31. Skou ST, Roos EM, Laursen MB, Rathleff MS, Arendt-Nielsen L, Simonsen O, et al. A randomized, controlled trial of total knee replacement. N Engl J Med. 2015;373(17):1597–606.
32. McAlindon TE, LaValley MP, Harvey WF, Price LL, Driban JB, Zhang M, et al. Effect of intra-articular triamcinolone vs saline on knee cartilage volume and pain in patients with knee osteoarthritis: a randomized clinical trial. JAMA. 2017;317(19):1967–75.
33. Hochberg MC, Altman RD, Brandt KD, Clark BM, Dieppe PA, Griffin MR, et al. Guidelines for the medical management of osteoarthritis. Part II. Osteoarthritis of the knee. American College of Rheumatology. Arthritis Rheum. 1995;38(11):1541–6.
34. Ahn YJ, Shin JS, Lee J, Lee YJ, Kim MR, Park KB, et al. Evaluation of use and cost of medical care of common lumbar disorders in Korea: cross-sectional study of Korean Health Insurance Review and Assessment Service National Patient Sample data. BMJ Open. 2016;6(9):e012432.
35. Specifics of National Cohort Sample database [https://nhiss.nhis.or.kr/bd/ab/bdaba002cv.do].

4

Comparison of semi-quantitative and quantitative dynamic contrast-enhanced MRI evaluations of vertebral marrow perfusion in a rat osteoporosis model

Jingqi Zhu[1,2], Zuogang Xiong[1], Jiulong Zhang[1], Yuyou Qiu[1], Ting Hua[1] and Guangyu Tang[1*]

Abstract

Background: This study aims to investigate the technical feasibility of semi-quantitative and quantitative dynamic contrast-enhanced magnetic resonance imaging (DCE-MRI) in the assessment of longitudinal changes of marrow perfusion in a rat osteoporosis model, using bone mineral density (BMD) measured by micro-computed tomography (micro-CT) and histopathology as the gold standards.

Methods: Fifty rats were randomly assigned to the control group (n=25) and ovariectomy (OVX) group whose bilateral ovaries were excised (n=25). Semi-quantitative and quantitative DCE-MRI, micro-CT, and histopathological examinations were performed on lumbar vertebrae at baseline and 3, 6, 9, and 12 weeks after operation. The differences between the two groups in terms of semi-quantitative DCE-MRI parameter (maximum enhancement, E_{max}), quantitative DCE-MRI parameters (volume transfer constant, K^{trans}; interstitial volume, V_e; and efflux rate constant, K_{ep}), micro-CT parameter (BMD), and histopathological parameter (microvessel density, MVD) were compared at each of the time points using an independent-sample t test. The differences in these parameters between baseline and other time points in each group were assessed via Bonferroni's multiple comparison test. A Pearson correlation analysis was applied to assess the relationships between DCE-MRI, micro-CT, and histopathological parameters.

Results: In the OVX group, the E_{max} values decreased significantly compared with those of the control group at weeks 6 and 9 (p=0.003 and 0.004, respectively). The K^{trans} values decreased significantly compared with those of the control group from week 3 ($p<0.05$). However, the V_e values decreased significantly only at week 9 (p=0.032), and no difference in the K_{ep} was found between two groups. The BMD values of the OVX group decreased significantly compared with those of the control group from week 3 ($p<0.05$). Transmission electron microscopy showed tighter gaps between vascular endothelial cells with swollen mitochondria in the OVX group from week 3. The MVD values of the OVX group decreased significantly compared with those of the control group only at week 12 (p=0.023). A weak positive correlation of E_{max} and a strong positive correlation of K^{trans} with MVD were found.

Conclusions: Compared with semi-quantitative DCE-MRI, the quantitative DCE-MRI parameter K^{trans} is a more sensitive and accurate index for detecting early reduced perfusion in osteoporotic bone.

Keywords: Osteoporosis, Dynamic contrast-enhanced magnetic resonance imaging, Micro-computed tomography, Vascular endothelial cell, Microvessel density

* Correspondence: tgy17@tongji.edu.cn
[1]Department of Radiology, Shanghai Tenth People's Hospital, Tongji University School of Medicine, 301 Middle Yanchang Road, Shanghai 200072, China
Full list of author information is available at the end of the article

Background

Osteoporosis (OP) is a chronic disorder, leading to an increased risk of fragile fractures. The pathophysiology of OP includes hormonal, microenvironmental, and genetic determinants which have been associated with a misbalance between bone formation and resorption.

Recently, a hypothetic pathophysiological mechanism for OP has been proposed involving reduced perfusion within the bone marrow which may affect the bone marrow microenvironment [1, 2]. More evidence from dynamic contrast-enhanced magnetic resonance imaging (DCE-MRI) indicates that compromised perfusion could be deleterious to the bone marrow [1–4]. However, the value of different DCE-MRI approaches such as semi-quantitative and quantitative analyses to assess the microcirculation in OP is unknown.

In this study, we aimed to compare the performances between semi-quantitative and quantitative DCE-MRI in the evaluation of bone marrow blood perfusion in a rat OP model after ovariectomy (OVX), regarding micro-computed tomography (micro-CT) and histopathological results as a referential gold standard. The effects of two techniques on early diagnosis of OP were also evaluated.

Methods

Animals

Fifty three-month-old female Sprague Dawley rats (weight, 250 to 290 g; Department of Laboratory Animal Science, Tongji University, Shanghai, China) were used in our study. Each cage housed five rats at 20 °C to 25 °C, with a 12 h light–dark cycle. Standard laboratory rat diet and water were available ad libitum. The experiment was approved by the animal review committee of Shanghai Tenth People's Hospital of Tongji University and the ethics committee of Science and Technology Commission of Shanghai Municipality [SYXK (Shanghai) 2011–0111], and was strictly in accordance with the guidelines for the care and use of laboratory animals as established by the Department of Science and Technology of China in 2006.

Rat OP model

Surgery was performed when all rats had been acclimatized to the new conditions for a week. The rats were randomly divided into a control group (n = 25) and OVX group (n = 25). All animals underwent operations while anesthetized by an intraperitoneal injection of 4% chloral hydrate (10 ml/kg). The rats in the control group underwent sham operation, defined as exteriorization but not removal of the ovaries. The OVX group underwent a bilateral OVX operation. After surgery, the two groups were fed a standard laboratory diets. Only two rats died in the process of conducting this study. One rat in the control group died of abdominal hemorrhage after the operation, whereas the other rat in the OVX group died of an anesthesia overdose at week 12. Hence, an additional two rats were provided to the corresponding groups as replacements. Each rat was weighted before surgery and the MRI scan. DCE-MRI and micro-CT examinations were performed at 0 (baseline), 3, 6, 9, and 12 weeks post operation on two groups of rats (five rats at each time point in each group).

DCE-MRI examination

DCE-MRI examination was performed on a 3.0-T MRI scanner (Magnetom Verio; Siemens Medical Solutions, Erlangen, Germany) with a gradient strength of 40 mT/m and a gradient slew rate of 200 mT/ms. A body coil was employed to transmit radio frequency signals. A small animal coil (C-MUC18-H300-AS; Shanghai Chenguang Medical Technology Co., Ltd., Shanghai, China) was used to receive signals.

Following a coronal scout scan, sagittal T1-weighted images of the lumbar vertebrae were obtained using the following protocol: three-dimensional volumetric interpolated breath-hold examination sequence; repetition time (msec)/echo time (msec), 7.1/2.05; field of view, 180 mm; slice thickness, 1.5 mm; averages, 1; flip angles, 5° and 15°; matrix, 69 × 192; and pixel size, 1.3 mm × 0.9 mm. Once the baseline scan was finished, a bolus of gadopentetate dimeglumine (Magnevist, Bayer Schering, Berlin, Germany; concentration, 0.5 mol/L) diluted in 0.9% saline to a final concentration of 0.06 mol/L was rapidly injected manually (injection time, 1–2 s; dose, 0.3 mmol/kg of body weight) into the tail vein through a 24-gauge intravenous catheter. Overall, the DCE-MRI scan required a total acquisition time of 493 s to acquire 592 dynamic images.

The DCE-MRI analysis was processed on an imaging workstation (Tissue 4D, Syngo multimodality workplace, software version B17_43.1_1.0, Siemens Healthcare). A region of interest (ROI) was drawn along the vertebral body of the fifth lumbar vertebra (L5), excluding the vertebral cortex. The signal intensity values in the locations of the ROI were plotted against time as time–signal intensity curve (TIC). One perfusion index of the semi-quantitative DCE-MRI analysis, maximum enhancement (E_{max}), defined as the maximum percentage increase in signal intensity from baseline, was acquired from the TIC according to the following eq. [1]: $E_{\max} = \frac{I_{\max} - I_{base}}{I_{base}} \times 100\%$, where $I_{\max}$ was defined as the peak signal intensity of the TIC, and I_{base} was calculated as the mean signal intensity of the baseline images. Three quantitative DCE-MRI indexes, K^{trans}, V_e, and K_{ep}, were calculated by arterial input function based on the Tofts model according to the following eqs. [5]:

$$K^{trans} = V_e \times K_{ep},$$

$$C_t = V_e \times C_e,$$

and $\frac{dC_t}{dt} = K^{trans}C_p - K^{trans}C_t/V_e,$

where C_t, C_e, and C_p are the concentrations of the contrast agent in the tissue, extravascular-extracellular space, and plasma, respectively. All DCE-MRI indexes were measured twice and the average values were taken.

Micro-CT examination

The rats were sacrificed with an overdose of 4% chloral hydrate (20 ml/kg) via an intraperitoneal injection after MRI examination. The L5 vertebrae were dissected, stored in 4% paraformaldehyde, and preserved at 4 °C for micro-CT (Explore locus, GE healthcare, Milwaukee, USA) examination. Each vertebra was imaged with the following protocol: tube voltage, 80 kV; tube current, 450 μA; exposure time, 400 ms; rotation step, 0.5°, a rotation of 360°; detector bin mode, 2 × 2; voxel size, 45 μm × 45 μm × 45 μm; frame averaging, 1; and scan time, 25 min. Cone beam reconstruction was performed on the projected files to acquire 4000 pixel × 4000 pixel two-dimensional images. Ring artifact correction, smoothing, and beam hardening correction were set at 10%, 1%, and 7%, respectively. Gaussian filtration ($\sigma = 0.8$, support = 1) was used to reduce signal noise and to maintain a sharp contrast between bone and marrow. A threshold of 800 was defined to isolate bone tissue. Axial, coronal, and sagittal micro-CT images showed that the ROI was a cuboid containing the cancellous bone 0.3 mm distal to the endplate within the L5 vertebral body, which was similar in size to that in the DCE-MRI to ensure that both ROIs matched. The bone mineral density (BMD, milligrams per cubic centimeter of trabeculae) value was calculated with GE Healthcare Microview V.2.1.1 software. Each L5 vertebral body was examined twice. The average values were taken as the final data.

Transmission electron microscopy (TEM) observation

One rat in the control group and two rats in the OVX group were randomly selected for TEM observation at each time point. The excised L4 vertebral body was cut into several pieces, quickly fixed in a mixture of 3% glutaraldehyde and 4% paraformaldehyde at 4 °C for one day, and decalcified in 4% ethylenediaminetetraacetic acid for 2–3 weeks at room temperature. Decalcified tissue was washed with 0.1 mol/L phosphate buffered saline (pH = 7.0), fixed in 1% osmium tetroxide, dehydrated through a series of ascending ethanol solutions, embedded in epoxy resin E51, and sectioned for double staining with 3% uranyl acetate and lead citrate. The mitochondria of vascular endothelial cells (VEC) and the gap between VECs in the bone marrow sample were observed using TEM (JEM-1230, JEOL, Tokyo, Japan).

Microvessel density (MVD) assessment

The L5 vertebral body was fixed in 10% buffered formalin for one day after micro-CT examination and decalcified in 4% ethylenediaminetetraacetic acid for 2–3 weeks. The decalcified sample was dehydrated in ethanol, embedded in paraffin, and cut into 4 μm-thick sections. Sections were dewaxed, microwaved, and rehydrated. Endogenous peroxidase and non-specific binding activity were blocked by incubation with 3% hydrogen peroxide and non-immune goat serum, respectively. VECs were stained with a rabbit-anti-rat CD34 (Wuhan Boster Biological Engineering Co., Ltd., Hubei, China; dilution 1:100). The immunochemical analysis was performed by an experienced pathologist without knowledge of the group allocation status. Three sections (the top, middle, and bottom levels of the specimen; eight 200× fields in hot spots per section) per vertebral body were selected for MVD assessment using a Leica Q-win Plus image analysis system (Leica Microsystems, Wetzlar, Germany). Care was taken to identify angiogenic CD34 positive VECs and to not count CD34-positive hematopoietic cells. The MVD value was determined as the mean microvessel number measured from three sections in each vertebra.

Statistical analysis

All statistical analyses were performed with SPSS 19.0 software (SPSS Inc., Chicago, IL, USA). Data were expressed as the means ± standard deviations. The differences between the two groups in terms of semi-quantitative DCE-MRI parameter (E_{max}), quantitative DCE-MRI parameters (K^{trans}, V_e, and K_{ep}), micro-CT parameter (BMD) and histopathological parameter (MVD) at the same time point were compared by using an independent-sample *t* test. The differences in those variables between baseline and the other time points in each group were assessed via Bonferroni's multiple comparison test. A Pearson correlation analysis was applied to assess the relationships between BMD, MVD, and DCE-MRI parameters. A p value <0.05 was considered to be statistical significance.

Results

Semi-quantitative DCE-MRI analysis

At baseline, no significant difference was found in the E_{max} between two groups ($p = 1.000$). The E_{max} values did not differ statistically over five time points in the two groups ($p > 0.05$ for all). Although the E_{max} values of the OVX group decreased compared with that of the control group from week 3 on, the only significant differences were at weeks 6 and 9 (p values were 0.003 and 0.004, respectively, for weeks 6 and 9).

Quantitative DCE-MRI analysis

At baseline, there was no significant difference in K^{trans}, V_e, and K_{ep} between the two groups ($p > 0.05$ for all). In the control group, these parameters did not differ statistically across the five time points ($p > 0.05$ for all). In contrast, in the OVX group, the K^{trans} values decreased significantly compared with those at baseline ($p < 0.001$ for all) and those of the control group at the same time points from week 3 on (p values were 0.029, 0.027, 0.039, and 0.041, respectively, for weeks 3, 6, 9, and 12). From week 3 on, the V_e values of the OVX group decreased compared with those at baseline and those of the control group. However, the difference reached statistical significance only at week 9 ($p = 0.018$ versus baseline, $p = 0.032$ versus control group at the same time point). The K_{ep} values of the OVX group did not differ statistically compared with those of the control group at the same time point ($p > 0.05$ for all). No significant differences were found for K_{ep} among the different time points in the OVX group ($p > 0.05$ for all). A comparison of semi-quantitative and quantitative DCE-MRI analysis between the two groups is shown in detail in Table 1.

Table 1 DCE-MRI parameters of L5 vertebral bodies at five time points

Time point	Control group	OVX group	t value	P value
E_{max}				
Baseline	1.51 ± 0.19	1.51 ± 0.06	0.000	1.000
Week 3	1.53 ± 0.34	1.35 ± 0.14	1.053	0.323
Week 6	1.69 ± 0.19	1.30 ± 0.09	4.182	0.003#
Week 9	1.58 ± 0.09	1.26 ± 0.16	3.971	0.004#
Week 12	1.39 ± 0.16	1.35 ± 0.16	0.313	0.762
K^{trans} (min^{-1})				
Baseline	0.29 ± 0.06	0.34 ± 0.03	−1.653	0.137
Week 3	0.28 ± 0.08	0.18 ± 0.03*	2.646	0.029#
Week 6	0.29 ± 0.07	0.20 ± 0.02*	2.691	0.027#
Week 9	0.26 ± 0.08	0.18 ± 0.01*	2.462	0.039#
Week 12	0.25 ± 0.06	0.16 ± 0.02*	2.724	0.041#
V_e (mL/100 mL)				
Baseline	0.36 ± 0.08	0.38 ± 0.09	−0.376	0.716
Week 3	0.41 ± 0.18	0.25 ± 0.07	1.825	0.105
Week 6	0.37 ± 0.08	0.29 ± 0.05	1.825	0.105
Week 9	0.33 ± 0.08	0.22 ± 0.05*	2.600	0.032#
Week 12	0.27 ± 0.05	0.25 ± 0.06	0.556	0.594
K_{ep} (min^{-1})				
Baseline	0.79 ± 0.08	0.94 ± 0.18	−1.667	0.134
Week 3	0.70 ± 0.29	0.84 ± 0.22	−0.868	0.410
Week 6	0.77 ± 0.15	0.71 ± 0.18	0.560	0.591
Week 9	0.80 ± 0.23	0.82 ± 0.24	−0.194	0.851
Week 12	0.86 ± 0.16	0.65 ± 0.15	2.224	0.057

Data are expressed as the means ± standard deviations. OVX group represents the rats underwent bilateral ovariectomy. Control group represents the rats underwent sham operation

*$P < 0$ .05, versus baseline in the same group

#$P < 0.05$, control group versus OVX group at the same time point

Micro-CT analysis

At baseline, there was no significant difference in BMD between the two groups ($p = 0.453$). In the control group, no significant difference in BMD was seen among the different time points ($p > 0.05$ for all). The BMD values of the OVX group decreased significantly compared with those of the baseline from week 6 on (p values were 0.013, 0.004, and <0.001, respectively, for weeks 6, 9, and 12) and compared with those of the control group at the same time points from week 3 on (p values were 0.008, 0.032, 0.007, and 0.002, respectively, for weeks 3, 6, 9, and 12) (Figs. 1 and 2).

TEM observation

In the control group, loose gaps between VECs with normal mitochondria were observed over five time points (Fig. 3a and b). However, tighter gaps between VECs with swollen mitochondria were seen in the OVX group compared to those in the control group from week 3 on (Fig. 3c and d).

MVD assessment

There was no significant difference in MVD between the two groups at baseline ($p = 0.230$). In the control group, the MVD values remained stable throughout the observation period ($p > 0.05$ for all). At week 12, the MVD values of the OVX group decreased significantly compared with those of the baseline ($p = 0.005$) and those of the control group at the same time point ($p = 0.023$) (Table 2, Fig. 4).

Correlations between BMD, MVD, and DCE-MRI parameters

There were significant positive correlations of BMD with E_{max} and K^{trans} ($r = 0.448$, $p = 0.001$; $r = 0.414$, $p = 0.003$, respectively). However, there were no correlations of BMD with V_e and K_{ep} ($r = 0.267$, $p = 0.061$; $r = 0.182$, $p = 0.205$, respectively). A weak positive correlation between MVD and E_{max} was found ($r = 0.289$, $p = 0.042$). However, there were strong positive correlations of MVD with K^{trans} and V_e ($r = 0.399$, $p = 0.004$; $r = 0.379$, $p = 0.007$, respectively). The relationship

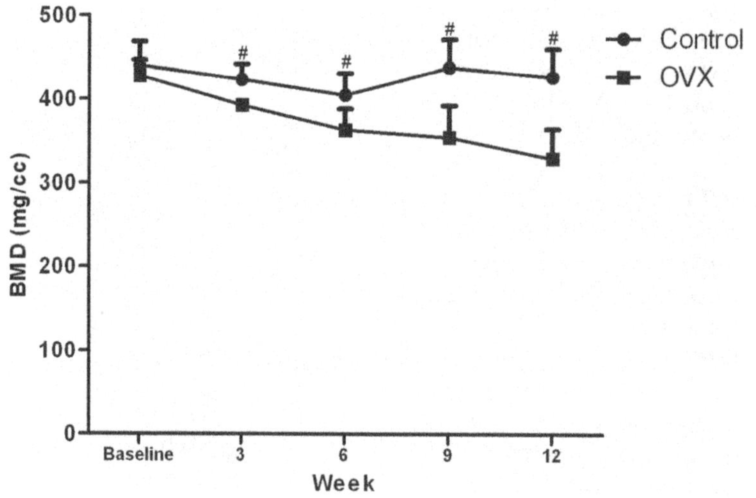

Fig. 1 Graph of BMD data in L5 vertebral bodies for the control and OVX groups. Data are expressed as the means ± standard deviations. # $P < 0.05$, control group versus OVX group at the same time point

between MVD and K_{ep} was not significant ($r = -0.035$, $p = 0.811$) (Table 3).

Discussion

OP is a significant public health problem that is characterized by a systemic impairment of bone mass and microarchitecture. This condition is most commonly reported among postmenopausal women. Bone loss in the OVX rat, which shares striking similarities with postmenopausal bone loss in aged women, is considered the "gold standard" animal model in postmenopausal OP studies [6]. Radiological assessment is mostly used in the detection of OP to prevent fragile fractures. However, BMD alone cannot predict fracture risk reliably or earlier [7]. Therefore, other aspects which may reflect the bone microenvironment have been investigated in the last two decades.

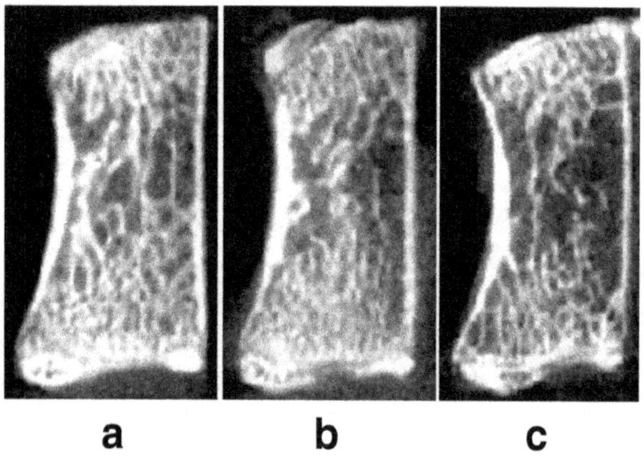

Fig. 2 Midsagittal micro-CT images of L5 vertebral bodies in the OVX group. The images show normal cancellous bone architecture at baseline (**a**) and continuously microarchitectural deterioration from week 3 (**b**) to week 12 (**c**)

Recently, a few studies have proposed the hypothesis that reduced bone perfusion is closely related to compromised BMD [1, 4, 8–10]. Our longitudinal observation showed a tendency of a decrease in the semi-quantitative perfusion parameter E_{max} accompanied with a decrease in BMD in the OVX group from week 6 on, which is consistent with other reports [1, 9]. Semi-quantitative DCE-MRI analysis consists of a group of

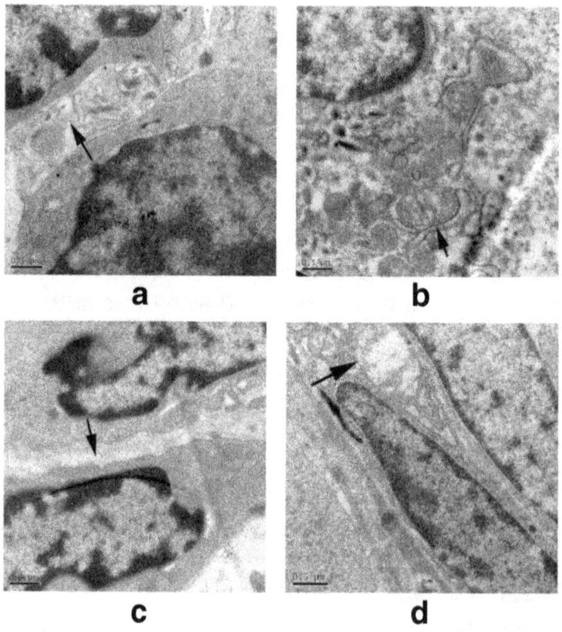

Fig. 3 TEM sections of L4 vertebral bodies show (**a**) loose gap between VECs (*arrow*) with (**b**) normal mitochondria (*arrow*) in the control group, and enhanced vasoconstriction appeared as (**c**) tight gap between VECs (*arrow*) with (**d**) swollen mitochondria (*arrow*) at week 3 after OVX (original magnification ×20,000)

Table 2 MVD of L5 vertebral bodies at five time points

Time point	Control group	OVX group	*t* value	*P* value
Baseline	4.80 ± 0.52	4.25 ± 0.80	1.299	0.230
Week 3	4.05 ± 0.49	3.84 ± 0.48	0.699	0.504
Week 6	4.29 ± 0.54	4.24 ± 0.33	0.183	0.859
Week 9	4.27 ± 0.60	3.52 ± 0.84	1.629	0.142
Week 12	3.79 ± 0.77	2.58 ± 0.57*	2.817	0.023#

Data are expressed as the means ± standard deviations. OVX group represents the rats underwent bilateral ovariectomy. Control group represents the rats underwent sham operation

*$P < 0$ .05, versus baseline in the same group

#$P < 0.05$, control group versus OVX group at the same time point

Table 3 Correlations between BMD, MVD, and DCE-MRI parameters

DCE-MRI parameters	BMD		MVD	
	r	*P*	*r*	*P*
E_{max}	0.448	**0.001**	0.289	**0.042**
K^{trans}	0.414	**0.003**	0.399	**0.004**
V_e	0.267	0.061	0.379	**0.007**
K_{ep}	0.182	0.205	−0.035	0.811

Bold fonts indicated statistical difference

BMD bone mineral density, *MVD* microvessel density

parameters such as E_{max} and enhancement slope that require calculation based on TIC, which allows for noninvasive evaluation of marrow perfusion in OP [1, 4, 11, 12]. Nonetheless, semi-quantitative DCE-MRI is more influenced by individual hemodynamic fluctuations and MRI protocols, and its hemodynamic parameters lacks a clear interpretation related to the underlying physiology [13, 14].

In the past decade, quantitative DCE-MRI parameters have been used to successfully reflect histological changes in vasculature. It is because of developments in pharmacokinetic models have enabled them to resolve those problems for semi-quantitative DCE-MRI [12, 15]. Therefore, a direct relationship between quantitative DCE-MRI parameters and bone marrow perfusion can be established. K^{trans} represents the volume transfer constant from the plasma space to the interstitial space. This physiological parameter is fully determined by plasma flow and the permeability-surface area product. K_{ep}, known as the interstitium-to-plasma rate constant, reflects the reverse transport of gadolinium back into the vascular space. V_e measures the interstitial volume, which is defined as the extravascular-extracellular volume fraction [15].

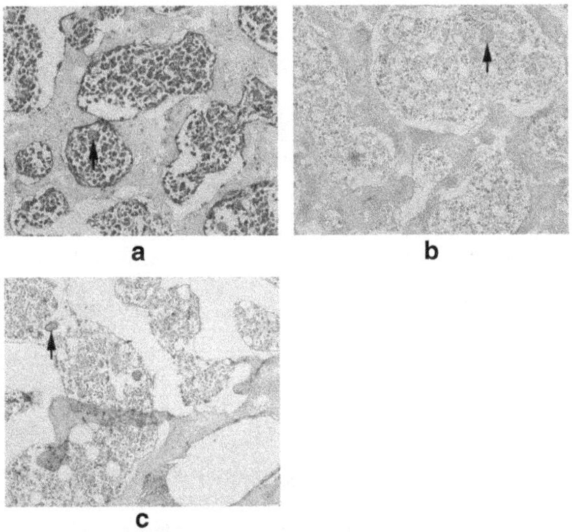

Fig. 4 Decalcified histopathologic sections of L5 vertebral bodies in the OVX group using endothelial marker CD34 stain (original magnification ×200). Microvessels (*arrows*) remain constant at baseline (**a**) and week 3 (**b**), and decrease at week 12 (**c**) after OVX operation

To the best of our knowledge, few longitudinal animal-based studies have compared semi-quantitative with quantitative DCE-MRI to determine which better reflects the perfusion condition in OP. In our study, acute estrogen deficiency caused a significant decrease in K^{trans} of the bone marrow from week 3 after OVX. It was identified by TEM observation, which showed vascular endothelial dysfunction appearing as tighter gaps between VECs with swollen mitochondria. Gulhan et al. [16] reported that postmenopausal women with OP may have an association with higher endothelin-1levels than those without OP. Animal studies indicated that the tendency of increased endothelin-1 serum levels in the OVX rats was one of the most likely causes of enhanced vasoconstriction and decreased permeability [2]. These findings strongly support the hypothesis that vascular endothelial dysfunction after OVX induced low bone marrow perfusion at an early stage [1]. It is notable that no significant change on MVD calculation was found between the OVX and control group until week 12. This phenomenon implies that the decrease in K^{trans} of the OVX group in the late stage may be attributed to the decrease of MVD in the bone marrow. Our study also found that the V_e values of the OVX group decreased significantly only at week 9 compared with those of the control group. It is obvious that the change of V_e values was later than that of the K^{trans} values in the OVX group. The increased and enlarged fat cells in the bone marrow of OVX rat occupied the trabecular space, which induced a reduction in extravascular-extracellular space [1, 17, 18]. This indicates that microvascular dysfunction may occur earlier than the accumulation of fat cells. K_{ep}, as the ratio of K^{trans} to V_e, was not significantly different throughout the observation period, which may be due to the reduction of K^{trans} and V_e in synchrony. Ma et al. [19] found that the two pharmacokinetic parameters (K^{trans} and V_e) showed a significant decrease in OP patients compared to normal subjects. In a few longitudinal animal-based studies, K^{trans} was reported to be a promising parameter to monitor acute ischemia in osteoporotic bone [2], while K_{ep} may be a sensitive index to reflect long-term chronic ischemia in OP due to vessel rarefication and maturation in the bone marrow [3]. Our results are consistent with these reports, which indicated that reduced bone marrow perfusion of OP could be directly reflected by quantitative DCE-MRI. However, no difference in E_{max} was found between the two groups until week 6 after the operation and the correlation coefficient of K^{trans} was the highest between MVD and DCE-MRI parameters. Together, these findings suggest that K^{trans} changes earlier and is more precise than E_{max}, although both of them have strong positive correlations with BMD and could reflect the reduced bone marrow perfusion in OP. In our study, DCE-MRI can be well performed on the vertebral body of the rat, which illustrates that this technique will be a feasible and reliable modality to quantify bone marrow perfusion in humans. Dual-energy X-ray absorptiometry (DXA) is a well-standardized, inexpensive, and convenient technique for BMD measurement, which has a low radiation dose. However, it is a two-dimensional measurement and is sensitive to degenerative diseases, which may alter the BMD value [20]. Compared with DXA, DCE-MRI is a relatively high-cost technique. However, lack of radiation and acquisition of compromised bone perfusion parameters in earlier stage of OP makes it more attractive in the clinical practice and more sensitive in monitoring the therapeutic effect. A comprehensive evaluation including BMD and bone metabolism should be performed for an OP patient regardless of whether it is for a precise diagnosis or the assessment of efficacy.

Our study has several limitations. First, the number of rats at each time point was relatively small, but it conforms to the statistical regulation. Experimental errors may affect the results because of individual differences. Second, only the L5 vertebral body was studied by DCE-MRI, micro-CT examination and immunochemical analysis. TEM observation were performed on L4 vertebral bodies of randomly selected rats: one in the control group and two in the OVX group at each time point. Differences in bone marrow perfusion and bone marrow microenvironment may exist at different points along the lumbar spine with varying BMD values [21, 22], The mismatch between imaging and TEM examination may affect the results. Third, only one semi-quantitative DCE-MRI parameter was selected to compare with the quantitative DCE-MRI parameters. However, E_{max} is one of the most common semi-quantitative indexes in the measurement of perfusion because of its relative stability and repeatability.

Conclusion

In comparison with semi-quantitative DCE-MRI, the quantitative DCE-MRI parameter K^{trans} is a sensitive and accurate index for demonstrating early reduced bone marrow perfusion in the OP.

Abbreviations

BMD: Bone mineral density; DCE-MRI: Dynamic contrast-enhanced magnetic resonance imaging; DXA: Dual-energy X-ray absorptiometry; E_{max}: Maximum enhancement; L5: The fifth lumbar vertebra; micro-CT: Micro-computed tomography; MVD: Microvessel density; OP: Osteoporosis; OVX: Ovariectomy; ROI: Region of interest; TEM: Transmission electron microscopy; TIC: Time–signal intensity curve; VEC: "Vascular endothelial cell

Acknowledgements

Not applicable.

Funding

This study was supported by National Natural Science Foundation of China ("81371517, 81071134), Shanghai Municipal Commission of Health and Family Planning (201640092), Shanghai Shenkang Hospital Development Center (SHDC22015026, 16CR4029A), and Shanghai Science and Technology Commission, International cooperation and exchange project (16410722200).

Authors' contributions

Zhu J and Tang G participated in the design of the study. Zhu J, Xiong Z, Zhang J, Qiu Y, and Hua T measured the data. Zhu J was responsible for the statistical analysis of the study and manuscript preparation. All authors read and approved the final manuscript.

Competing interests

The authors declare that they have no competing interests.

Author details

[1]Department of Radiology, Shanghai Tenth People's Hospital, Tongji University School of Medicine, 301 Middle Yanchang Road, Shanghai 200072, China. [2]Department of Radiology, East Hospital, Tongji University School of Medicine, Shanghai 200120, China.

References

1. Griffith JF, Wang YX, Zhou H, Kwong WH, Wong WT, Sun YL, et al. Reduced bone perfusion in osteoporosis: likely causes in an ovariectomy rat model. Radiology. 2010;254(3):739–46.
2. Zhu J, Zhang L, Wu X, Xiong Z, Qiu Y, Hua T, et al. Reduction of longitudinal vertebral blood perfusion and its likely causes: a quantitative dynamic contrast-enhanced MR imaging study of a rat osteoporosis model. Radiology. 2017;282(2):369–80.
3. Liu Y, Cao L, Hillengass J, Delorme S, Schlewitz G, Govindarajan P, et al. Quantitative assessment of microcirculation and diffusion in the bone marrow of osteoporotic rats using VCT, DCE-MRI, DW-MRI, and histology. Acta Radiol. 2013;54(2):205–13.
4. Griffith JF, Yeung DK, Tsang PH, Choi KC, Kwok TC, Ahuja AT, et al. Compromised bone marrow perfusion in osteoporosis. J Bone Miner Res. 2008;23(7):1068–75.
5. Tofts PS, Brix G, Buckley DL, Evelhoch JL, Henderson E, Knopp MV, et al. Estimating kinetic parameters from dynamic contrast-enhanced T(1)-weighted MRI of a diffusable tracer: standardized quantities and symbols. J Magn Reson Imaging. 1999;10(3):223–32.
6. Lelovas PP, Xanthos TT, Thoma SE, Lyritis GP, Dontas IA. The laboratory rat as an animal model for osteoporosis research. Comp Med. 2008;58(5):424–30.
7. Damilakis J, Maris TG, Karantanas AH. An update on the assessment of osteoporosis using radiologic techniques. Eur Radiol. 2007;17(6):1591–602.
8. Griffith JF, Yeung DK, Antonio GE, Wong SY, Kwok TC, Woo J, et al. Vertebral marrow fat content and diffusion and perfusion indexes in women with varying bone density: MR evaluation. Radiology. 2006;241(3):831–8.
9. Wang YX, Zhang YF, Griffith JF, Zhou H, Yeung DK, Kwok TC, et al. Vertebral blood perfusion reduction associated with vertebral bone mineral density reduction: a dynamic contrast-enhanced MRI study in a rat orchiectomy model. J Magn Reson Imaging. 2008;28(6):1515–8.

10. Wáng YX, Griffith JF, Deng M, Yeung DK, Yuan J. Rapid increase in marrow fat content and decrease in marrow perfusion in lumbar vertebra following bilateral oophorectomy: an MR imaging-based prospective longitudinal study. Korean J Radiol. 2015;16(1):154–9.
11. Wang YX, Zhou H, Griffith JF, Zhang YF, Yeung DK, Ahuja AT. An in vivo magnetic resonance imaging technique for measurement of rat lumbar vertebral body blood perfusion. Lab Anim. 2009;43(3):261–5.
12. Barnes SL, Whisenant JG, Loveless ME, Yankeelov TE. Practical dynamic contrast enhanced MRI in small animal of cancer: data acquisition, data analysis, and interpretation. Pharmaceutics. 2012;4(3):442–78.
13. Biffar A, Dietrich O, Sourbron S, Duerr HR, Reiser MF, Baur-Melnyk A. Diffusion and perfusion imaging of bone marrow. Eur J Radiol. 2010;76(3):323–8.
14. Biffar A, Sourbron S, Dietrich O, Schmidt G, Ingrisch M, Reiser MF, et al. Combined diffusion-weighted and dynamic contrast-enhanced imaging of patients with acute osteoporotic vertebral fractures. Eur J Radiol. 2010;76(3): 298–303.
15. Sourbron SP, Buckley DL. Classic models for dynamic contrast-enhanced MRI. NMR Biomed. 2013;26(8):1004–27.
16. Gulhan I, Kebapcilar L, Alacacioglu A, Bilgili S, Kume T, Aytac B, et al. Postmenopausal women with osteoporosis may be associated with high endothelin-1. Gynecol Endocrinol. 2009;25(10):674–8.
17. Qiu Y, Yao J, Wu X, Zhou B, Shao H, Hua T, et al. Longitudinal assessment of oxytocin efficacy on bone and bone marrow fat masses in a rabbit osteoporosis model through 3.0-T magnetic resonance spectroscopy and micro-CT. Osteoporos Int. 2015;26(3):1081–92.
18. Li GW, Tang GY, Liu Y, Tang RB, Peng YF, Li WMR. Spectroscopy and micro-CT in evaluation of osteoporosis model in rabbits: comparison with histopathology. Eur Radiol. 2012;22(4):923–9.
19. Ma HT, Griffith JF, Zhao X, Lv H, Yeung DK, Leung PC. Relationship between marrow perfusion and bone mineral density: a pharmacokinetic study of DCE-MRI. Conf Proc IEEE Eng Med Biol Soc. 2012;2012:377–9.
20. Link TM. Osteoporosis imaging: state of the art and advanced imaging. Radiology. 2012;263(1):3–17.
21. Ma HT, Lv H, Griffith JF, Li AF, Yeung DK, Leung J, et al. Perfusion and bone mineral density as function of vertebral level at lumbar spine. Conf Proc IEEE Eng Med Biol Soc. 2012;2012:3488–91.
22. Savvopoulou V, Maris TG, Vlahos L, Moulopoulos LA. Differences in perfusion parameters between upper and lower lumbar vertebral segments with dynamic contrast-enhanced MRI (DCE MRI). Eur Radiol. 2008;18(9): 1876–83.

5

Differences in vertebral morphology around the apical vertebrae between neuromuscular scoliosis and idiopathic scoliosis in skeletally immature patients: a three-dimensional morphometric analysis

Takahiro Makino[1], Yusuke Sakai[1], Masafumi Kashii[1], Shota Takenaka[1], Kazuomi Sugamoto[2], Hideki Yoshikawa[1] and Takashi Kaito[1*]

Abstract

Background: Recent morphological analyses of vertebrae in patients with scoliosis have revealed three-dimensional (3D) deformities in the vertebral bodies. However, it remains controversial whether these deformities are secondary changes caused by asymmetrical vertebral loading or primary changes caused by aberrant asymmetrical vertebral growth. Furthermore, the difference in vertebral morphology between scoliosis with different pathogeneses remains unclear. This study was aimed to investigate the difference in the coronal asymmetry of vertebral bodies between neuromuscular scoliosis (NS) in Duchenne muscular dystrophy (DMD) and idiopathic scoliosis (IS) using in vivo 3D analysis.

Methods: Twelve male skeletally immature patients with NS in DMD and 13 female skeletally immature patients with IS who underwent corrective fusion at our institution were included retrospectively. 3D bone models of the apical and adjacent upper and lower vertebrae in the major curve in the NS patients and in the main and compensatory curves in the IS patients were constructed using an image processing workstation. The heights of the concave and convex sides of the vertebral bodies were measured at the anterior, middle, and posterior and the concave-to-convex vertebral height ratios (VHR) were calculated.

Results: The mean VHRs (anterior/middle/posterior) for the main curve for IS (0.897 ± 0.072/0.832 ± 0.086/0.883 ± 0.059) were significantly smaller than those for NS (0.970 ± 0.048/0.934 ± 0.081/0.958 ± 0.043) in all three parts ($p < 0.001$). Those of the compensatory curve in IS (0.968 ± 0.045/0.942 ± 0.067/0.967 ± 0.046) did not differ significantly from the NS values in any part.

Conclusions: When compared to the wedging of the vertebral bodies around apical vertebrae in the major curve in NS, which was caused by asymmetric loading, the wedge deformities in both the main and compensatory curves in IS were more severe than would be expected. Our results indicated that morphometric characteristics of vertebral bodies differed according to the pathogenesis of scoliosis and that the pathology of the wedging of vertebral bodies in IS could not be a result only of asymmetric loading to the vertebral bodies.

Keywords: Wedging, Vertebral body, Asymmetry, Idiopathic scoliosis, Neuromuscular scoliosis

* Correspondence: takashikaito@gmail.com
[1]Department of Orthopaedic Surgery, Osaka University Graduate School of Medicine, 2-2, Yamadaoka, Suita, Osaka 565-0871, Japan
Full list of author information is available at the end of the article

Background

Recent morphological analyses of vertebrae in patients with idiopathic scoliosis (IS) have revealed three-dimensional (3D) deformities in the vertebral bodies such as wedging and torsion [1–4]. However, it remains controversial whether these deformities are secondary changes caused by asymmetrical vertebral loading or primary changes caused by aberrant asymmetrical vertebral growth [5]. Furthermore, how the vertebral morphology differs between scoliosis with different pathogeneses remains unclear. We hypothesized that morphometric characteristics of the vertebral bodies differed according to the pathogenesis of scoliosis.

Duchenne muscular dystrophy (DMD) is one of the causes of neuromuscular scoliosis (NS). The muscle weakness and pelvic imbalance that arise in the natural history of DMD induce the development of secondary scoliosis [6, 7]. The progression of scoliosis in DMD involves the whole thoracic and lumbar spine, and so the shape is often described as "C-type" [6]. Because the scoliotic change in patients with DMD is not caused by primary vertebral wedging, establishing the differences in the morphometric characteristics of vertebral bodies between IS and NS in DMD could help to clarify the pathology of vertebral deformities in patients with IS.

Scoliosis is a 3D deformity with vertebral rotation in an axial plane that increases with curve progression. Because of this, morphological analyses of vertebrae by conventional two-dimensional (2D) radiographs in scoliotic patients can be misleading because these cannot show true frontal (coronal) or lateral (sagittal) views of each vertebra [8]. We previously established an in vivo method using computed tomography (CT) scans for the 3D morphological analysis of vertebral bodies in patients with scoliosis [9]. The purpose of the present study was to investigate the difference in the wedging of vertebral bodies between NS in DMD and IS in skeletally immature patients using this in vivo 3D analysis.

Methods

Subjects

This study was a retrospective review of a radiological database of patients with IS and NS in DMD who underwent corrective surgery, and was approved by the Research Ethics Committee of Osaka University Hospital (no. 15098–2).

Twelve consecutive patients with NS in DMD who underwent corrective spinal fusion surgery between 2010 and 2015 were included in this study (the NS Group). All patients in the NS Group were male. The mean age at the time of the surgery was 12.9 years (range, 12–15 years) and the mean Risser grade was 0.6 (range, 0–3). Thirteen consecutive skeletally immature patients (Risser grades ≤3) with IS who underwent corrective spinal fusion surgery between 2008 and 2015 were also included (the IS Group). All patients in the IS Group were female. Their mean age at the time of the surgery was 12.1 years (range, 10–14 years) and the mean Risser grade was 1.7 (range, 0–3).

The periods between the loss of ambulation and surgery and the use of steroids in the NS Group were obtained from the medical charts.

Radiographic assessments

From preoperative full-length posteroanterior radiographs obtained in the sitting (NS Group) or standing (IS Group) position, the apical vertebrae were determined for the major curve in the NS Group and for the main thoracic (MT) and thoracolumbar/lumbar (TL/L) curves in the IS Group. Cobb angles of the major curve in the NS Group and of the MT and TL/L curves in the IS Group were digitally measured on a flat-panel monitor at our hospital using built-in imaging software (Centricity WebDX; GE Healthcare Japan, Tokyo, Japan). These Cobb angles were also measured from preoperative supine bending posteroanterior radiographs. The flexibility of each curve was evaluated and the type of scoliosis was classified as a structural or non-structural curve according to the Lenke classification [10]. In the IS Group, the structural curve was defined as the main curve and the non-structural curve as the compensatory curve; if both curves were flexible (non-structural), the greater curve when in the standing position was defined as the main curve. The flexibility index (FI, %) of each curve was calculated from the following formula:

$$\mathrm{FI}(\%) = ([\textit{Preoperative standing or sitting Cobb angle}] - [\textit{Preoperative supine bending Cobb angle}]) / (\textit{Preoperative standing or sitting Cobb angle}) \times 100\%.$$

Computed tomography assessments

The patients underwent CT scans within 3 months preoperatively using Discovery CT750HD (GE Healthcare Japan, Tokyo, Japan) or Aquilion ONE (Toshiba Medical Systems Corporation, Tochigi, Japan) scanners. The settings used for the scans were a slice thickness of 0.625 mm with the Discovery CT750HD and 0.5 mm with the Aquilion ONE, and a tube voltage of 120 kVp. The tube current was maintained between 50 and 250 mA by an automatic exposure control system. Hounsfield unit (HU) values of the vertebral bodies of the apical vertebrae and the adjacent upper and lower vertebrae were measured from the CT scans to assess the bone mineral density (BMD) by the following method (Fig. 1). First, the largest possible spherical region of interest (ROI) that excluded the cortical margin was placed on each vertebral body, with its center set to

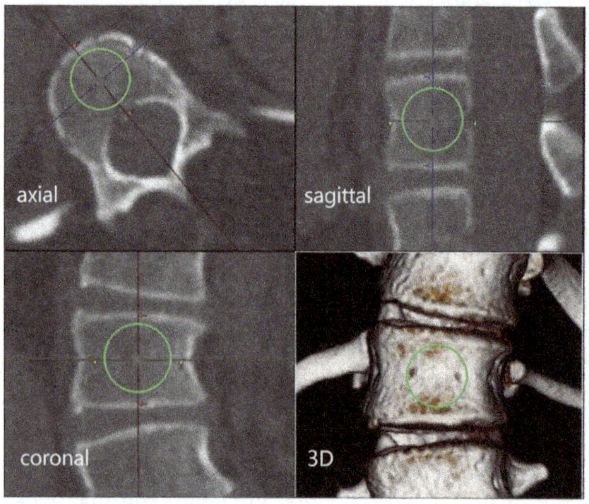

Fig. 1 An example of the measurement of the Hounsfield Unit (HU) value for a vertebral body to assess bone mineral density. The largest possible spherical region of interest (ROI, *green line*) that excluded the cortical margin was placed on the vertebral body. The center of the spherical ROI was set to be the center of the vertebral body on the axial, coronal, and sagittal planes. The HU value of the ROI was then calculated automatically

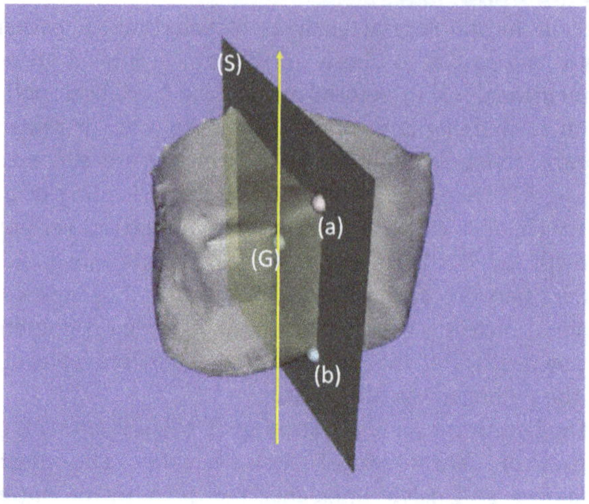

Fig. 2 The vertical axis (arrow) was defined as the line passing through the center of gravity (**G**) parallel to the line connecting the anterior edges of the vertebral foramen on the upper and lower vertebral end plates (**a**, **b**). The sagittal plane (**S**) contained the center of gravity (**G**) and the anterior edges of the vertebral foramen on the upper and lower end plates (**a**, **b**)

be the center of the vertebral body on the axial, coronal, and sagittal planes. The HU value of the ROI was then calculated automatically by built-in imaging software (Synapse Vincent; Fujifilm Holdings Corporation, Tokyo, Japan). The mean HU values for each curve were calculated.

Segmentation and creation of a 3D bone surface model and measurement of vertebral height

A 3D bone surface model of each vertebra was segmented and created semi-automatically by our previously reported method using a 3D image processing workstation (Synapse Vincent; Fujifilm Holdings Corporation, Tokyo, Japan) [9]. From these, 3D models of the apical vertebrae and the adjacent upper and lower vertebrae in the major curve in the NS Group and in both MT and TL/L curves in the IS Group were constructed, resulting in 36 3D models of vertebrae in the NS Group and 78 in the IS Group. The vertebral bodies were then extracted semi-automatically from the 3D models of the vertebrae by removing the posterior elements at the transitions between the vertebral bodies and pedicles. From the 3D models, vertebral height was measured semi-automatically using the original digital viewer (Orthopedic Viewer; Osaka University, Osaka, Japan), as described in our previous report in detail (Figs. 2, 3 and 4) [9]. Then, vertebral height ratio (VHR: the ratio of the vertebral height of the concave side to that of the convex side) was calculated as the index of wedge deformity of the vertebral bodies in the coronal plane. VHR was assessed at the anterior, middle, and posterior of each vertebral body. A value of VHR close to 1.0 indicated that the upper and lower endplates of the vertebral body in the frontal plane were nearly parallel.

Statistical analysis

The statistical analysis was performed using IBM SPSS Statistics Version 22 (IBM, Armonk, NY, USA). The Mann–Whitney U-test was used to compare variables. Differences in age between the NS and IS Groups were considered statistically significant at $p < 0.05$. Statistical

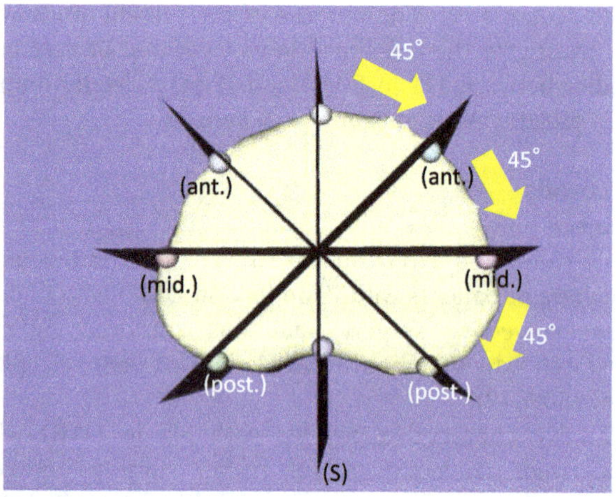

Fig. 3 The sagittal plane (S) was rotated about the vertical axis at 45° intervals. The two anterior intersection points (ant.) between the rotated sagittal planes and the lower endplate were used for assessing the anterior part of the vertebral body, the middle two intersection points (mid.) for assessing the middle part, and the posterior two intersection points (post.) for assessing the posterior part

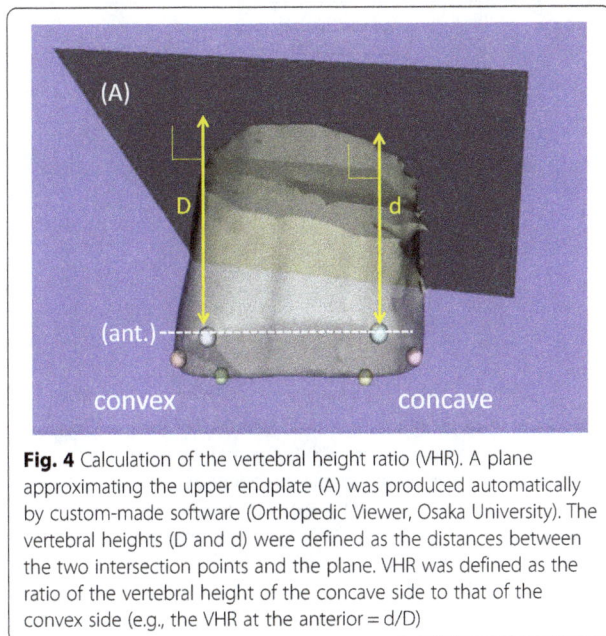

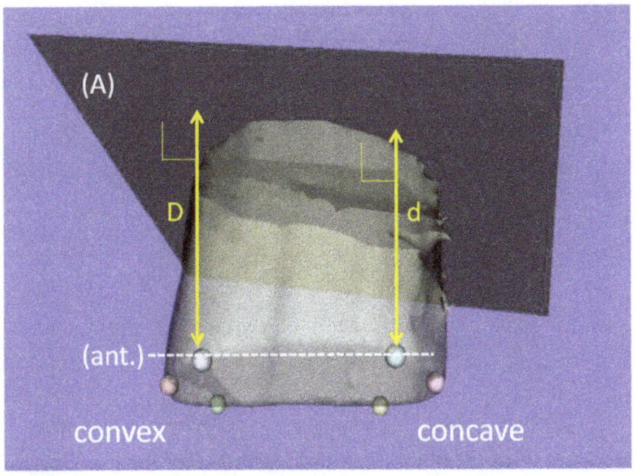

Fig. 4 Calculation of the vertebral height ratio (VHR). A plane approximating the upper endplate (A) was produced automatically by custom-made software (Orthopedic Viewer, Osaka University). The vertebral heights (D and d) were defined as the distances between the two intersection points and the plane. VHR was defined as the ratio of the vertebral height of the concave side to that of the convex side (e.g., the VHR at the anterior = d/D)

significance for the other variables related to the curves (the major curve in the NS Group and the main curve and compensatory curves in the IS Group) was set as $p < 0.017$ after applying the Bonferroni correction.

Results

The demographic and radiographic data of each group are shown Tables 1 and 2. The mean age did not differ significantly between the Groups ($p = 0.20$). All patients in the NS Group exhibited "C-type" coronal curves. In the IS Group, three patients exhibited Lenke type 1 curves, seven patients, type 2, and three patients, type 5. There was no significant difference between the Cobb angles of the major curve in the NS Group in the sitting position and the main curve in the IS Group in the standing position ($p = 0.26$); however, the Cobb angle of the compensatory curve in the IS Group was significantly smaller than that of the major curve in the NS Group ($p < 0.001$) (Fig. 5). In the IS Group, the Cobb angle of the main curve was greater than that of the compensatory curve ($p < 0.001$) (Fig. 5). The FI of the major curve in the NS Group did not differ significantly from that of the main curve in the IS Group ($p = 0.19$); however, the FI of the compensatory curve in the IS

Table 1 Demographic and radiographic data for the neuromuscular scoliosis group ($n = 12$)

Characteristic	
Age (years)	12.9 ± 1.1
Risser grade (0:1:2:3)	9:0:2:1
Period between loss of ambulation and surgery (month)	45.0 ± 18.4
Steroid use (yes: no)	3: 9
Configuration of major curve	
Apical vertebra (no. of patients)	T12, 1; L1, 4; L2, 4; L3, 3
Cobb angle (°) in the sitting position	73.0 ± 16.8
Cobb angle (°) in the supine bending position	31.8 ± 13.9
Flexibility index (%)	56.4 ± 16.1
Hounsfield unit (HU)	139.0 ± 33.3

Values are expressed as means ± standard deviations

Table 2 Demographic and radiographic data for the idiopathic scoliosis group ($n = 13$)

Characteristic	
Age (years)	12.1 ± 1.3
Risser grade (0:1:2:3)	3:2:4:4
Lenke classification (no. of patients)	Type 1, 3; Type 2, 7; Type 5, 3
Configuration of main and compensatory curves	
Main curve	
Apical vertebra (no. of patients)	T8, 3; T9, 5; T10, 2; T12, 2; L1, 1
Cobb angle (°) in the standing position	64.2 ± 16.1
Cobb angle (°) in the supine bending position	31.5 ± 8.8
Flexibility index (%)	49.5 ± 13.3
Hounsfield unit (HU)	220.1 ± 25.2
Compensatory curve	
Apical vertebra (no. of patients)	T3, 1; T6, 1; T7, 1; L2, 2; L3, 5; L4, 3
Cobb angle (°) in the standing position	36.8 ± 13.3
Cobb angle (°) in the supine bending position	4.5 ± 10.8
Flexibility index (%)	93.0 ± 37.6
Hounsfield unit (HU)	209.5 ± 23.5

Values are expressed as means ± standard deviations

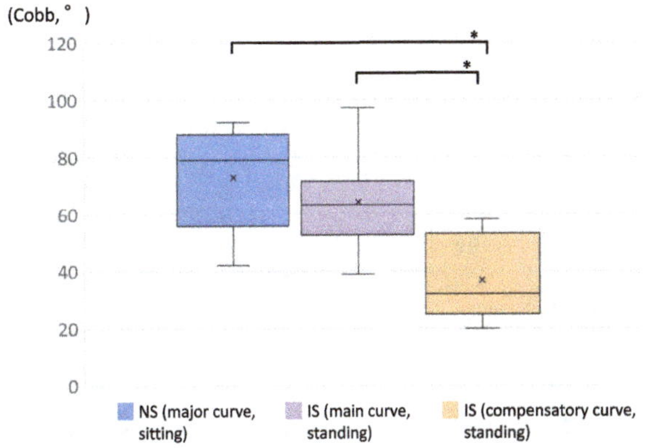

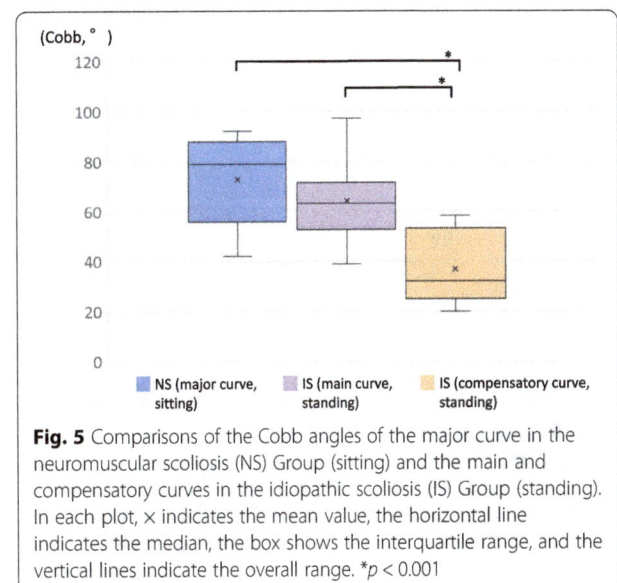

Fig. 5 Comparisons of the Cobb angles of the major curve in the neuromuscular scoliosis (NS) Group (sitting) and the main and compensatory curves in the idiopathic scoliosis (IS) Group (standing). In each plot, × indicates the mean value, the horizontal line indicates the median, the box shows the interquartile range, and the vertical lines indicate the overall range. *$p < 0.001$

Group was significantly greater than that of the major curve in the NS Group ($p = 0.005$) (Fig. 6). In the IS Group, the FI of the main curve was smaller than that of the compensatory curve ($p < 0.001$) (Fig. 6). The HU values of the major curve in the NS Group were smaller than those of the main and compensatory curves in the IS Group ($p < 0.001$) (Fig. 7). In the IS Group, the HU values did not differ between the main curve and the compensatory curve ($p = 0.34$) (Fig. 7).

The VHRs for the major curve in the NS Group and the main and compensatory curves in the IS Group are presented in Table 3. The VHR for the main curve in the IS Group was significantly smaller (further from 1.0) than that for the major curve in the NS Group and the compensatory curve in the IS Group at the anterior, middle, and posterior of the vertebral bodies (all $p < 0.001$) (Fig. 8). In contrast, there was no significant difference in the VHRs for the compensatory curve in the IS Group and the major curve in the NS Group for any part of the vertebral bodies (anterior, $p = 0.54$; middle, $p = 0.87$; posterior, $p = 0.64$) (Fig. 8).

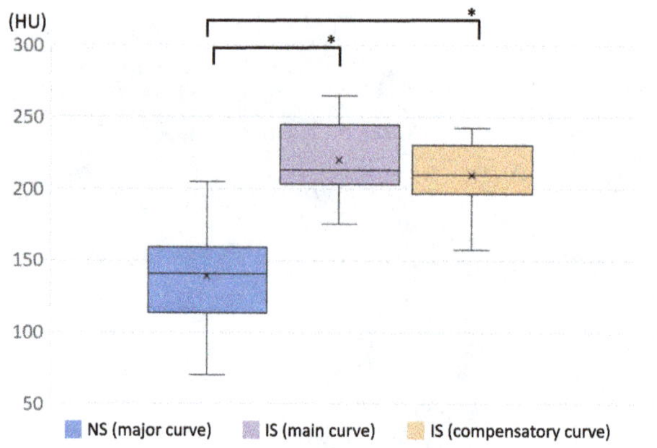

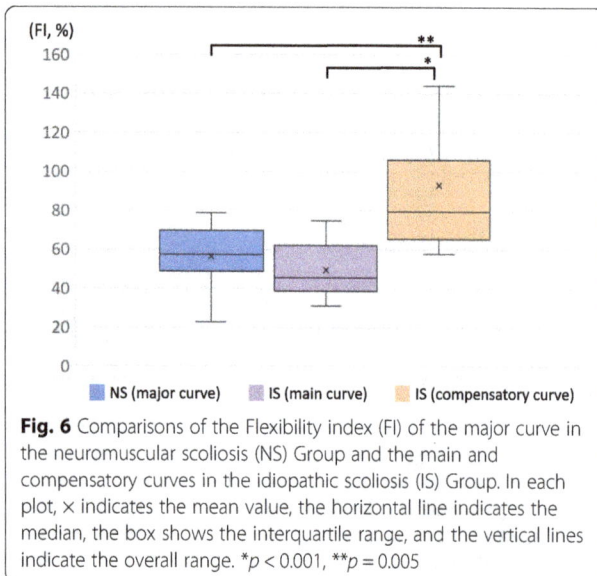

Fig. 7 Comparisons of the Hounsfield Unit (HU) of the major curve in the neuromuscular scoliosis (NS) Group and the main and compensatory curves in the idiopathic scoliosis (IS) Group. In each plot, × indicates the mean value, the horizontal line indicates the median, the box shows the interquartile range, and the vertical lines indicate the overall range. *$p < 0.001$

Discussion

This study revealed that the morphology of vertebral bodies differed according to the pathogenesis of scoliosis, in accordance with our hypothesis. First, the wedging of vertebral bodies in the main curve in the IS Group was more severe than that in the major curve in the NS Group across the whole vertebral body (anterior, middle, and posterior), although the severity and flexibility of scoliosis did not differ between the curves. Second, the wedge deformity in the compensatory curve in the IS Group was similar to that in the major curve in the NS Group across the whole vertebral body, although the curve of the compensatory curve in the IS Group was less severe and more flexible than that of the major curve in the NS Group. To the best of our knowledge, this is the first study to compare vertebral morphology between patients with NS in DMD and patients with IS.

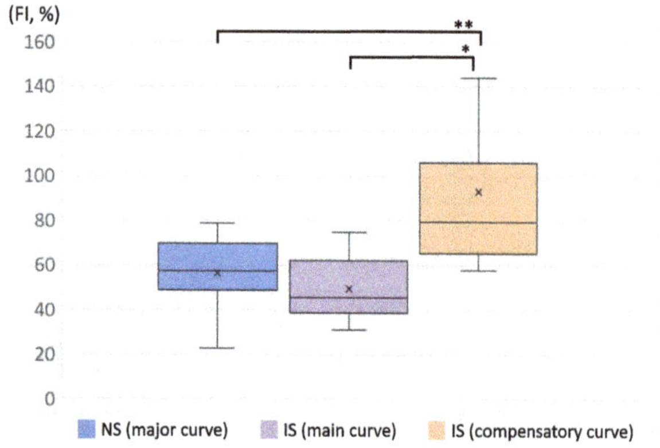

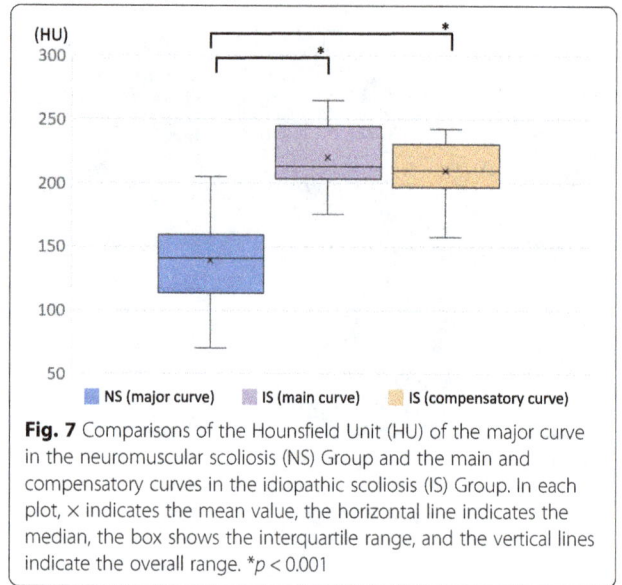

Fig. 6 Comparisons of the Flexibility index (FI) of the major curve in the neuromuscular scoliosis (NS) Group and the main and compensatory curves in the idiopathic scoliosis (IS) Group. In each plot, × indicates the mean value, the horizontal line indicates the median, the box shows the interquartile range, and the vertical lines indicate the overall range. *$p < 0.001$, **$p = 0.005$

It has been well known that vertebral wedge deformities can occur in patients with scoliosis [1–4, 11], and these deformities can be primarily obvious in the frontal plane [1, 12]. Several authors have shown that the deformities became more severe according to increase in Cobb angle and that this deformities was greatest in the apical region by 3D morphometric analyses [1, 11]. We therefore, investigated the morphology of vertebral bodies in the frontal plane around apical lesions. We showed in our previous report that intra-class correlation coefficients for intra-observer and inter-observer reliabilities for the calculation of vertebral heights were 0.996 (95% confidence interval, 0.994–0.997) and 0.990 (0.986–0.993) [9].

It is well established that mechanical loading influences the longitudinal growth of the long bones and vertebrae. This phenomenon is known as the Hueter–Volkmann Law, which explains that growth is retarded by increased

Table 3 Vertebral height ratios for the major curve in the neuromuscular scoliosis (NS) group and the main and compensatory curves in the idiopathic scoliosis (IS) group

Characteristic	Anterior	Middle	Posterior
NS Group			
Major curve	0.970 ± 0.048	0.934 ± 0.081	0.958 ± 0.043
IS Group			
Main curve	0.897 ± 0.072	0.832 ± 0.086	0.883 ± 0.059
Compensatory curve	0.968 ± 0.045	0.942 ± 0.067	0.967 ± 0.046

Values are expressed as means ± standard deviations

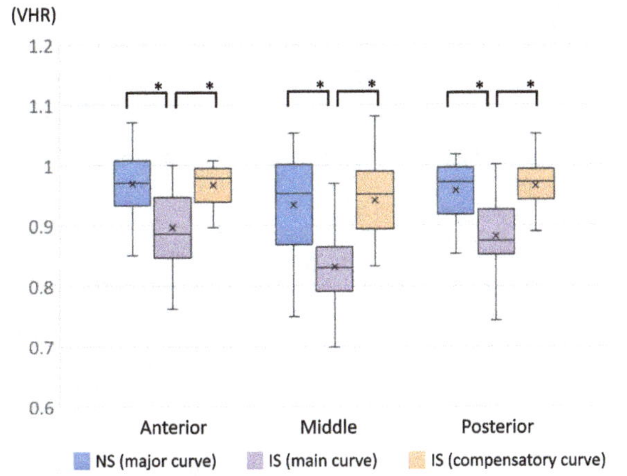

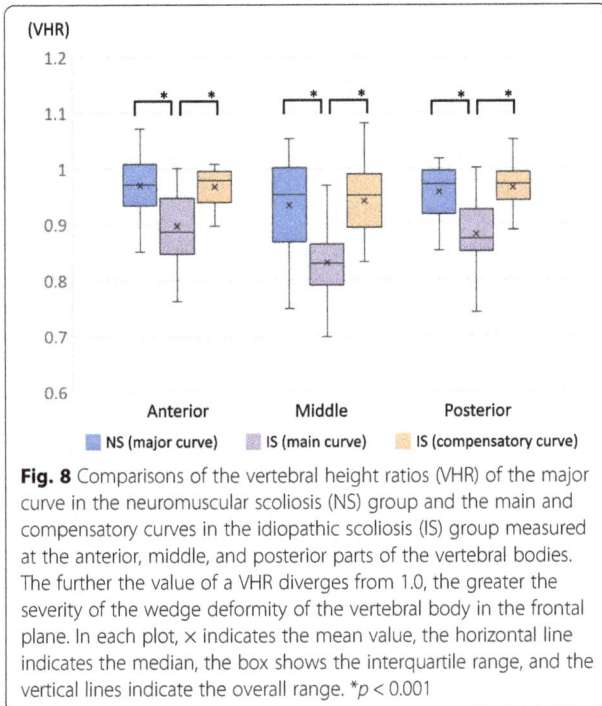

Fig. 8 Comparisons of the vertebral height ratios (VHR) of the major curve in the neuromuscular scoliosis (NS) group and the main and compensatory curves in the idiopathic scoliosis (IS) group measured at the anterior, middle, and posterior parts of the vertebral bodies. The further the value of a VHR diverges from 1.0, the greater the severity of the wedge deformity of the vertebral body in the frontal plane. In each plot, × indicates the mean value, the horizontal line indicates the median, the box shows the interquartile range, and the vertical lines indicate the overall range. *$p < 0.001$

mechanical compression and accelerated by decreased loading [13]. Stokes et al. [14] revealed that a compression force could suppress the longitudinal growth of vertebrae and a distraction force could accelerate it by using a rat-tail model. Meir et al. [15, 16] demonstrated that the loading in the intervertebral disc in the concave annulus was greater than that in the convex annulus in patients with scoliosis in vivo. The vicious cycle of asymmetrical loading to the intervertebral disc and vertebral wedge deformities can continue in patients with scoliosis [5, 14]. The effect of asymmetrical loading and severity of vertebral wedge deformities can be influenced by the BMD of the vertebral bodies. However, it is difficult to measure BMD of each vertebral body from thoracic to lumbar spine by conventional dual-energy X-ray absorptiometry measurements. Thus, we measured HU values of the vertebral bodies directly from the CT scans because the HU values reportedly correlate with BMD [17].

It has been recognized in the natural history of patients with NS in DMD that the loss of function for maintaining their posture due to muscle weakness and pelvic imbalance results in the development of their scoliosis [6, 7]. Thus, scoliosis in patients with NS in DMD does not originate from the wedging of vertebral bodies; these wedge changes of the vertebral bodies are secondary to asymmetric loading. The progression of scoliosis in patients with NS in DMD reportedly begins after the loss of ambulation [18]. In the present study, the mean period between loss of ambulation and surgery was about 45 months. Thus, our present data for the NS Group represent the natural course of the wedging of vertebral bodies induced by asymmetric loading over several years.

In comparison to this wedging of vertebral bodies in the NS Group, the wedging in the main curve in the IS Group was more severe, although the severity and flexibility of the curves were similar between both types of patient. Furthermore, the wedge deformity of vertebral bodies was similar between the compensatory curve in the IS Group and the major curve in the NS Group despite there being less severity and greater flexibility in the compensatory curve in the IS Group. The wedge deformities in both the main and compensatory curves in the IS Group were more severe than would be expected, because the BMD of vertebral bodies in the NS group was lower than in the IS group and thus the wedging of vertebral bodies was more likely to occur in the NS group only from the perspective of bone quality. These discrepancies in the progression of asymmetry in the vertebral bodies could relate to the difference between NS in DMD and IS in the progression of scoliosis. The scoliosis in NS often progresses rapidly [6, 7], so the asymmetric deformity secondary to asymmetric loading by scoliosis may not be as severe in patients with NS.

The primary factors that affect the vertebral morphology in IS could also contribute to the difference in the asymmetric changes of vertebral bodies between NS in DMD and IS. Several candidate susceptibility genes for adolescent IS have been reported since the development of a genome-wide association study [19–23]. *GPR126* knockdown and *BNC2* overexpression in zebrafish have been shown to cause delayed ossification of the developing spine and scoliosis [19, 20]. Growth arrest at the epiphyseal growth plates at the concave side of the apical vertebrae in patients with IS can be induced by the asymmetrical expression of these genes regulating spine ossification.

There were some limitations to the present study. Because of the retrospective nature of our study, it was not clear when the curves of the patients appeared. Furthermore, the male-to-female ratio was different between the two patient groups because DMD is more likely to occur in male and IS in female. These factors could affect the difference between the patients in the wedging of vertebral bodies. However, we think the effect of the difference in sex on vertebral morphology is relatively small in our study, because age and skeletal maturity did not differ between the groups and both the major curve in the NS Group and the main curve in the IS Group had already equally developed.

Conclusions

In conclusion, when compared to the frontal wedging of the vertebral bodies around apical vertebrae in the major curve in the patients with NS, which was caused by asymmetric loading, the wedge deformities in both the main and compensatory curves in patients with IS were more severe than would be expected. Our results indicated that morphometric characteristics of vertebral bodies differed according to the pathogenesis of scoliosis and that the pathology of the wedging of vertebral bodies in patients with IS could not be a result only of asymmetric loading to the vertebral bodies. With regard to the clinical relevance of our findings, the evaluation of vertebral wedge deformities can be an index to distinguish idiopathic scoliosis and syndromic scoliosis in adolescent patients.

Abbreviations

2D: Two-dimensional; 3D: Three-dimensional; BMD: Bone mineral density; CT: Computed tomography; DMD: Duchenne muscular dystrophy; FI: Flexibility index; HU: Hounsfield unit; IS: Idiopathic scoliosis; MT: Main thoracic; NS: Neuromuscular scoliosis; ROI: Region of interest; TL/L: Thoracolumbar/lumbar; VHR: Vertebral height ratio

Acknowledgements

The authors would like to thank Dr. Tsuyoshi Murase (Department of Orthopaedic Surgery, Osaka University Graduate School of Medicine) for permission to use Orthopedic Viewer.

Funding

This work was supported by a JSPS Grant-in-Aid for Young Scientists (B) (Grant Number 15 K19994).

Authors' contributions

TM and KS designed the study. TM, YS, MK, and TK contributed to data collection. TM, MK, and TK interpreted the acquired data. ST advised and supervised the statistical analysis. TM drafted the manuscript. All authors reviewed and edited the manuscript. KS and HY contributed to supervision of this study. All authors read and approved the final manuscript.

Competing interests

All authors report no conflict of interest concerning the materials or methods used in this study or the findings specified in this paper.

Author details

[1]Department of Orthopaedic Surgery, Osaka University Graduate School of Medicine, 2-2, Yamadaoka, Suita, Osaka 565-0871, Japan. [2]Department of Orthopedic Biomaterial Science, Osaka University Graduate School of Medicine, 2-2, Yamadaoka, Suita, Osaka 565-0871, Japan.

References

1. Schlösser TP, van Stralen M, Brink RC, Chu WC, Lam TP, Vincken KL, et al. Three-dimensional characterization of torsion and asymmetry of the intervertebral discs versus vertebral bodies in adolescent idiopathic scoliosis. Spine (Phila Pa 1976). 2014;39:E1159–66. doi:10.1097/BRS.0000000000000467.
2. Scherrer SA, Begon M, Leardini A, Coillard C, Rivard CH, Allard P. Three-dimensional vertebral wedging in mild and moderate adolescent idiopathic scoliosis. PLoS One. 2013;8:e71504. doi:10.1371/journal.pone.0071504.
3. Begon M, Scherrer SA, Coillard C, Rivard CH, Allard P. Three-dimensional vertebral wedging and pelvic asymmetries in the early stages of adolescent idiopathic scoliosis. Spine J. 2015;15:477–86. doi:10.1016/j.spinee.2014.10.004.
4. Nault ML, Mac-Thiong JM, Roy-Beaudry M, deGuise J, Labelle H, Parent S. Three-dimensional spine parameters can differentiate between progressive and nonprogressive patients with AIS at the initial visit: a retrospective analysis. J Pediatr Orthop. 2013;33:618–23. doi:10.1097/BPO.0b013e318292462a.
5. Sarwark J, Aubin CE. Growth considerations of the immature spine. J Bone Joint Surg Am. 2007;89(Suppl 1):8–13.
6. Hsu JD, Quinlivan R. Scoliosis in Duchenne muscular dystrophy (DMD). Neuromuscul Disord. 2013;23:611–7. doi:10.1016/j.nmd.2013.05.003.
7. Archer JE, Gardner AC, Roper HP, Chikermane AA, Tatman AJ. Duchenne muscular dystrophy: the management of scoliosis. J Spine Surg. 2016;2:185–94.
8. Newton PO, Fujimori T, Doan J, Reighard FG, Bastrom TP, Misaghi A. Defining the "three-dimensional sagittal plane" in thoracic adolescent idiopathic scoliosis. J Bone Joint Surg Am. 2015;97:1694–701. doi:10.2106/JBJS.O.00148.
9. Makino T, Kaito T, Sakai Y, Takenaka S, Sugamoto K, Yoshikawa H. Plasticity of vertebral wedge deformities in skeletally immature patients with adolescent idiopathic scoliosis after posterior corrective surgery. BMC Musculoskelet Disord. 2016;17:424.
10. Lenke LG, Betz RR, Harms J, Bridwell KH, Clements DH, Lowe TG, et al. Adolescent idiopathic scoliosis: a new classification to determine extent of spinal arthrodesis. J Bone Joint Surg Am. 2001;83-A:1169–81.
11. Modi HN, Suh SW, Song HR, Yang JH, Kim HJ, Modi CH. Differential wedging of vertebral body and intervertebral disc in thoracic and lumbar spine in adolescent idiopathic scoliosis - a cross sectional study in 150 patients. Scoliosis. 2008;3:11. doi:10.1186/1748-7161-3-11.
12. Parent S, Labelle H, Skalli W, de Guise J. Vertebral wedging characteristic changes in scoliotic spines. Spine (Phila Pa 1976). 2004;29:E455–62.
13. Stokes IA. Mechanical effects on skeletal growth. J Musculoskelet Neuronal Interact. 2002;2:277–80.
14. Stokes IA, Spence H, Aronsson DD, Kilmer N. Mechanical modulation of vertebral body growth. Implications for scoliosis progression. Spine (Phila Pa 1976). 1996;21:1162–7.
15. Meir AR, Fairbank JC, Jones DA, McNally DS, Urban JP. High pressures and asymmetrical stresses in the scoliotic disc in the absence of muscle loading. Scoliosis. 2007;2:4.
16. Meir A, McNally DS, Fairbank JC, Jones D, Urban JP. The internal pressure and stress environment of the scoliotic intervertebral disc–a review. Proc Inst Mech Eng H. 2008;222:209–19.
17. Schreiber JJ, Anderson PA, Rosas HG, Buchholz AL, Au AG. Hounsfield units for assessing bone mineral density and strength: a tool for osteoporosis management. J Bone Joint Surg Am. 2011;93:1057–63. doi:10.2106/JBJS.J.00160.
18. Shapiro F, Zurakowski D, Bui T, Darras BT. Progression of spinal deformity in wheelchair-dependent patients with Duchenne muscular dystrophy who are not treated with steroids: coronal plane (scoliosis) and sagittal plane (kyphosis, lordosis) deformity. Bone Joint J. 2014;96-B(1):100–5. doi:10.1302/0301-620X.96B1.32117.
19. Kou I, Takahashi Y, Johnson TA, Takahashi A, Guo L, Dai J, et al. Genetic variants in GPR126 are associated with adolescent idiopathic scoliosis. Nat Genet. 2013;45:676–9. doi:10.1038/ng.2639.
20. Ogura Y, Kou I, Miura S, Takahashi A, Xu L, Takeda K, et al. A functional SNP in BNC2 is associated with adolescent idiopathic scoliosis. Am J Hum Genet. 2015;97:337–42. doi:10.1016/j.ajhg.2015.06.012.
21. Guo L, Yamashita H, Kou I, Takimoto A, Meguro-Horike M, Horike S, et al. Functional investigation of a non-coding variant associated with adolescent idiopathic scoliosis in Zebrafish: elevated expression of the ladybird Homeobox gene causes body Axis deformation. PLoS Genet. 2016;12:e1005802. doi:10.1371/journal.pgen.1005802.
22. Ikegawa S. Genomic study of adolescent idiopathic scoliosis in Japan. Scoliosis Spinal Disord. 2016;11:5. doi:10.1186/s13013-016-0067-x.
23. Zhu Z, Xu L, Leung-Sang Tang N, Qin X, Feng Z, Sun W, et al. Genome-wide association study identifies novel susceptible loci and highlights Wnt/beta-catenin pathway in the development of adolescent idiopathic scoliosis. Hum Mol Genet. 2017;26:1577–83. doi:10.1093/hmg/ddx045.

6

Association between sarcopenia and low back pain in local residents prospective cohort study from the GAINA study

Shinji Tanishima[1*], Hiroshi Hagino[2,3], Hiromi Matsumoto[3], Chika Tanimura[2] and Hideki Nagashima[1]

Abstract

Background: Low back pain (LBP) is one of the most common ailments that people experience in their lifetime. On the other hands, Sarcopenia also leads to several physical symptoms and contributes to reducing the quality of life of elderly people.The purpose of this study is to investigate the association between sarcopenia and low back pain among the general population.

Methods: The subjects included 216 adults (79 men and 137 women; mean age, 73.5 years) undergoing a general medical examination in Hino, Japan. Skeletal muscle index (SMI), The percentage of young adults' mean (%YAM) of the calcaneal bone mass using with quantitative ultrasound (QUS) method and walking speed were measured, and subjects who met the criteria of the Asian Working Group for Sarcopenia were assigned to the sarcopenia group. Subjects with decreased muscle mass only were assigned to the pre-sarcopenia group, and all other subjects were assigned to the normal group. Then, we compared the correlations with low back pain physical finding. The Oswestry Disability Index (ODI) and the low back pain visual analogue scale (VAS) were used as indices of low back pain. Statistical analysis was performed among three groups with respect their characteristic, demographics, data of sarcopenia determining factor, VAS and ODI. We also analysed prevalence of LBP and sarcopenia. We investigated the correlations between ODI and the sarcopenia-determining factors of walking speed, muscle mass and grip strength.

Results: Sarcopenia was noted in 12 subjects (5.5%). The pre-sarcopenia group included 38 subjects (17.6%), and the normal group included 166 subjects (76.9%). The mean ODI score was significantly higher in the sarcopenia group (25. 2% ± 12.3%; $P < 0.05$) than in the pre-sarcopenia group (11.2% ± 10.0%) and the normal group (11.9% ± 12.3%). %YAM and BMI were significantly lower in the sarcopenia group than in other groups ($P < 0.05$). A negative correlation existed between walking speed and ODI ($r = -0.32$, $P < 0.001$).

Conclusions: The results of this study suggested that decreased physical ability due to quality of life in residents with LBP may be related to sarcopenia.

Keywords: Sarcopenia, Low back pain, Muscle strength, Osteoporosis

Background

Low back pain (LBP) is one of the most common ailments that people experience in their lifetime. The lifetime prevalence of LBP is approximately 84% [1]. LBP is caused by many factors. Wan et al. reported that muscle atrophy may lead to chronic LBP at multiple levels of the lumbar spine [2]. Several studies have reported that atrophy of the back muscles is a factor that causes LBP [2–4]; however, no consensus has been reached on an association between sarcopenia and LBP. Sarcopenia is defined as the pathophysiology caused by decreased muscle strength accompanying ageing [5]. Sarcopenia results in several disorders, such as hypertension, obesity, osteoporosis and diabetes mellitus [6, 7]. Sarcopenia also leads to several physical symptoms and contributes to reducing the quality of life of elderly people [8, 9].

The relationship between sarcopenia and LBP is unclear, and has been explored by only few studies. The

* Correspondence: shinji@sanmedia.or.jp
[1]Department of Orthopedic Surgery,Faculty of Medicine, Tottori University, 36-1 Nishi-cho, Yonago, Tottori 683-8504, Japan
Full list of author information is available at the end of the article

current study aimed to clarify the association between sarcopenia and LBP.

Methods

Subjects

This study was based on the results obtained from a prospective cohort of subjects enrolled in the Good Ageing and Intervention Against Nursing Care and Activity Decline (GAINA) study. The GAINA study, which began in 2014, is a population-based study of cohorts from Hino, Tottori Prefecture, Japan. The population comprised 3352 subjects in September 2016, with an ageing rate of approximately 45%. The subjects were recruited from individuals who underwent an annual town-sponsored medical check-up. A self-administered questionnaire was sent to 1450 subjects aged >40 years who were eligible to receive the medical check-up. We sent the consent form for The GAINA study together with medical check-up form to all subjects before an annual town-sponsored medical check-up. We enrolled the subjects who agreed The GAINA study. The baseline assessment was performed between May and June 2014 on 273 individuals undergoing the medical check-up. The inclusion criteria for subjects in the study were 1) living independently, 2) the ability to walk to where the survey was performed and 3) agreement to provide self-reported data. Fifty-seven subjects were excluded for lack of data because of omission of recording of medical check-up form. A total of 216 subjects (79 men and 137 women) participated in the baseline assessment. All subjects provided written informed consent, and the study was approved by the local ethics committee of the Faculty of Medicine, Tottori University (No. 2354).

Baseline measurements

Baseline characteristics, such as age, sex, height, body weight, body mass index (BMI), smoking habit and alcohol habit were recorded. We regarded the subjects who answered "yes" against this question "Do you feel low back pain in your daily life lately?" were LBP subjects. The position of low back was defined by each subject. Subjects were asked to make a vertical mark through a 100-mm horizontal VAS Scale.

We also used the Oswestry Disability Index (ODI) to assess functional outcomes associated with LBP. The results of the self-administered questionnaire were then checked for accuracy by researchers who personally interviewed each subject.

Assessment of sarcopenia

The participants were classified as having sarcopenia based on muscle mass, muscle strength and physical performance. The classification was based on the recommendations of the Asian Working Group for Sarcopenia [10]. The Recommendations of the Asian Working Group for Sarcopenia defined Sarcopenia as the Subjects were classified as having sarcopenia if they were aged >60 years and had a low handgrip strength (<26 kg in men and <18 kg in women) and/or a lower walking speed (<0.8 m/s) with a low muscle mass (<7.0 kg/m^2 in men and 5.7 kg/m^2 in women).

In this study, some subjects had low muscle mass under 60 years, so we defined subjects were classified as having sarcopenia if they were aged >40 years and had a low handgrip strength (<26 kg in men and <18 kg in women) and/or a lower gait speed (<0.8 m/s) with a low muscle mass (<7.0 kg/m^2 in men and 5.7 kg/m^2 in women). Subjects were classified as having pre-sarcopenia if they were aged >40 years and had a low handgrip strength (<26 kg in men and <18 kg in women) and/or a lower walking speed (<0.8 m/s) without a low muscle mass (<7.0 kg/m^2 in men and 5.7 kg/m^2 in women). Subjects without low muscle mass or strength or low physical performance were classified as normal (Fig. 1).

Body function and structure measurements

Handgrip strength was measured using a TKK 5401 dynamometer (Takei Co, Niigata City, Japan). The subjects were asked to squeeze the dynamometer twice with each hand. The highest scores for the left and right hands were summed. Muscle mass was measured by bioelectrical impedance analysis (BIA) with a MC-780A Body Composition Analyzer (Tanita Co., Tokyo, Japan). The BIA method requires the subjects onto a platform and remain in the standing position for approximately 30 s. Skeletal mass index was calculated by dividing the limb muscle mass (kg) by the square of the height (m). We used quantitative ultrasound (QUS) to assess the calcaneal bone mass [11, 12]. The speed of sound through the calcaneus was evaluated using a CM-200 sonometer (Furuno Co., Nishinomiya City, Japan). The subject was seated and was asked to place the right heel on the QUS device. Coupling gel was applied to the heel to facilitate the transmission of ultrasound to the skeletal site being examined. The sum of the percentage of young adult mean was calculated. Gait parameters were obtained using the Opto Gait (Microgate Co., Bolzano, Italy) designed for optical-sensitive gait analysis. We prepared a 10-m walking line. Walking section and measurement section were set respectively. The subjects completed a single trial at free speed with the instruction to 'walk at your normal speed '. Walking speed was calculated with specific software (OPTO Gait analysis software, version 1.6.4.0, Microgate S.r.L, Italy).

Statistical analysis

All data were expressed as mean ± standard deviation. The subjects were divided into normal, pre-sarcopenia and sarcopenia groups. Differences characteristic, demographics, data of sarcopenia determining factor, VAS and

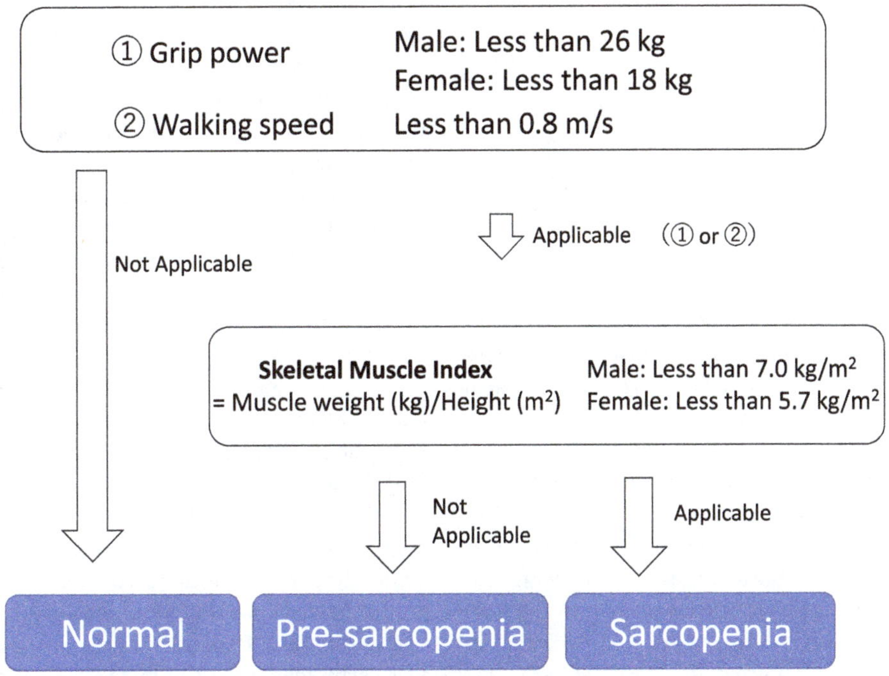

Fig. 1 Classification of study subjects. The subjects were divided into three groups by the Asian Working Group for Sarcopenia. Subjects with decreased muscle mass only were assigned to the pre-sarcopenia group and all other subjects were assigned to the normal group

ODI of the subjects among three groups were examined using Steel-Dwass test. The differences of prevalence of LBP among three groups analysed with Chi-square for independence test, m × n contingency table.

The differences of prevalence of LBP between men and women analysed with the Pearson's chi-square test or Fisher's exact test. We performed Fisher's exact test when expected cell size is <5. To investigate the correlations between ODI and the sarcopenia-determining factors, we used a partial correlation analysis with controlling the age and BMI available.

Data were analysed with StatMate for windows, version 4.01 (ATMS Corporation, Tokyo, Japan).

Results

Prevalence of sarcopenia

The prevalence of sarcopenia was approximately 5.5% (12 subjects; 5 men and 7 women). %YAM and BMI were significantly lower in the sarcopenia group than in the Normal groups. BMI in the Pre-sarcopenia group were significantly lower in the other groups (Table 1). The prevalence of sarcopenia in men and women were 8.4% in men and 4.3% in women. There was not significantly different in gender (Chi-square test; $P = 0.32$, data not shown).

Prevalence of LBP

One hundred-forty out of 216 subjects complained LBP. The overall prevalence of complaints of LBP was 64.8% (140/216 subjects). More than 60% of the subjects in each group complained of LBP. The prevalence of LBP was not significantly different among the three groups (Table 2). The prevalence LBP in men and women were 72.2% (52/79 subjects) and 65.0% (88/137 subjects). There was not significantly different in gender (Chi-square test; $P = 0.89$, data not shown).

Table 1 Characteristic and demographics of the subjects

	Normal ($n = 166$)	Pre-sarcopenia ($n = 38$)	Sarcopenia ($n = 12$)
Age (years)	73.0 ± 7.8	72.2 ± 8.5	84.9 ± 5.0 **
Gender (M:F)	63:103	11:27	5:7
%YAM (%)	78.9 ± 13.7	78.3 ± 15.9	63.8 ± 8.7 **
BMI (Kg/m^2)	22.8 ± 2.3	18.9 ± 2.0**	20.6 ± 2.4*
Smoking habit (%)	25.6	26.3	8.3
Alcohol habit (%)	30.1	42.1	25.0

(Mean ± SD)
Steel-Dwass *$P < 0.05$,**$P < 0.01$
%YAM: the percentage of young adult mean
BMI: Body mass index
M:male
F: female
Sarcopenia was noted in 12 of 216 subjects (5.5%). %YAM and BMI were significantly lower in the sarcopenia group than in the Normal groups. BMI in the Pre-sarcopenia group were significantly lower in the other groups. %YAM and BMI were significantly lower in the sarcopenia group than in the other groups (Steel-Dwass test, *: $P < 0.05$, **:$P < 0.01$). There were no significant differences among the three groups about smoking habit and alcohol habit (Chi-square for independence test, m × n contingency table)

Table 2 Prevalence of low back pain

	LBP(−)	LBP(+)	Prevalence of LBP (%)
Normal ($n = 166$)	61	105	60.1 (105/166)
Pre-sarcopenia ($n = 38$)	13	25	65.8 (25/38)
Sarcopenia ($n = 12$)	2	10	83.3 (10/12)
Total ($n = 216$)	76	140	64.8 (140/216)

There were no significant differences among the three groups

Sarcopenia and LBP

The mean VAS score was the highest in the sarcopenia group, although there were no significant differences among the groups. The mean ODI score in sarcopenia group was 24.3%. This score was significantly higher in the Sarcopenia group than in the other groups. The mean walking speed in the sarcopenia group was significantly lower than in the other groups. Grip power in the Pre-sarcopenia and Sarcopenia group were significantly lower than in the normal group. SMI in the Pre-sarcopenia and Sarcopenia group were significantly lower than in the normal group (6.9kg/m^2 in Pre-sarcopenia and 6.5kg/m^2 in Sarcopenia vs 6.9kg/m^2 in Normal, $P < 0.05$) (Table 3).

Association between sarcopenia and ODI

We investigated the correlations between ODI and the sarcopenia-determining factors of walking speed, muscle mass and grip strength. The only correlation was a negative correlation with walking speed (correlation confident −0.32, $P < 0.001$) (Table 4).

Discussion

We investigated the association between sarcopenia and LBP in local residents, focussing on elderly people. Sarcopenia was defined as 'age-related loss of muscle mass and function' by Rosenberg [5]. Musculoskeletal disorders are greatly influenced by sarcopenia. Baumgartner et al. reported that the prevalence of sarcopenia was more than 50% in people aged >80 years in Mexico and that more people with sarcopenia had physical disabilities [13]. Janssen et al. reported that fifth decades people begin to start decreasing their muscle volume [14] and people with low skeletal muscle mass index existed in third to sixth decades with same prevalence of over six decades in their study for 4504 American adults [15]. We included residents who are around fifth decades in this study for this reason.

The prevalence of sarcopenia was only 12% in this study, this was lower than other study. The inclusion criteria for subjects in the study were 1) living independently, 2) the ability to walk to where the survey was performed.

This criterion might affect that low prevalence of sarcopenia in this study.

LBP is one of the most common symptoms treated in daily medical practice. Park et al. investigated the prevalence of sarcopenia and lumbar spinal stenosis in Korea [16]. The prevalence of sarcopenia was higher in people with lumbar spinal stenosis than in normal people. They suggested that LBP with lumbar spinal stenosis led to low physical activity, causing sarcopenia. Although the present study showed that the prevalence of LBP was not significantly different among the three groups, the ODI scores were significantly higher in the sarcopenia group than in the other groups. The mean VAS score in the sarcopenia group was the highest among the three groups, although there were no significant differences among the groups.

The overall prevalence rate of LBP was 64.8%. Suka et al. performed a big survey for 3048 men and 1885 women in Japan to investigate the prevalence rate of LBP. They reported the prevalence rate of LBP was 26.5%. This prevalence was lower than our study [17]. In this study, most subjects over seventies and work as a former in this study, this situation might have relationship with high prevalence rate of LBP.

We consider that sarcopenia is not the cause of LBP. However, we focused on LBP in this study. LBP is induced by many factors, such as osteoporosis and muscle disorders [18]. The sarcopenia group in this study had low %YAM and BMI. The average %YAM in the sarcopenia group was 63.8% ± 8.7%. Verschueren et al. reported that sarcopenia was associated with low BMD in

Table 3 Sarcopenia and low back pain

	Normal ($n = 166$)	Pre-sarcopenia ($n = 38$)	Sarcopenia ($n = 12$)
VAS (mm)	20.5 ± 25.4	21.3 ± 25.8	23.5 ± 22.0
ODI (%)	11.9 ± 12.3	11.2 ± 10.0	25.2 ± 12.3 **
Walking speed (m/s)	1.2 ± 0.3	1.3 ± 0.3	0.9 ± 0.4**
Grip power (kg)	29.8 ± 8.3	26.3 ± 6.4*	20.7 ± 6.0**
SMI (Kg/m^2)	7.0 ± 0.9	5.8±0.7**	6.1±0.6**

(Mean ± SD)
Steel-Dwass
*$P < 0.05$ **$P < 0.01$
Oswestry Disability Index scores were significantly higher in the sarcopenia group than in the other groups ($P < 0.05$). The mean visual analogue scale score in the sarcopenia group was the highest among the three groups, although there were no significant differences among the groups. The mean walking speed in the sarcopenia group was significantly lower than in the other groups. Grip power in the Pre-sarcopenia and Sarcopenia group were significantly lower than in the normal group. SMI in the Pre-sarcopenia and Sarcopenia group were significantly lower than in the normal group

Table 4 Association between sarcopenia and Oswestry Disability Index (ODI)

	Correlation coefficient	*P* Value
Walking speed	−0.32	<0.001
Grip power	−0.26	0.05
Skeletal muscle index	−0.26	0.70

(Partial correlation analysis: control the age and BMI variable)
BMI:Body mass index
The only relationship was a negative correlation between walking speed and ODI. (Partial correlation analysis: control the age and BMI variable)

middle-aged and elderly European men [19]. In Japan, under 70% YAM is one of the criteria for osteoporosis [20]. Based on this criterion, most subjects with sarcopenia in our study may have had osteoporosis. Generally, the prevalence of osteoporosis is higher in elderly women than in men [21, 22]. The fact that more than 50% of the subjects in this study were women may affect these results. It is a well-known fact that osteoclasts are highly active in osteoporosis. The relationship between bone cancer pain and osteoclast activity is well known [23, 24]. There are no reports showing a relationship between osteoclast activity and osteoporotic bone pain.

In the periosteum, the A-delta and C-sensory nerve fibres are arranged in a fishnet-like pattern, which appears to be designed to act as a "neural net" to detect mechanical injury or distortion of the underlying cortical bone [25]. Park et al. mentioned that the following mechanisms contribute to generating and maintaining pain in osteoporosis: 1) the increasing density of the bone sensory nerve fibres in the elderly; 2) the expression of nociceptors by sensory nerve fibres sensitised by lower pH (as observed during osteoclastic activity) and 3) pathological modifications of bone sensory nerve fibres. The periosteum receives more sensory innervation than any other part of the skeleton [26]. We did not investigate the mechanism of LBP induced by osteoporosis in this study. As most subjects were elderly women, the presence of osteoporosis could not be neglected. We consider that the subjects who complained of LBP had low bone mineral density (BMD)-induced bone pain, especially elderly women.

We also investigated correlations between ODI and the sarcopenia-determining factors of walking speed, muscle mass and grip strength. ODI was associated with walking speed. Muscle power and volume did not affect LBP. Previous studies reported that exercising the lumbar muscles improved chronic LBP [27, 28].

We did not assess the volume and strength of the lumbar muscles and the effect of lumbar exercise of local residents. The relationship between the strength of these muscles and LBP is unclear. Among the sarcopenia-determining factors, only walking speed correlated with ODI.

Low walking speed associated ODI. We consider that low walking speed equates to low physical ability. Low physical activity might have association with low muscle volume and %YAM. We consider that low physical ability may associate with sarcopenia. In this study, although we could not be determined whether low physical activity is a cause or a result of sarcopenia and osteoporosis, measures against low physical ability, such as exercise and osteoporosis therapy, may help prevent sarcopenia.

This study had several limitations. First, being a cross-sectional study, it did not reveal the causal relationships between sarcopenia and LBP. We did not investigate the causes of LBP without sarcopenia, such as disc herniation, lumbar spinal stenosis and spinal deformity. Second, the study may have had a subject selection bias because the subjects voluntarily participated in the medical check-up. We performed this study in a small town in mountains and most of subject who were recruited were over 70's. Our inclusion criteria were living independently and the ability to walk to where the survey was performed. As a result, subjects who could attend the check-up may have had higher levels of activities of daily living. These factors affect the result of our research as a selection bias. Especially, this bias may have relationship with the low prevalence of sarcopenia in this study. Third, sample size was too small.

Conclusion

Low back pain was associated with osteoporosis and cause low physical activity. As a result, these situations caused sarcopenia. We consider that exercise against low physical activity and osteoporosis therapy may affect sarcopenia.

Abbreviations

%YAM: The percentage of young adult mean; BIA: Bioelectrical impedance analysis; BMD: Bone mineral density; GAINA: Good Ageing and Intervention Against Nursing Care and Activity Decline; LBP: Low back pain; ODI: Oswestry Disability Index; QUS: Quantitative ultrasound; SMI: Skeletal muscle index; VAS: Visual analogue scale

Acknowledgements

The authors sincerely acknowledge all staff members of the GAINA study involved in this study. The authors also acknowledge Shinichi Taniguchi, Eri Kobayashi, Kyohei Nakata, Takeshi Sota, Taro Omori, Takashi Wada, Tetsuji Morita, Naoyuki Nakaso, Tomoko Akita, Nao Nakata, Takuya Sugimura and Naoko Ikuta for their support and Ryoko Ikehara for her secretarial assistance.

Funding

This study was supported by a Ministry of Education, Culture, Sports, Science and Technology Grant (Chi-no kyoten seibi jigyou) and a Japanese Society for Musculoskeletal Medicine Grant.

Authors' contributions

ST designed the study and participated in this study, and did the acquisition, analysis, and interpretation of data of the work and drafting of the manuscript. HH, CT and HM help designed the study and participated in this study, and did the acquisition, analysis, and interpretation of data of the work. HN contributed to the designs and drafted the manuscript. All authors read and approved the final version of the manuscript.

Competing interests

HN received research funding from Nippon Zoki Pharmaceutical Co.,ltd(Osaka, Japan), TEIJIN PHARMA LIMITED (Tokyo, Japan) and Taisho Toyama Pharmaceutical Co., Ltd.(Tokyo, Japan).
HM received grant from Ministry of Education,Culture,Sports,Scince and Technology Grant and Japanese Society for Musculoskeletal Medicine Grant. Other authors have non-financial competing interests.

Author details

[1]Department of Orthopedic Surgery,Faculty of Medicine, Tottori University, 36-1 Nishi-cho, Yonago, Tottori 683-8504, Japan. [2]School of Health Science, Tottori University Faculty of Medicine, 86 Nishi-cho, Yonago, Tottori 683-8503, Japan. [3]Rehabilitation Division, Tottori University Hospital, 36-1 Nishi-cho, Yonago, Tottori 683-8504, Japan.

References

1. Airaksinen O, Brox JI, Cedraschi C, Hildebrandt J, Klaber-Moffett J, Kovacs F, Mannion AF, Reis S, Staal JB, Ursin H, et al. Chapter 4. European guidelines for the management of chronic nonspecific low back pain. European spine journal : official publication of the European Spine Society, the European Spinal Deformity Society, and the European Section of the Cervical Spine Research Society. 2006;15(Suppl 2):S192–300.
2. Wan Q, Lin C, Li X, Zeng W, Ma C. MRI assessment of paraspinal muscles in patients with acute and chronic unilateral low back pain. Br J Radiol. 2015; 88(1053):20140546.
3. Goubert D, Oosterwijck JV, Meeus M, Danneels L. Structural changes of lumbar muscles in non-specific low back pain: a systematic review. Pain Physician. 2016;19(7):E985–E1000.
4. Teichtahl AJ, Urquhart DM, Wang Y, Wluka AE, Wijethilake P, O'Sullivan R, Cicuttini FM. Fat infiltration of paraspinal muscles is associated with low back pain, disability, and structural abnormalities in community-based adults. Spine J. 2015;15(7):1593–601.
5. Rosenberg IH. Sarcopenia: origins and clinical relevance. J Nutr. 1997;127(5 Suppl):990S–1S.
6. Aagaard T, Roed C, Dahl B, Obel N. Long-term prognosis and causes of death after spondylodiscitis: a Danish nationwide cohort study. Infectious diseases. 2016;48(3):201–8.
7. Kalyani RR, Tra Y, Yeh HC, Egan JM, Ferrucci L, Brancati FL. Quadriceps strength, quadriceps power, and gait speed in older U.S. adults with diabetes mellitus: results from the National Health and nutrition examination survey, 1999-2002. J Am Geriatr Soc. 2013;61(5):769–75.
8. Hida T, Shimokata H, Sakai Y, Ito S, Matsui Y, Takemura M, Kasai T, Ishiguro N, Harada A. Sarcopenia and sarcopenic leg as potential risk factors for acute osteoporotic vertebral fracture among older women. European spine journal : official publication of the European Spine Society, the European Spinal Deformity Society, and the European Section of the Cervical Spine Research Society. 2016;25(11):3424–31.
9. Kim SH, Kim TH, Hwang HJ. The relationship of physical activity (PA) and walking with sarcopenia in Korean males aged 60 years and older using the fourth Korean National Health and nutrition examination survey (KNHANES IV-2, 3), 2008-2009. Arch Gerontol Geriatr. 2013;56(3):472–7.
10. Chen LK, Liu LK, Woo J, Assantachai P, Auyeung TW, Bahyah KS, Chou MY, Chen LY, Hsu PS, Krairit O, et al. Sarcopenia in Asia: consensus report of the Asian working Group for Sarcopenia. J Am Med Dir Assoc. 2014; 15(2):95–101.
11. Camozzi V, De Terlizzi F, Zangari M, Luisetto G. Quantitative bone ultrasound at phalanges and calcaneus in osteoporotic postmenopausal women: influence of age and measurement site. Ultrasound Med Biol. 2007;33(7):1039–45.
12. Pisani P, Renna MD, Conversano F, Casciaro E, Muratore M, Quarta E, Paola MD, Casciaro S. Screening and early diagnosis of osteoporosis through X-ray and ultrasound based techniques. World J Radiol. 2013;5(11):398–410.
13. Baumgartner RN, Koehler KM, Gallagher D, Romero L, Heymsfield SB, Ross RR, Garry PJ, Lindeman RD. Epidemiology of sarcopenia among the elderly in New Mexico. Am J Epidemiol. 1998;147(8):755–63.
14. Janssen I, Heymsfield SB, Wang ZM, Ross R. Skeletal muscle mass and distribution in 468 men and women aged 18-88 yr. J Appl Physiol. 2000; 89(1):81–8.
15. Janssen I, Heymsfield SB, Ross R. Low relative skeletal muscle mass (sarcopenia) in older persons is associated with functional impairment and physical disability. J Am Geriatr Soc. 2002;50(5):889–96.
16. Park S, Kim HJ, Ko BG, Chung JW, Kim SH, Park SH, Lee MH, Yeom JS. The prevalence and impact of sarcopenia on degenerative lumbar spinal stenosis. The bone & joint journal. 2016;98-B(8):1093–8.
17. Suka M, Yoshida K. The national burden of musculoskeletal pain in Japan: projections to the year 2055. Clin J Pain. 2009;25(4):313–9.
18. Chou R, Qaseem A, Snow V, Casey D, Cross JT Jr, Shekelle P, Owens DK. Clinical efficacy assessment Subcommittee of the American College of P, American College of P, American pain society low back pain guidelines P: diagnosis and treatment of low back pain: a joint clinical practice guideline from the American College of Physicians and the American pain society. Ann Intern Med. 2007;147(7):478–91.
19. Verschueren S, Gielen E, O'Neill TW, Pye SR, Adams JE, Ward KA, FC W, Szulc P, Laurent M, Claessens F, et al. Sarcopenia and its relationship with bone mineral density in middle-aged and elderly European men. Osteoporos Int. 2013;24(1):87–98.
20. Soen S, Fukunaga M, Sugimoto T, Sone T, Fujiwara S, Endo N, Gorai I, Shiraki M, Hagino H, Hosoi T, et al. Diagnostic criteria for primary osteoporosis: year 2012 revision. J Bone Miner Metab. 2013;31(3):247–57.
21. Yoshimura N, Muraki S, Oka H, Kawaguchi H, Nakamura K, Akune T. Cohort profile: research on osteoarthritis/osteoporosis against disability study. Int J Epidemiol. 2010;39(4):988–95.
22. Yoshimura N, Muraki S, Oka H, Mabuchi A, En-Yo Y, Yoshida M, Saika A, Yoshida H, Suzuki T, Yamamoto S, et al. Prevalence of knee osteoarthritis, lumbar spondylosis, and osteoporosis in Japanese men and women: the research on osteoarthritis/osteoporosis against disability study. J Bone Miner Metab. 2009;27(5):620–8.
23. Campbell MK, James A, Hudson MA, Carr C, Jackson E, Oakes V, Demissie S, Farrell D, Tessaro I. Improving multiple behaviors for colorectal cancer prevention among african american church members. Health Psychol. 2004;23(5):492–502.
24. Clohisy DR, Perkins SL, Ramnaraine ML. Review of cellular mechanisms of tumor osteolysis. Clin Orthop Relat Res. 2000;373:104–14.
25. Martin CD, Jimenez-Andrade JM, Ghilardi JR, Mantyh PW. Organization of a unique net-like meshwork of CGRP+ sensory fibers in the mouse periosteum: implications for the generation and maintenance of bone fracture pain. Neurosci Lett. 2007;427(3):148–52.
26. Mattia C, Coluzzi F, Celidonio L, Vellucci R. Bone pain mechanism in osteoporosis: a narrative review. Clinical cases in mineral and bone metabolism : the official journal of the Italian Society of Osteoporosis, Mineral Metabolism, and Skeletal Diseases. 2016;13(2):97–100.
27. Deutsch FE. Isolated lumbar strengthening in the rehabilitation of chronic low back pain. J Manip Physiol Ther. 1996;19(2):124–33.
28. Jeong UC, Sim JH, Kim CY, Hwang-Bo G, Nam CW. The effects of gluteus muscle strengthening exercise and lumbar stabilization exercise on lumbar muscle strength and balance in chronic low back pain patients. J Phys Ther Sci. 2015;27(12):3813–6.

7

Treatment of Charcot Neuroarthropathy and osteomyelitis of the same foot: a retrospective cohort study

Martin Berli*, Lazaros Vlachopoulos, Sabra Leupi, Thomas Böni and Charlotte Baltin

Abstract

Background: We evaluated treatment of osteomyelitis in the foot in the presence of Charcot neuroarthropathy, a devastating condition with progressive degeneration and joint destruction. We hypothesized that there was a difference in (1) amputation rate, (2) amputation level, (3) duration of antibiotic therapy, and (4) duration of immobilization for treatment of osteomyelitis within versus outside the Charcot zone.

Methods: Forty patients (43 ft) diagnosed with Charcot neuroarthropathy and osteomyelitis of the same foot were retrospectively analyzed. Some patients were successfully treated for osteomyelitis at different sites on the same foot at different times, thus 60 cases of osteomyelitis were identified in 40 treated patients. Cases were divided according to osteomyelitis localization: Group 1 had osteomyelitis outside the active Charcot region; Group 2 had osteomyelitis within the active Charcot region.

Results: Male patients ($n = 29$; mean age 58.2, range 40.1 to 77.5 years) were younger than female patients ($n = 11$; mean age 70.4, range 51.4 to 87.5, $p = 0.02$ years). Amputation rate was 52% overall (26/40 patients; 26/43 ft): 63% of 30 Group 1 cases and 40% of 30 Group 2 cases ($p = 0.09$). Amputation level ($p = 0.009$), duration of antibiotic treatment ($p = 0.045$) and duration of immobilization ($p = 0.01$) differed significantly between the groups.

Conclusions: Osteomyelitis within the Charcot region is associated with a higher level of amputation and longer durations of antibiotic therapy and immobilization. Osteomyelitis outside and within the Charcot affected region should be considered separately. If osteomyelitis occurs outside the active Charcot region, primary amputation may be preferred to internal resection.

Level of Evidence: Retrospective cohort chart review study.

Keywords: Charcot, Osteomyelitis, Amputation, Antibiotic, Treatment

Background

Charcot neuroarthropathy (CN), or diabetic neuropathic osteoarthropathy with progressive degeneration and joint destruction as a consequence of any condition resulting in decreased peripheral sensation [1], is a rare but devastating complication. The most common cause of CN is diabetes mellitus; other causes include alcoholism, vitamin B12 or folic acid deficiency, intravenous drug use, late stage syphilis, syringomyelia, and multiple sclerosis. While the precise pathogenesis of CN remains controversial, it is undoubtedly multifactorial [2, 3]. The current theory of Charcot pathogenesis combines both neurotraumatic and neurovascular aspects [3–6].

Elements of osteopenia, bone hyperemia, instability, muscle weakness, and loss of protective sensation place the limb at risk for developing neuropathic bone and joint changes [7]. When the compromised foot experiences trauma and the injury remains unrecognized, the cascade of events that subsequently ensues will often result in neuropathic fractures, subluxation or osteoarthropathy [8], and severe foot deformity. If an ulcer is also present, and the bone can be palpated through the ulcer, osteomyelitis may be an aggravating complication. An infection can spread into the bone of the foot of a patient with diabetes and/or CN from any infection of adjacent soft tissue

* Correspondence: martin.berli@balgrist.ch
Department of Orthopedics, Balgrist University Hospital, University of Zurich, Forchstrasse 340, -8008 Zurich, CH, Switzerland

that is complicated by an ulcer [9]. Risk factors for osteomyelitis include peripheral neuropathy, vascular disease, limited joint mobility, foot deformities, abnormal foot pressures, minor trauma, a history of ulceration or amputation, and immunosuppression [9–12].

Treatment of early stage CN with the use of crutches and/or immobilization (i.e., total contact cast and/or orthosis) may stop the progression of deformity and reduce the occurrence of complications [13–16]. However, if the diagnosis is initially missed, or if treatment is not initiated, the neuro-osteoarthropathy results in progressive deformities, consecutive ulcers and osteomyelitis, and is accompanied by a high risk of amputation [17].

Several studies have recently demonstrated that the location of diabetic foot ulcers or osteomyelitis affects prognosis and healing time [18–24]. However, there is a paucity of data on healing outcomes of osteomyelitis in the presence of CN. Dalla Paola et al. [25] evaluated the rate of limb salvage and time to recovery in 33 patients affected by CN complicated by diffuse osteomyelitis. However, their study focused on outcomes of surgical treatment to stabilize and correct bone deformity, rather than on outcomes of treating the osteomyelitis. The purpose of this study was to evaluate the treatment of osteomyelitis of the foot in the presence of CN. We hypothesized that there was a difference in (1) amputation rate, (2) level of amputation, (3) duration of antibiotic therapy, and (4) duration of immobilization after treatment in a CN foot with osteomyelitis within versus outside the Charcot zone. The potential effects of the initial surgical treatment, duration of insulin dependency, and patient compliance with treatment on these outcomes were also evaluated.

Methods

A retrospective analysis of all medical records of patients treated for a diagnosis of CN and osteomyelitis of the same foot between 2002 and 2012 at the outpatient clinic of a large, urban, orthopedic, university-affiliated research hospital was performed. Inclusion criteria were: a diagnosis of CN according to the definition and diagnostic criteria of the French neurologist J.M. Charcot [26], radiographs of the affected foot, and osteomyelitis of the same side with radiological findings of osteomyelitis on MRI and/or positive bone biopsy cultures. Exclusion criteria were: primary treatment at another institution, or a previous fracture due to trauma of the same foot. This study was approved by the Research Ethics Committee of our institution.

Cases were divided into two groups according to whether the osteomyelitis was localized outside the active Charcot region of the foot (Group 1), or within the active Charcot region of the foot (Group 2). The region of the foot (i.e., forefoot, midfoot or hindfoot) where the osteomyelitis was localized was also recorded. To evaluate the effectiveness of the initial surgical treatment, the surgical management was divided into four categories: 1) "limited resection" was defined as resection of the infected bone, leaving the surrounding soft tissue in place, 2) "amputation" was defined as surgical removal of part of the lower limb (bone and soft tissue), 3) "arthrodesis" was defined as removal of the infected bone combined with external (Ilizarov fixateur) or internal fixation, and 4) "debridement" was defined as surgical removal of the infected or necrotic tissue around the wound with underlying osteomyelitis. Successful treatment was defined as the absence of clinical or radiological signs of a recurrence of osteomyelitis at the initially affected region. Duration of treatment was defined as the time from the first clinic visit to the last clinic visit for a single case of osteomyelitis. Antibiotic therapy was discontinued based on the recommendations of in-house infectious disease specialists, the elimination of clinical signs of infection (e.g. redness, warmth and swelling), C-reactive protein level and MRI results. The duration of antibiotic treatment, duration of immobilization, and duration of treatment were calculated in days, separately for each case of osteomyelitis. Other factors likely to influence outcome were recorded, including duration of diabetic treatment, insulin dependency, duration of surgery, smoking status, immunosuppressive therapy, peripheral arterial occlusive disease, obesity, age, gender, incidence of bilateral CN, and patient compliance.

Statistical analysis

Continuous data are reported as means and standard deviations. Categorical data are reported as numbers and percentages. Statistical analysis was performed using the software R (The R Foundation for Statistical Computing, Version 3.1.0, Vienna, Austria). Differences in categorical baseline characteristics were evaluated using the Mann-Whitney U test and the chi-square test. To address clustering of cases within patients, logistic regression analysis was performed, with amputation as the dependent variable and localization of osteomyelitis as the independent variable with robust standard error (patient identification as a cluster). Duration of antibiotic therapy and duration of immobilization were analyzed as logarithmic transformed dependent variables in linear regression with robust standard error (patient identification as a cluster). Categorical data (i.e., amputation level) were assessed using Fisher's exact test. The significance level was set at $p < 0.05$. For graphical visualization, Tukey boxplots were depicted with whiskers maximum of 1.5 interquartile ranges (IQR).

Results

Study population

This retrospective chart review identified 70 patients diagnosed with CN and osteomyelitis of the same foot between 2002 and 2012. Thirty patients were excluded from the study due to incomplete medical reports (n = 26) or absence of reliable evidence of osteomyelitis (n = 4). Three patients (#7, #26, and #34) had bilateral osteomyelitis combined with CN. Thus, 40 patients (43 ft) were included in the study (Table 1).

Due to the progressive nature of CN, some patients were successfully treated for multiple episodes of osteomyelitis, which occurred independently of each other, at different sites on the same foot, or at different time points, months or years apart. One patient (#22) presented with osteomyelitis within the Charcot region, and then one month later presented with a separate case of osteomyelitis outside the Charcot region. Ten patients (#1, #4, #7 right foot, #11, #18, #25, #26 left foot, #27, #28, #39) had 2 separately treated and resolved cases of osteomyelitis on the same foot, months apart. Three patients (#6, #7 left foot, #21) had 3 separately treated and resolved cases of osteomyelitis on the same foot, months apart. The mean duration between independent cases of osteomyelitis in a single patient, measured as the date treatment ended for the first case to the date of diagnosis of the second case, was 16.3 months (range: 2.4 to 33.5 months).Thus, in total, we identified 60 cases of osteomyelitis for the 40 patients included in this study. The 60 cases were divided into two groups according to the localization of the osteomyelitis and CN, with 30 cases in Group 1 (i.e., osteomyelitis outside the active Charcot region), and 30 cases in Group 2 (i.e., osteomyelitis within the active Charcot region of the foot).

Patient demographic characteristics and individual treatments are summarized in Table 1. There were 29 (73%) male and 11 female patients; 44/60 (73%) cases of osteomyelitis were in male patients. Mean age was 61.6 ± 12.4 (range, 40.1 to 87.5) years. Male patients (mean age 58.2 ± 10.5; range, 40.1 to 77.5 years) were significantly younger than female patients (mean age 70.4 ± 13.4; range 51.4 to 87.5 years; $p = 0.02$). Twenty-three (58%) patients were between 50 and 70 years of age at initial diagnosis of CN; 8 (20%) were over 70 years of age, and 9 (23%) were under 50 years of age. No female patient was under 50 years of age at initial diagnosis of CN.

Twenty-five of 40 (63%) patients had insulin-dependent diabetes and 15 had non-insulin-dependent diabetes. The mean duration of treatment for diabetes at the time of initial treatment for osteomyelitis was 17.7 ± 13.2 (range: 0.2 to 52.9) years. The mean duration of treatment for diabetes at the time of initial diagnosis of CN was 15.5 ± 13.8 (range: 0.6 to 52.9) years. In Group 1, 16/30 (53%) cases were insulin-dependent; in Group 2, 19/30 (63%) cases were insulin-dependent.

There was no significant difference in age, gender, and duration of treatment for diabetes between the groups ($p = 0.81$, $p = 0.82$, and $p = 0.30$, respectively) (Table 2).

Amputation rate

An amputation was performed in 31/60 (52%) cases of osteomyelitis (26/40 patients; 26/43 ft). In the 44 male cases, 21 (48%) amputations were performed. In the 16 female cases, 10 (63%) amputations were performed.

The amputation rate was similar for Group 1 with osteomyelitis outside the Charcot region (19 amputations; 63%) and Group 2 with osteomyelitis within the Charcot region (12 amputations; 40%) ($p = 0.09$). Amputation rate did not differ significantly based on insulin dependency or compliance with treatment.

Level of amputation

The 31 amputations included 16 toe, 4 transmetatarsal, 1 Lisfranc, 1 Chopart, 8 transtibial and 1 transfemoral amputation. A major amputation (i.e., above the level of the ankle) was performed in 3/30 (10%) cases in Group 1 with osteomyelitis outside the active Charcot region and 6/30 (20%) cases in Group 2 with osteomyelitis within the active Charcot region ($p = 0.009$) (Fig. 1). The level of amputation did not differ significantly based on insulin dependency or compliance with treatment (Fig. 2).

Duration of antibiotic treatment

The duration of antibiotic treatment was significantly shorter in Group 1 (mean 55.7 ± 48.9, range: 9 to 228 days) compared to Group 2 (mean 84.1 ± 51.2, range: 6 to 238 days, $p = 0.045$). Within Group 1, the mean duration of antibiotic treatment was 43.9 days shorter in cases initially treated with amputation compared to cases initially treated with internal resection ($p = 0.02$). Within Group 2,

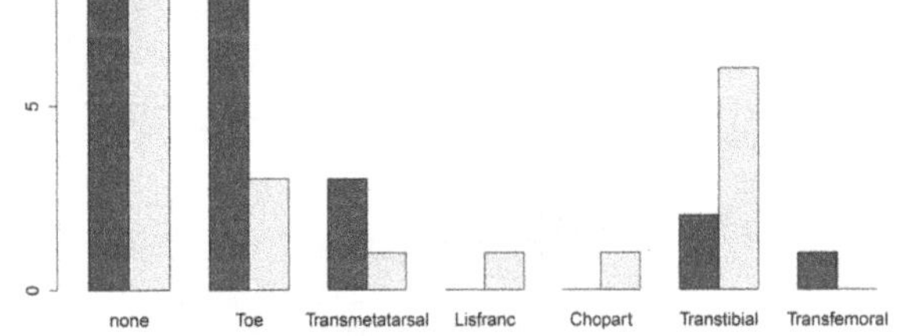

Fig. 1 Histogram showing the level of amputation in Group 1 with osteomyelitis outside the Charcot region ($n = 30$) and in Group 2 with osteomyelitis within the Charcot region ($n = 30$) when treatment was successfully completed, and in the absence of recurrence of osteomyelitis

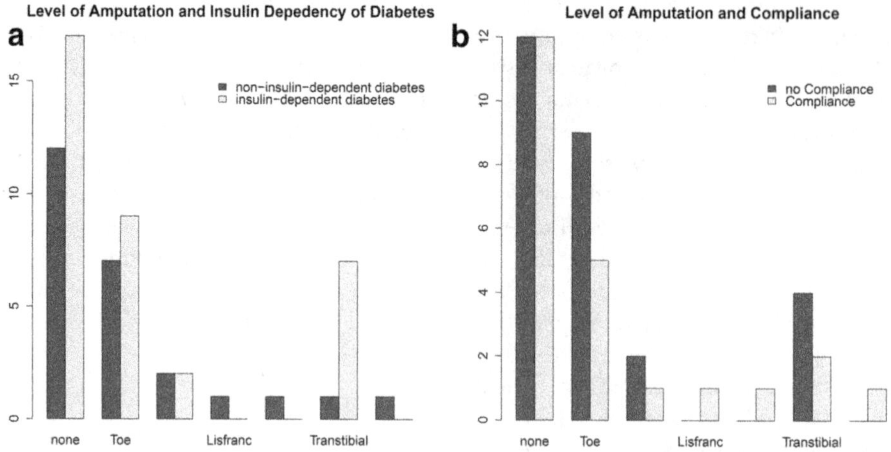

Fig. 2 Histograms showing the level of amputation in relation to (**a**) insulin dependency ($n = 35$ insulin-dependent diabetes, $n = 25$ non-insulin-dependent diabetes) and (**b**) compliance with treatment for osteomyelitis and Charcot arthropathy ($n = 23$ compliant, $n = 27$ non-compliant, $n = 10$ not recorded)

the duration of antibiotic treatment was similar across all initial surgical treatments ($p = 0.09$) (Fig. 3).

Duration of immobilization

The duration of immobilization was 61.4 days shorter in Group 1 where osteomyelitis outside the active Charcot region (mean 83.1 ± 70.5, range 19 to 304 days), compared to Group 2 with osteomyelitis within the active Charcot region (mean 144 ± 91.8, range 17 to 389 days, $p = 0.01$). There was no significant difference in the duration of immobilization between the different initial surgical treatments within each group ($p = 0.40$ and $p = 0.90$, respectively) (Fig. 4).

Discussion

Treatment of CN complicated by osteomyelitis is a complex, long-lasting procedure, demanding considerable perseverance from patients and physicians. Multiple surgical procedures, including a high rate of amputations, as well as prolonged antibiotic therapy and immobilization are often required [27]. This study demonstrated that patients treated for osteomyelitis within the Charcot region on the foot underwent more high level amputations and had longer durations of antibiotic treatment and immobilization than patients treated for osteomyelitis outside the Charcot region. However, the amputation rate was statistically similar for both groups.

Amputation was required during the course of treatment in 31/60 cases treated for CN and osteomyelitis of the same foot, whereas 29/60 cases were successfully treated with a combination of conservative surgery and antibiotic medication. The overall amputation rate did not differ significantly between the patients treated for osteomyelitis outside the Charcot region and those

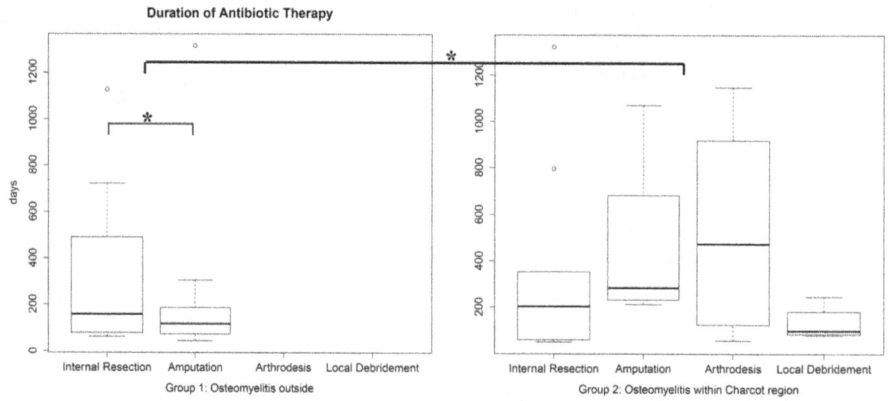

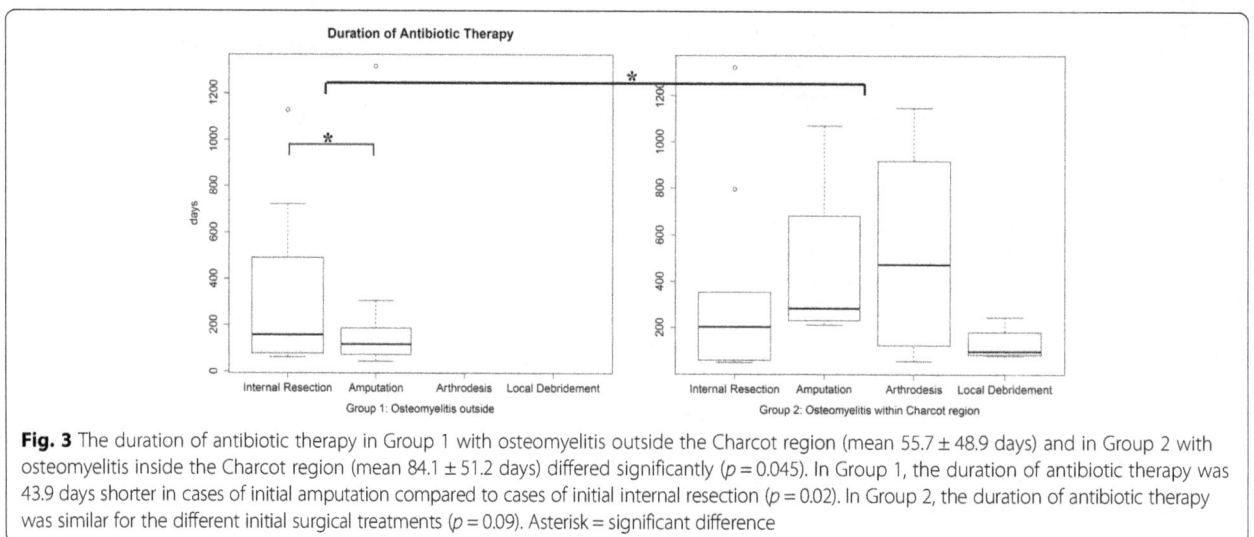

Fig. 3 The duration of antibiotic therapy in Group 1 with osteomyelitis outside the Charcot region (mean 55.7 ± 48.9 days) and in Group 2 with osteomyelitis inside the Charcot region (mean 84.1 ± 51.2 days) differed significantly ($p = 0.045$). In Group 1, the duration of antibiotic therapy was 43.9 days shorter in cases of initial amputation compared to cases of initial internal resection ($p = 0.02$). In Group 2, the duration of antibiotic therapy was similar for the different initial surgical treatments ($p = 0.09$). Asterisk = significant difference

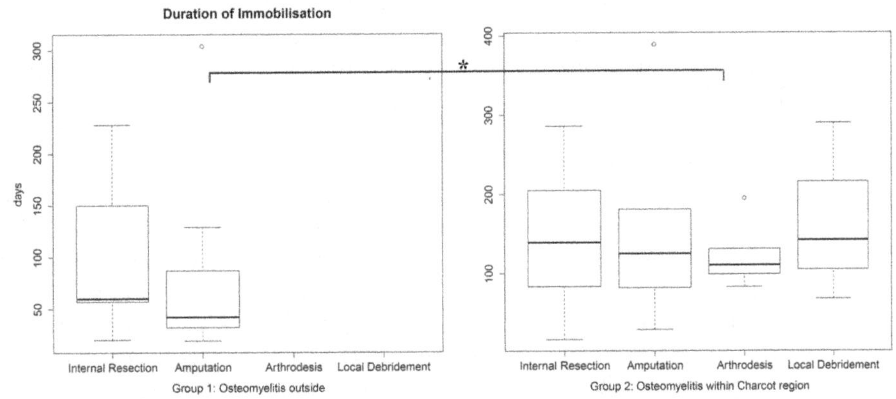

Fig. 4 The duration of immobilization in Group 1 with osteomyelitis outside the Charcot region (mean 83.1 ± 70.5, range 19 to 304 days) and in Group 2 with osteomyelitis inside the Charcot region (mean 144 ± 91.8, range 17 to 389 days, $p = 0.01$) differed significantly ($p = 0.01$). The duration of immobilization was similar for the different initial surgical treatments within each group. Asterisk = significant difference

treated for osteomyelitis within the Charcot region. Wukich et al. [28] recently reported 16 of 43 patients (37.2%) with CN hospitalized for osteomyelitis underwent major amputation, but this rate can be expected to be lower in less severe cases that can be effectively managed in an outpatient setting such as ours. When considering the level of amputation, the 20% rate of major amputations we reported in cases of osteomyelitis within the Charcot region is comparable to the 23% rate of major amputations reported by Gazis et al. [29] in 47 patients with CN managed by a specialist diabetic foot clinic. However, our 10% amputation rate in cases of osteomyelitis outside the active Charcot region was significantly lower.

The mean duration of antibiotic treatment in this study ranged from 56 to 84 days, where patients with osteomyelitis within the active Charcot region required a longer duration of treatment. Two recent studies reported similar mean durations of antibiotic treatment of 76 days [30] and 77 days [31] for the nonsurgical management of diabetic foot osteomyelitis. Mutluoglu et al. [32] reported a mean of 47 days of antibiotic treatment in 37 patients with diabetic foot osteomyelitis, of whom 22 underwent minor amputation. In 2008, the International Working Group on the Diabetic Foot determined that there are no data to inform the optimal duration of antibiotic therapy [4].

In this study, the mean duration of immobilization ranged from 83 to 144 days, with patients with osteomyelitis within the active Charcot region requiring a longer period of immobilization. Several clinical trials evaluated different off-loading techniques for the treatment of diabetic foot ulcers and reported the duration of immobilization with a total contact cast ranged from 35 to 69 days [33–36]. However, these trials excluded patients with osteomyelitis. In a study of 288 patients with acute Charcot foot that included 81 cases of ulceration and 20 cases of osteomyelitis, the median duration of immobilization for resolution of symptoms was 273 days [37]. Literature reporting specifically on immobilization of the Charcot foot with osteomyelitis is notably lacking.

The region of the foot on which the osteomyelitis was located likely contributed to the significant differences in the amputation level ($p < 0.001$), duration of antibiotic treatment ($p = 0.045$), and duration of immobilization ($p = 0.01$) observed between the groups who presented with osteomyelitis within the Charcot region versus outside the Charcot region. In the group with osteomyelitis within the Charcot region, a major amputation was performed in 3/8 cases with osteomyelitis in the hindfoot, 3/13 cases with osteomyelitis in the midfoot, and none of the cases with osteomyelitis in the forefoot. In the group with osteomyelitis outside the Charcot region, the osteomyelitis was almost exclusively (29/30 cases) located in the forefoot, thus elimination of infection by internal resection or amputation could be achieved more reliably. Diabetic foot ulcers and osteomyelitis located in the forefoot have been demonstrated to have a shorter healing time compared to those in the hindfoot [18, 20–22, 24]. We therefore recommend that patients with osteomyelitis of the foot within versus outside the Charcot region should be analyzed separately in future research evaluating the outcome and treatment of CN and osteomyelitis.

The initial surgical treatment provided in this study did not affect the duration of antibiotic therapy or immobilization in the group with osteomyelitis in the Charcot region, but this may be due to the small sample sizes for each type of surgery. In the group with osteomyelitis outside the Charcot region, the duration of antibiotic therapy was 6 weeks shorter ($p = 0.02$) in those who initially underwent amputation compared to those who initially underwent internal resection, indicating that internal resection may not be sufficient to eliminate the infected tissue.

Four studies recently evaluated limb salvage procedures as alternatives to amputation in Charcot foot and ankle osteomyelitis. Farber et al. [38] reported that none of the 11 patients with midfoot CN and ulceration who underwent operative debridement and corrective osteotomy as a limb salvage procedure needed an amputation. Dalla Paola et al. [39] reported four (9%) major amputations for failed infection control in 43 patients who underwent arthrodesis [40] and external fixation as a limb salvage procedure for CN and ankle osteomyelitis. Pinzur et al. [41] reported 3 amputations (4.2%) in a cohort of 71 patients who underwent single-stage resection of infection and correction of deformity with a ring fixateur. Ramanujam et al. [42] reported one lower extremity amputation (3.7%) in 27 patients with diabetic CN and osteomyelitis who underwent surgical reconstruction using circular external fixation.

A long-standing history (>10 years) of diabetes at the time of initial diagnosis of CN is common [43, 44]. The mean duration of treatment for diabetes in our study was 15 (range: 0.6 to 53) years. No patient with insulin-dependent diabetes received the diagnosis of diabetes less than one year before the diagnosis of CN. However, two patients with non–insulin-dependent diabetes had an almost synchronous diagnosis of CN and diabetes, suggesting that the initial occurrence of Charcot may have guided the diagnosis of diabetes. There were less patients (62%) with insulin-dependent diabetes compared to the 75% previously reported in another study of CN [45]. However, insulin dependency did not appear to influence the amputation rate or amputation level.

In previous studies, noncompliance with treatment of CN was determined to be the strongest predictor for recurrence of CN, with an odds ratio of 19.7 [46, 47]. While the rate of noncompliance as recorded in patient charts was high in the present study (38%), noncompliance with treatment of the osteomyelitis did not appear to influence the amputation rate or level of amputation.

The large number of patients excluded from this study due to incomplete patient charts may have resulted in selection bias. Typically, CN patients do not come in for follow-up visits because they are poorly compliant with treatment (i.e., total contact cast) or they do not understand that they have a disease. The less complex cases are often followed for longer durations than the severe cases, to monitor their feet and their special shoes. Thus, to minimize the potential selection bias for more severe cases, we evaluated the effect of compliance with treatment on amputation rate and amputation level.

Limitations of this study include the retrospective study design, such that some pertinent factors that could potentially affect treatment outcomes may not have been recorded, and data collection at a single site, which limits the generalizability of the conclusions. Another limitation is the lack of recorded reasons for the initial surgical treatment that was elected. Finally, the heterogeneity of initial surgical treatments performed in Group 2 patients and the relatively small sample sizes did not allow further subgroup analysis.

Strengths of this study include the relatively large sample size compared to other studies of CN, and the detailed information available about the treatment regimens. However, the heterogeneity of patients with this disease and initial surgical treatment options limited may require prospective trials with larger samples to better elucidate the best treatment option for osteomyelitis in the presence of CN.

Conclusions

Patients treated for osteomyelitis within the Charcot region on the foot underwent more high level amputations and had longer durations of antibiotic treatment and immobilization than patients treated for osteomyelitis outside the Charcot region, although the amputation rate was similar for both groups. We recommend that. osteomyelitis outside and within the Charcot affected region should be regarded as separate entities when considering treatment protocols and in future research evaluating the outcome and treatment of CN and osteomyelitis. If osteomyelitis occurs outside the active Charcot region, primary amputation may be preferred to internal resection.

Abbreviations

CN: Charcot neuroarthropathy; IQR: interquartile range; MRI: magnetic resonance imaging

Acknowledgements

The authors thank Dagmar Gross for assistance with preparation of this manuscript.

Funding

The authors received no financial support for the research, authorship, and/or publication of this article.

Authors' contributions

CB and SL carried out the data collection from patient records and, together with MB, drafted the manuscript. TB helped with drafting the manuscript, gave helpful input during writing of the manuscript, and gave substantial input in revising the manuscript. LV participated in the design of the study, performed the statistical analysis, and helped design all figures and tables. All authors read and approved the final manuscript and all revisions.

Authors' information

CB and SL are residents in orthopedic surgery; LV, TB, and MB are board-certified orthopedic surgeons; additionally, the senior authors TB and MB are specialized in the treatment of the diabetic foot.

Competing interests

The authors declare that they have no potential conflicts of interest or competing interests with respect to the research, authorship, and/or publication of this article.

References

1. Frykberg RG, Bevilacqua NJ, Habershaw G. Surgical off-loading of the diabetic foot. J Vasc Surg. 2010;52(3 Suppl):44S–58S.
2. Wukich DK, Sung W. Charcot arthropathy of the foot and ankle: modern concepts and management review. J Diabetes Complicat. 2009;23(6):409–26.
3. Strotman PK, Reif TJ, Pinzur MS. Charcot Arthropathy of the foot and ankle. Foot Ankle Int. 2016;37(11):1255–63.
4. Berendt AR, Peters EJ, Bakker K, Embil JM, Eneroth M, Hinchliffe RJ, Jeffcoate WJ, Lipsky BA, Senneville E, Teh J, et al. Diabetic foot osteomyelitis: a progress report on diagnosis and a systematic review of treatment. Diabetes Metab Res Rev. 2008;24(Suppl 1):S145–61.
5. Rajbhandari SM, Jenkins RC, Davies C, Tesfaye S. Charcot neuroarthropathy in diabetes mellitus. Diabetologia. 2002;45(8):1085–96.
6. Chisholm KA, Gilchrist JM. The Charcot joint: a modern neurologic perspective. J Clin Neuromuscul Dis. 2011;13(1):1–13.
7. Herbst SA, Jones KB, Saltzman CL. Pattern of diabetic neuropathic arthropathy associated with the peripheral bone mineral density. J Bone Joint Surg Br. 2004;86(3):378–83.
8. Frykberg RG, Mendeszoon E. Management of the diabetic Charcot foot. Diabetes Metab Res Rev. 2000;16(Suppl 1):S59–65.
9. Game FL. Osteomyelitis in the diabetic foot: diagnosis and management. Med Clin North Am. 2013;97(5):947–56.
10. Boulton AJ, Kirsner RS, Vileikyte L. Clinical practice. Neuropathic diabetic foot ulcers. N Engl J Med. 2004;351(1):48–55.
11. Ciampolini J, Harding KG. Pathophysiology of chronic bacterial osteomyelitis. Why do antibiotics fail so often? Postgrad Med J. 2000;76(898):479–83.
12. Frykberg RG. Diabetic foot ulcers: pathogenesis and management. Am Fam Physician. 2002;66(9):1655–62.
13. Chantelau E. The perils of procrastination: effects of early vs. delayed detection and treatment of incipient Charcot fracture. Diabet Med. 2005; 22(12):1707–12.
14. Sanders LJFR. Diabetic neuropathic osteoarthropathy: the Charcot foot. In: The high risk foot in diabetes mellitus; 1991. p. 325–33.
15. Petrova NL, Edmonds ME. Charcot neuro-osteoarthropathy-current standards. Diabetes Metab Res Rev. 2008;24(Suppl 1):S58–61.
16. Ruotolo V, Di Pietro B, Giurato L, Masala S, Meloni M, Schillaci O, Bergamini A, Uccioli L. A new natural history of Charcot foot: clinical evolution and final outcome of stage 0 Charcot neuroarthropathy in a tertiary referral diabetic foot clinic. Clin Nucl Med. 2013;38(7):506–9.
17. Illgner U, Podella M, Rummler M, Wuhr J, Busch HG, Wetz HH. Reconstructive surgery for Charcot foot. Long-term 5-year outcome. Orthopade. 2009;38(12): 1180–6.
18. van Asten SA, Jupiter DC, Mithani M, La Fontaine J, Davis KE, Lavery LA. Erythrocyte sedimentation rate and C-reactive protein to monitor treatment outcomes in diabetic foot osteomyelitis. Int Wound J. 2017;14(1):142–8.
19. Aragon-Sanchez J, Lazaro-Martinez JL, Alvaro-Afonso FJ, Molines-Barroso R. Conservative surgery of diabetic forefoot osteomyelitis: how can I operate on this patient without amputation? Int J Low Extrem Wounds. 2015;14(2): 108–31.
20. Vaseenon T, Thitiboonsuwan S, Cheewawattanachai C, Pimchoo P, Phanphaisarn A. Off-loading total contact cast in combination with hydrogel and foam dressing for management of diabetic plantar ulcer of the foot. J Med Assoc Thail. 2014;97(12):1319–24.
21. Cull DL, Manos G, Hartley MC, Taylor SM, Langan EM, Eidt JF, Johnson BL. An early validation of the Society for Vascular Surgery lower extremity threatened limb classification system. J Vasc Surg. 2014;60(6):1535–41.
22. Wang A, Sun X, Wang W, Jiang K. A study of prognostic factors in Chinese patients with diabetic foot ulcers. Diabet Foot Ankle. 2014;5
23. Cecilia-Matilla A, Lazaro-Martinez JL, Aragon-Sanchez J, Garcia-Alvarez Y, Chana-Valero P, Beneit-Montesinos JV. Influence of the location of nonischemic diabetic forefoot osteomyelitis on time to healing after undergoing surgery. Int J Low Extrem Wounds. 2013;12(3):184–8.
24. Pickwell KM, Siersma VD, Kars M, Holstein PE, Schaper NC, Eurodiale c. Diabetic foot disease: impact of ulcer location on ulcer healing. Diabetes Metab Res Rev. 2013;29(5):377–83.
25. Dalla Paola L, Carone A, Baglioni M, Boscarino G, Vasilache L. Extension and grading of osteomyelitis are not related to limb salvage in Charcot neuropathic osteoarthropathy: a cohort prospective study. J Diabetes Complicat. 2016;30(4):608–12.
26. Charcot J. Lectures on the diseases of the nervous system: delivered at la Salpêtrière. HC Lea. 1879;
27. Dalla Paola L. Confronting a dramatic situation: the charcot foot complicated by osteomyelitis. Int J Low Extrem Wounds. 2014;13(4):247–62.
28. Wukich DK, Hobizal KB, Sambenedetto TL, Kirby K, Rosario BL. Outcomes of osteomyelitis in patients hospitalized with diabetic foot infections. Foot Ankle Int. 2016;37(12):1285–91.
29. Gazis A, Pound N, Macfarlane R, Treece K, Game F, Jeffcoate W. Mortality in patients with diabetic neuropathic osteoarthropathy (Charcot foot). Diabet Med. 2004;21(11):1243–6.
30. Zeun P, Gooday C, Nunney I, Dhatariya K. Predictors of outcomes in diabetic foot osteomyelitis treated initially with conservative (nonsurgical) medical management: a retrospective study. Int J Low Extrem Wounds. 2016;15(1):19–25.
31. Lesens O, Desbiez F, Theis C, Ferry T, Bensalem M, Laurichesse H, Tauveron I, Beytout J, Aragon Sanchez J. Working group on diabetic O: Staphylococcus Aureus-related diabetic osteomyelitis: medical or surgical management? A French and Spanish retrospective cohort. Int J Low Extrem Wounds. 2015; 14(3):284–90.
32. Mutluoglu M, Sivrioglu AK, Eroglu M, Uzun G, Turhan V, Ay H, Lipsky BA. The implications of the presence of osteomyelitis on outcomes of infected diabetic foot wounds. Scand J Infect Dis. 2013;45(7):497–503.
33. Faglia E, Caravaggi C, Clerici G, Sganzaroli A, Curci V, Vailati W, Simonetti D, Sommalvico F. Effectiveness of removable walker cast versus nonremovable fiberglass off-bearing cast in the healing of diabetic plantar foot ulcer: a randomized controlled trial. Diabetes Care. 2010;33(7):1419–23.
34. Lavery LA, Higgins KR, La Fontaine J, Zamorano RG, Constantinides GP, Kim PJ. Randomised clinical trial to compare total contact casts, healing sandals and a shear-reducing removable boot to heal diabetic foot ulcers. Int Wound J. 2015;12(6):710–5.
35. Armstrong DG, Lavery LA, Wu S, Boulton AJ. Evaluation of removable and irremovable cast walkers in the healing of diabetic foot wounds: a randomized controlled trial. Diabetes Care. 2005;28(3):551–4.
36. Ha Van G, Siney H, Hartmann-Heurtier A, Jacqueminet S, Greau F, Grimaldi A. Nonremovable, windowed, fiberglass cast boot in the treatment of diabetic plantar ulcers: efficacy, safety, and compliance. Diabetes Care. 2003; 26(10):2848–52.
37. Game FL, Catlow R, Jones GR, Edmonds ME, Jude EB, Rayman G, Jeffcoate WJ. Audit of acute Charcot's disease in the UK: the CDUK study. Diabetologia. 2012;55(1):32–5.
38. Farber DC, Juliano PJ, Cavanagh PR, Ulbrecht J, Caputo G. Single stage correction with external fixation of the ulcerated foot in individuals with Charcot neuroarthropathy. Foot Ankle Int. 2002;23(2):130–4.
39. Dalla Paola L, Brocco E, Ceccacci T, Ninkovic S, Sorgentone S, Marinescu MG, Volpe A. Limb salvage in Charcot foot and ankle osteomyelitis: combined use single stage/double stage of arthrodesis and external fixation. Foot Ankle Int. 2009;30(11):1065–70.
40. Biz C, Hoxhaj B, Aldegheri R, Iacobellis C. Minimally invasive surgery for Tibiotalocalcaneal arthrodesis using a retrograde intramedullary nail: preliminary results of an innovative modified technique. J Foot Ankle Surg. 2016;55(6):1130–8.
41. Pinzur MS, Gil J, Belmares J. Treatment of osteomyelitis in charcot foot with single-stage resection of infection, correction of deformity, and maintenance with ring fixation. Foot Ankle Int. 2012;33(12):1069–74.
42. Ramanujam CL, Han D, Zgonis T. Lower extremity amputation and mortality rates in the reconstructed diabetic Charcot foot and ankle with external fixation: data analysis of 116 patients. Foot Ankle Spec. 2016;9(2):113–26.
43. Fabrin J, Larsen K, Holstein PE. Long-term follow-up in diabetic Charcot feet with spontaneous onset. Diabetes Care. 2000;23(6):796–800.
44. Pakarinen TK, Laine HJ, Honkonen SE, Peltonen J, Oksala H, Lahtela J. Charcot arthropathy of the diabetic foot. Current concepts and review of 36 cases. Scand J Surg. 2002;91(2):195–201.
45. Myerson MS, Henderson MR, Saxby T, Short KW. Management of midfoot diabetic neuroarthropathy. Foot Ankle Int. 1994;15(5):233–41.
46. Osterhoff G, Boni T, Berli M. Recurrence of acute Charcot neuropathic osteoarthropathy after conservative treatment. Foot Ankle Int. 2013;34(3): 359–64.
47. Renner N, Wirth SH, Osterhoff G, Boni T, Berli M. Outcome after protected full weightbearing treatment in an orthopedic device in diabetic neuropathic arthropathy (Charcot arthropathy): a comparison of unilaterally and bilaterally affected patients. BMC Musculoskelet Disord. 2016;17(1):504.

8

L161982 alleviates collagen-induced arthritis in mice by increasing Treg cells and down-regulating Interleukin-17 and monocyte-chemoattractant protein-1 levels

Liang Chen[1], Xianglei Wu[2], Jun Zhong[1] and Dongqing Li[3*]

Abstract

Background: To investigate the effects and potential mechanism of L161982 (a kind of EP4 antagonist) on the collagen-induced arthritis (CIA) mice model.

Methods: The CIA mice model were first established by immunizing with Chicken Type II Collagen on DBA/1 mice. The CIA groups were administered once a day for 2 weeks with either 5 mg/kg L161982 by intraperitoneal injections (IP), 200 U celecoxib by intragastrical injections, or 100 μl PBS (IP). At the end of the study, total arthritis score and histopathologic examination were assessed to determine CIA severity. The plasma and tissue expressions of IL-17 and monocyte chemoattractant protein-1 (MCP-1) were detected by enzyme-linked immunosorbent assay (ELISA) and Immunohistochemical staining (IHC) respectively; The number of $CD4^{+}CD25^{+}Foxp3^{+}$ regulatory T cells (Treg) determined as a proportion of total $CD4^{+}$ cells in the lymph nodes and spleen. We also tested the proliferation of isolated Tregs and the ratio of Th17 polarization of Naïve T cells under the treatment of L161982 by BrdU assay and flow cytometry respectively.

Results: CIA mice treated with L161982 showed reduced arthritis scores, joint swellings, cracked cartilage surface, and less hyperplasia in the connective tissue of the articular cavity. Plasma and tissue IL-17 and MCP-1 decreased, while the proportion of Treg cells is increased both in the spleen and lymph nodes of CIA mice. Otherwise, L161982 have no direct effect on Tregs proliferation; a decreased tendency of Th17 polarization in vitro were observed in L161982-treated naïve T cells.

Conclusion: Although less effective than Celecoxib, L161982 also resulted in a reduction of ankle joint inflammation in CIA mice. L161982 reduces the RA severity in CIA mice through inhibition of IL-17 and MCP-1, increasing Treg cells, and reducing inflammation. The mechanism of the reduction of IL-17 in plasma or tissue after administration of L161982 might be potentially derived from the suppression of $CD4^{+}$ T cells differentiation into Th-17 cells.

Keywords: Collagen-induced arthritis, Interleukin-17, Monocyte chemotactic protein-1, EP4 antagonist, Rheumatoid arthritis

* Correspondence: lidongqing@whu.edu.cn
[3]Department of Microbiology, School of Basic Medical Science, Wuhan University, 185 Donghu Road, Wuhan, Hubei 430071, People's Republic of China
Full list of author information is available at the end of the article

Background

Rheumatoid arthritis (RA) is a chronic debilitating autoimmune disorder that results in long-lasting joints injuries and pain [1, 2]. Various randomized controlled trials have been conducted with an aim to find an effective treatment, but some questions remain to be resolved, especially with regards to pathogenic factors, targeted compounds, or drugs [3, 4].

The activation of naïve helper T cells (Th0) can differentiate into a variety of phenotypes depending on cytokine environment: Th1, Th17, Th2, and regulatory T cells (Treg) [5]. Th1 and Th17 cells may be involved in promoting the development of RA and Treg cells may have a protective effect, while the role of Th2 cells, which are associated with immune regulation, is not fully understood [6–9].

In the pathogenesis of RA, the imbalanced secretion of cytokines results in increased inflammatory mediators, including the arachidonic acid metabolite prostaglandin E2 (PGE2) [10]. PGE2 is synthesized from arachidonic acid by cyclooxygenase (COX) and prostaglandin E synthase. PGE2 has been identified as having an immunoregulatory role in the differentiation of Th1 and Th2 cells [11, 12]. The numerous biological effects of PGE2 are mediated by four G protein-coupled receptors (EP1, 2, 3, 4). The activation of the EP4 receptors [10] may promote both inflammatory or anti-inflammatory effects, with an inflammatory role in Th17 cell-dependent diseases [13]. Of note, EP4 knock-out mice have been found to be resistant to type-II collagen antibody-induced arthritis [14].

In this paper, we investigated the effects of blocking PGE2 signaling using an EP4-receptor antagonist on disease severity in a mouse model of CIA. Additionally, we examined changes in the cytokines IL-17 and MCP-1 and resulting changes in the proportions of regulatory T cell, through which EP4-receptor antagonism can potentially modulate CIA disease progression.

Methods

Animals and reagents

Female DBA/1 mice of 6 to 8 weeks old were provided by the Center for Animal Experiment and ABSL-3 Laboratory, Wuhan University School of Medicine, Hubei, China. The following reagents were used in this study: EP4 receptor antagonist L161982 (*N*-[[4′-[[3-Butyl-1,5-dihydro-5-oxo-1-[2-(trifluoromethyl)phenyl]-4*H*-1,2,4-triazol-4-yl]methyl] [1,1′-biphenyl]-2-yl]sulfonyl]-3-methyl-2-thiophenecarboxamide) (Tocris, UK); Chicken Type II Collagen (Sigma, USA); Celecoxib, PGE2 and BrdU Cell Proliferation ELISA Kit (Abcam, USA); Dimethyl sulfoxide (DMSO, Sigma, USA); Freund's Complete Adjuvant (Chondrex, USA); Interleukin-17 (IL-17), monocyte chemoattractant protein-1 (MCP-1), and ELISA kit (eBioscience, USA); Mouse antibodies: FITC-anti-CD4, PE-anti-CD25, PeCY5-anti-Foxp3, PE-CD62L and PeCY5-anti-IL-17, anti-IL-17, anti-MCP-1, anti-cleaved-caspas 3, soluble anti-CD3 and soluble anti-CD28 (eBioscience, USA); EasySep mouse $CD4^{+}CD62L^{+}$ naïve T cells isolation kit (Milenyi biotec, USA); Th17 cells inducement: mouse TGF-β1, IL-6, IL-23, anti-IFNγ and anti-IL-4 (Milenyi biotec, USA).

Establishment of CIA mouse model and dosing regimen

Forty mice were randomly divided into five groups, 8 mice per group: the control group and four CIA groups. For CIA groups, 200 μg of chicken type II collagen dissolved in DMSO was mixed with an equal volume of Freund's Complete Adjuvant and emulsified in ice bath. Of this emulsion, 100 μl was administrated through intradermal injection at the base of the tail and this immunization was boosted 3 weeks later [15]. For the model control group, the emulsion with Freund's Complete Adjuvant but without chicken type II collagen was injected according to the same protocol. For the remaining CIA treatment groups, mice were treated firstly as the CIA group and then administered with 5 mg/kg of L161982 by intraperitoneal injections (IP), 200 U celecoxib by intragastrical injections (IA) or 100 μl PBS (IP) respectively [16, 17] as the previous studies. All injections were administered once per day for 2 weeks.

Evaluation of arthritis lesions

The degree of arthritis was evaluated using scores from 0 to 4 points per foot, with a maximum of 16 points as the total arthritis score (AS) of four feet. 0 point: no joint swelling; 1 point: detectable swelling in one or more toe joints; 2 points: swelling in toe and tarsometatarsal joints; 3 points: swelling inferior the ankle line; 4 points: swelling of the entire paw or ankylosis. These evaluations were conducted on day 35 after the first immunization.

Pathological evaluation of lesion severity on mouse model of arthritis

Mice were sacrificed by CO2 asphyxiation at the peak phase of pathological changes (34 days after the primary immunization) and the hind limbs, the ankle joints, and the toes were taken. Tissues were fixed for 2 days in 10% neutral formalin, decalcification was carried out using ethylenediaminetetraacetic acid (EDTA), and then paraffin-cut sections were stained with hematoxylin and eosin and assessed for pathological evaluation. Synovitis score was evaluated by following criteria: Grade 0 = absence of inflammatory lesions; Grade 1 = mild focal infiltrations; Grade 2 = moderate infiltrations; Grade 3 = severe infiltrations but no cartilage damages or pannus formations; Grade 4 = extremely serious inflammatory infiltrations, pannus formations and/or cartilage damages.

Elisa

After the sacrifice, the eyeballs of mice were quickly removed and blood was collected from the orbital sinus. The quantitative measurements of IL-17 and MCP-1 levels in plasma were detected according to commercial ELISA kit protocol.

Immunohistochemical staining

Immunohistochemical staining was performed on slides. Briefly, the slides were deparaffinized, blocked with hydrogen peroxide at the concentration of 3% and antigen retrieval was then performed in in a steam cooker for 1.5 min in 1 mM EDTA, pH 9.0. Mice IL-17, MCP-1 and Caspase 3 monoclonal antibody were applied at 1:150 diluents for 1 h. The HRP (horseradishpero xidase) labeled secondary antibody was applied for 15 min. Diaminobenzidine was used as chromogens and slides were counterstained with haematoxylin before mounting.

Flow cytometry analysis

To test the percentage of Treg cells in vivo, mice spleen and inguinal draining lymph nodes were dissected under sterile conditions, rinsed by phosphate buffered saline (PBS), polished using a 200 mesh, and then harvested with a 30 μm filter. Approximately 1×10^6 cells were stained with the mosue FITC-CD4, PE-CD25, PeCY5-Foxp3 antibodies in together; To assess Th17 cells polarization level in vitro, naïve T cells were first isolated from mice splenocytes by using of the aforementioned CD4 + CD62L+ naïve T cells isolation kit, and then cultured in the presence of cytokines including 10 ng/ml TGF-β1, 80 ng/ml IL-6, 20 ng/ml IL-23, 10 μg/ml anti-IFNγ, 10 μg/ml anti-IL-4 and 700 pg/ml PGE2 with or without 150 pg/ml of L161982. Seven days after incubation, Cells were stained with mouse FITC-anti-CD4, PE-CD62L and PeCY5-anti-IL-17 after fixation/perm to test Th17 cells polarization. All analysis were perforemed on a Gallios™ Flow Cytometer (Beckman Coulter, USA). Data were analyzed with Kaluza® software (Beckman Coulter, USA).

In vitro proliferation assay

$CD4^+CD25^+$ cells were purified from mice splenocytes by using the $CD4^+CD25^+$ Regulatory T Cell Isolation Kit by a negative selection procedure. Cells were cultured at a density of 2 x 10^3cells per well, and were stimulated with 0.5 μg/ml soluble mouse anti-CD3, 1 μg/ml anti-CD28 and 700 pg/ml PEG2 with or without 150 pg/ml L161982. After five days incubation at 37 ° C and 5% CO_2, the cells were pulsed with BrdU (100 μM) and were assessed for BrdU incorporation 4 h later. Results are expressed as optical density (OD) at 405 nm.

Statistical analysis

Statistical analysis was performed using SigmaPlot Version 12 (Systat Software Inc., USA). All measured variables were normally distributed. Data is presented as mean ± standard deviation. Multiple group means were tested firstly for homoscedasticity and were then compared using one-way analysis of variance (one-way ANOVA). Where significant effects were reported, post hoc evaluations were performed using Tukey's Honestly Significant Difference (HSD) test. *P* values less than 0.05 were considered statistically significant. All statistical analyses were completed using SPSS statistical package (SPSS Inc.).

Results

Incidence of CIA

Three weeks after primary immunization, total 24 mice in 35 collagen induced mice were showed joint swelling with progressive worsening of symptoms compared to mice in the model- control group.The incidence of CIA is 69%. Arthritis score on day 35 were showed in Table 1.

L161982 treatment reduced arthritis lesions and lesion progression in CIA mice

CIA mice were treated with L161982 showed less joint swelling and lower AS after 35 days post immunization compared with the PBS-treated mice ($P < 0.01$) and blank CIA mice ($P < 0.01$) (Fig. 1). However, the reduction in joint swelling was greater in celecoxib-treated mice than L161982-treated mice. Anatomopathological analysis showed that CIA mice treated with L161982 presented with significantly less inflammatory cells infiltration, tissue necrosis, and joint swellings in comparison to blank and PBS-treated mice (Fig. 2). These results showed that the CIA immunization model successfully produced arthritis in these DBA/1 mice.

L161982 reduced plasma and tissue IL-17 and MCP-1 expression in CIA mice

Plasma IL-17 and MCP-1 increased ($p < 0.01$) in the CIA mice compared to the CIA control mice (Table 1). In comparison to the PBS treated mice, plasma IL-17 and MCP-1 was significantly reduced in L161982-treated mice. Celecoxib-treated mice showed a greater reduction in IL-17 and MCP-1 than L161982-treated mice (Table 1). IHC staining for IL-17 and MCP-1 on tissue section confirmed our findings from plasma ELISA (Fig.3). More importantly, Cleaved-caspase-3 immunohistochemical staining of each group showed the tissues in each group have the similar cell apoptosis level (Fig.3).

Table 1 Arthritis score, plasma cytokines, and Treg proportions in CIA mice in response to treatment with celecoxib or L161982

	Mouse groups ($n = 6$)				
	Model Control	CIA-model			
		Blank	PBS	Celecoxib	L161982
Arthritis score(day 35)	0	7.00 ± 2.90	6.67 ± 2.34	3.67 ± 1.21	4.83 ± 1.17
Synovitis score	0	3.50 ± 0.54	3.83 ± 1.17	1.56 ± 0.8	1.83 ± 0.75
Il-17 (pg/ml)	14.38 ± 3.2	27.51 ± 8.1*	28.51 ± 6.4	10.65 ± 4.8#	13.52 ± 3.9#
MCP-1 (pg/ml)	13.1 ± 2.8	30.2 ± 3.4*	30.2 ± 3.4	14.98 ± 3.8#	15.80 ± 2.1#
Treg/ CD4+ T cell (%)					
Lymph node	4.7 ± 0.5	3.31 ± 0.36*	3.01 ± 0.96	3.25 ± 1.6	4.21 ± 0.52#
Spleen	2.8 ± 0.5	1.67 ± 0.14*	1.7 ± 0.33	1.75 ± 0.73	2.63 ± 0.41#

Data are mean ± SD; "CIA" means collagen induced arthritis; "Blank" means CIA model without any drug treatment; "PBS" means phosphate buffered saline. "*" means $p < 0.01$ compared to Model control group; "#" means $p < 0.01$ compared to PBS group; Additional file 1

L161982 increased the ratio of Treg cells in CIA mice but could not promote the growth of Treg cells directly

The proportion of $CD4^+CD25^+Foxp3^+$ Treg cells among the $CD4^+$ T lymphocytes from the lymph nodes and spleen was significantly increased in L161982-treated mice compared to CIA mice, PBS-treated mice, and celecoxib-treated mice (Table 1, Fig. 4a). However, L161982 could not enhance the proliferation of purified Treg cells directly in vitro (Fig. 4b).

L161982 suppress Th 17 differentiation of Naïve T cells in vitro

To explore the mechanism of the lower IL-17 level in CIA mice. Purified $CD4^+CD62L^+$ naïve T cells were cultured in vitro with the treatment of L161982. By measuring the ratio of IL-17 produced cell, we found Th17 cells polarization were reduced by L161982 (Fig. 4c).

Discussion

In this study, the EP4 antagonist L161982 were uesd in treating a classic CIA model [18] to reduce arthritis scores, joint swellings, and cracked cartilage surface of the mice. All pathological feature in vivo were consistent with a previous report that L161982 could mitigate connective tissue inflammation through the inhibition of PGE2-EP4 signaling [19].

EP4 is one of the PGE2 receptor sub-types, which is a G-protein-coupled receptor involved in reproductive system and expressed on the cell surface of macrophages [20]. PGE2 receptor antagonists have been studied in many fields, including tumor and some pain treatments, and have the potential to suppress tumor-associated lymph angiogenesis and, consequently, lymphatic metastasis in breast cancer [21, 22]. Furthermore, co-administration of

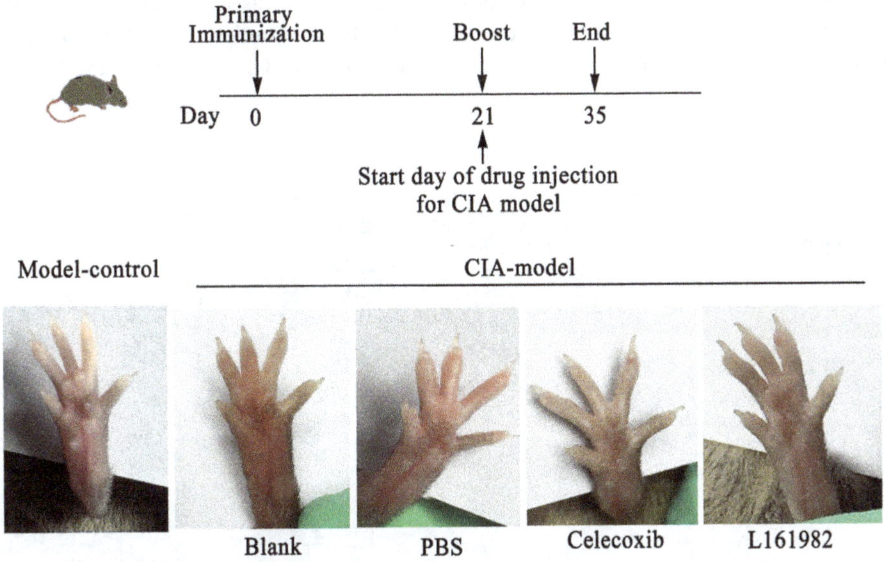

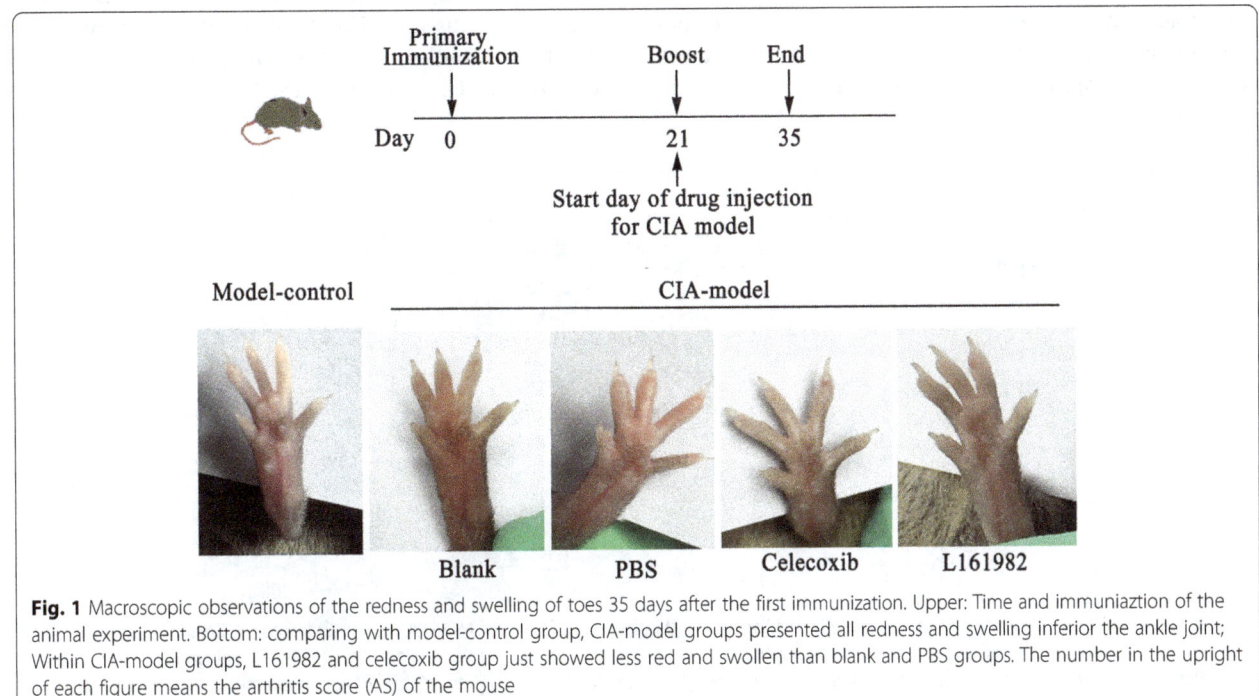

Fig. 1 Macroscopic observations of the redness and swelling of toes 35 days after the first immunization. Upper: Time and immuniaztion of the animal experiment. Bottom: comparing with model-control group, CIA-model groups presented all redness and swelling inferior the ankle joint; Within CIA-model groups, L161982 and celecoxib group just showed less red and swollen than blank and PBS groups. The number in the upright of each figure means the arthritis score (AS) of the mouse

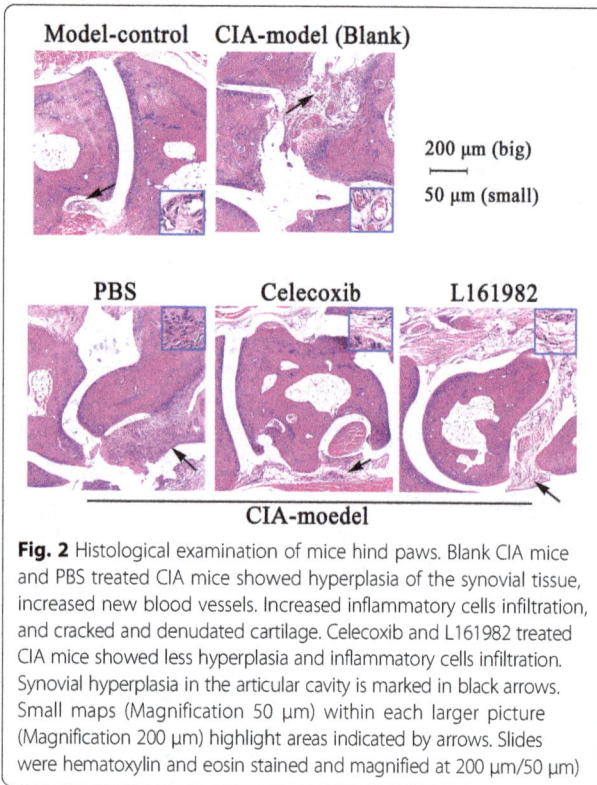

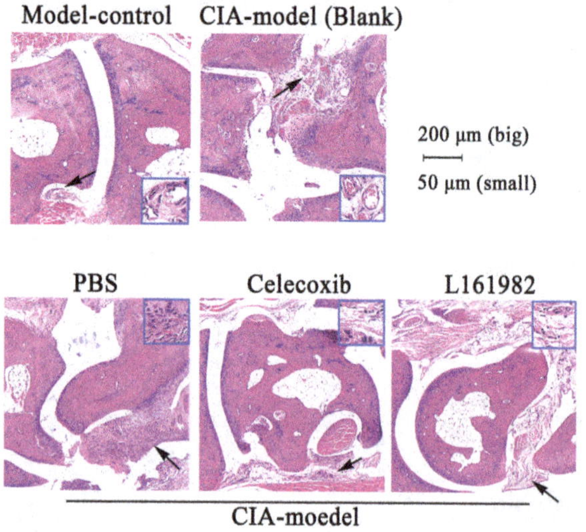

Fig. 2 Histological examination of mice hind paws. Blank CIA mice and PBS treated CIA mice showed hyperplasia of the synovial tissue, increased new blood vessels. Increased inflammatory cells infiltration, and cracked and denudated cartilage. Celecoxib and L161982 treated CIA mice showed less hyperplasia and inflammatory cells infiltration. Synovial hyperplasia in the articular cavity is marked in black arrows. Small maps (Magnification 50 μm) within each larger picture (Magnification 200 μm) highlight areas indicated by arrows. Slides were hematoxylin and eosin stained and magnified at 200 μm/50 μm)

EP4 antagonists CJ-023423 and RO3244019 also showed an analgesic effect in a rat model [23]. This also indicated that EP4 antagonists may be therapeutically useful for RA, but the specific EP4 receptor antagonist L161982 still lacks evidence.

Although the pathological mechanisms in RA are not fully understood, dysfunction and imbalance of T-cell types are important factors. PGE2-EP4 signaling has been shown to promote inflammation through Th1 differentiation and Th17 cell expansion [24]. EP4 receptor antagonists may help alleviate RA symptoms including pain and tissue damage, potentially due to the inhibition of Th17 cell differentiation and reduced cytokine expression [25, 26]. While previous evidence has suggested that EP4 receptor antagonists may be beneficial in the CIA mouse, the mechanism of action is currently not well understood [27, 28].

Here we show that the plasma IL-17, secreted principally by Th17 cells, was higher in the CIA mice compared with the control mice, while plasma IL-17 was reduced in L161982-treated mice compared to PBS-treated mice. We further confirm this results by testing tissue IL-17 level via immunohistochemistry staining. The alleviations of RA symptoms resulting from L161982 administration were related to reductions in IL-17 [29, 30]. Low concentrations of PGE2 can increase IL-17A expression through binding to EP4 receptors and activation of EP4-cAMP signaling pathways [31]. We also observed a decreased tendency of Th17 polarization in naïve T cells in vitro, it indicates that the reduction of IL-17 in plasma or tissue after administration of L161982 might be potentially derived from the suppression of $CD4^{+}$ T cell differentiation into Th-17 cells.

MCP-1 is derived principally from endothelial cells, fibroblasts, and monocytes, which can bind to a variety of chemokine receptors to induce lymphocyte differentiation. A previous study reported MCP-1 is an important indicator for evaluating RA disease activity [32]. Increased MCP-I level in rheumatoid arthritis is prone to endothelial dysfunction which is also indicate poor prognosis of disease [33]. Our results are compatible with these studies, however, whether the effects of L161892 on CIA are primarily by MCP-1 or other

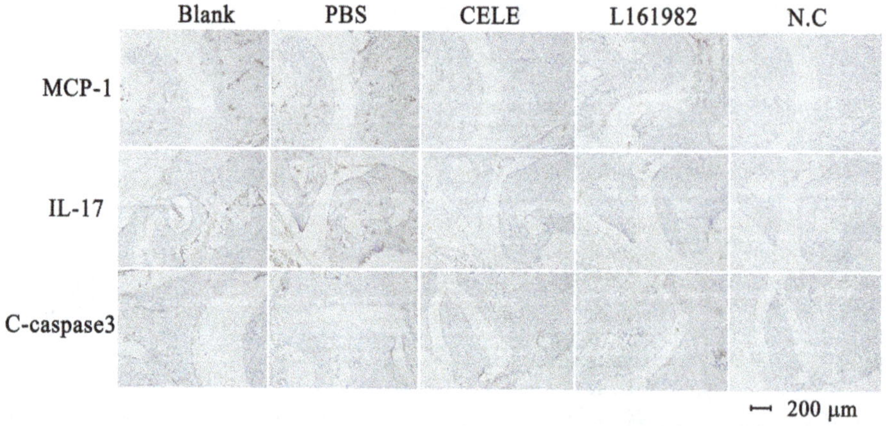

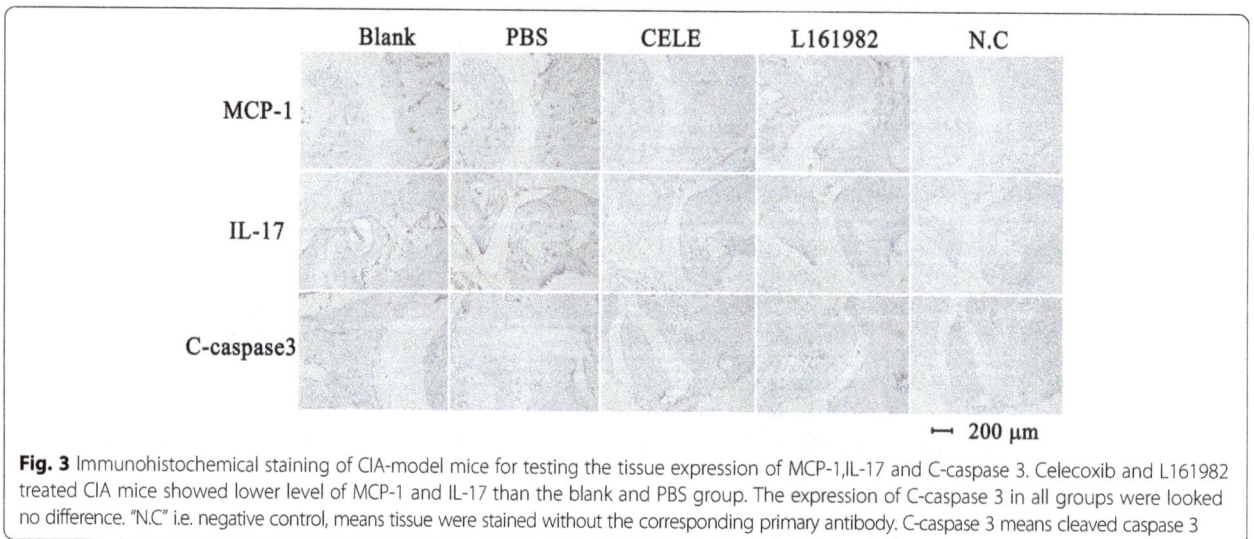

Fig. 3 Immunohistochemical staining of CIA-model mice for testing the tissue expression of MCP-1,IL-17 and C-caspase 3. Celecoxib and L161982 treated CIA mice showed lower level of MCP-1 and IL-17 than the blank and PBS group. The expression of C-caspase 3 in all groups were looked no difference. "N.C" i.e. negative control, means tissue were stained without the corresponding primary antibody. C-caspase 3 means cleaved caspase 3

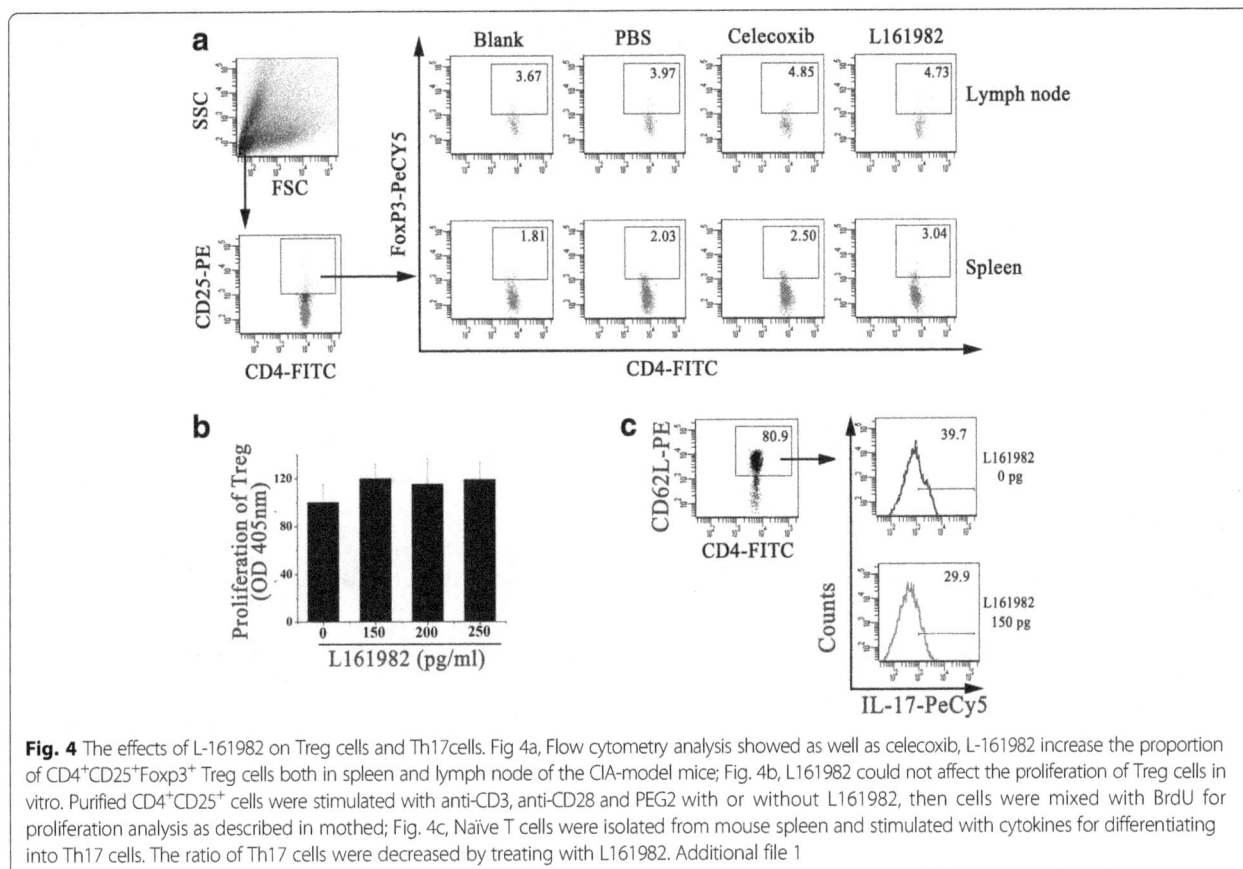

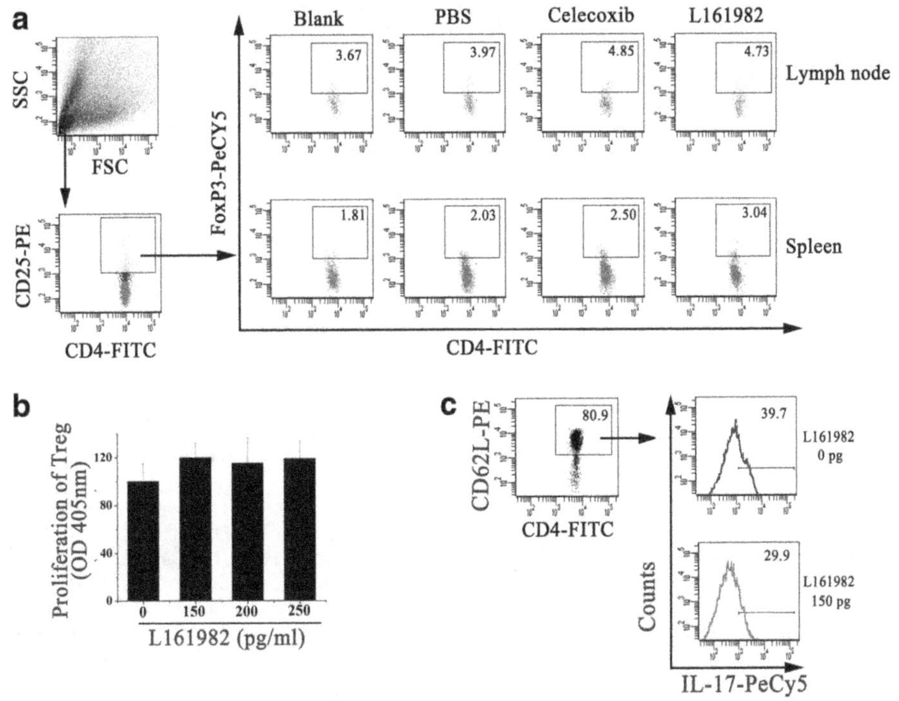

Fig. 4 The effects of L-161982 on Treg cells and Th17cells. Fig 4a, Flow cytometry analysis showed as well as celecoxib, L-161982 increase the proportion of $CD4^+CD25^+Foxp3^+$ Treg cells both in spleen and lymph node of the CIA-model mice; Fig. 4b, L161982 could not affect the proliferation of Treg cells in vitro. Purified $CD4^+CD25^+$ cells were stimulated with anti-CD3, anti-CD28 and PEG2 with or without L161982, then cells were mixed with BrdU for proliferation analysis as described in mothed; Fig. 4c, Naïve T cells were isolated from mouse spleen and stimulated with cytokines for differentiating into Th17 cells. The ratio of Th17 cells were decreased by treating with L161982. Additional file 1

important cytokines need to be further confirmed. Importantly, higher PGE2 level in trauma can facilitate the apoptosis of cells. We verified tissue cleaved-caspase-3 level also by IHC to confirm all groups have the similar cells apoptosis level. Therefore, the reduction of IL-17 and MCP-1 are due to the effects of L161982 rather than the apoptosis of the cells.

PGE2 can also modulate the secretion of IL-12 and IL-23 through EP4 receptor activation, ultimately affecting the differentiation of $CD4^+$ T cells [24]. In our study, the increased proportion of $CD4^+CD25^+Foxp3^+$ Treg cells in L161982-treated CIA mice and BrdU incorporation assay in vitro indicated that L161982 might somehow affect the differentiation rather than proliferation of Treg cells.

Current therapeutic treatments for RA include the widely used COX-2 inhibitors, NSAIDs, and methylprednisolone. These drugs can be effective but a major limitation to their use, is the damage they cause to the gastrointestinal (GI) trac. Thus, a selective antagonist (s) of one or more critical downstream prostaglandin receptors may be more effective than broad inhibition of COX activity. Some reports had demonstrated EP4 antagonist did not cause any damage in the arthritic rat stomach, even did not worsen the gastric ulcerogenic response to stress or aspirin in normal rats. Thus, it would be an ideal therapeutic agent for the treatment of inflammatory pain [34]. However, little envidence of L161982 in related areas can be found. Therefore, the saftey of L161982 need to be further confirmed.

In short, L161982 has a beneficial effect on the pathogenesis of RA, and it might be developed as a new therapeutic treatment for RA. However, further research will be required to understand the mechanism through which L161982 acts on T cells, to identify potential side effects, and to determine the most effective therapeutic dose.

Conclusion

Although less effective than Celecoxib, L161982 also resulted in a reduction of ankle joint inflammation in CIA mice via inhibiting IL-17 and MCP-1 expression, and increasing the ratio of Treg cells. The mechanism of the reduction of IL-17 in plasma or tissue after administration of L161982 might be potentially derived from the suppression of $CD4^+$ T cells differentiation into Th-17 cells.

Abbreviations
AS: Arthritis score; CIA: Collagen-induced arthritis; EDTA: Ethylenediaminetetraacetic acid; ELISA: Enzyme-linked immunosorbent assay; IA: Intragastrical injections; IHC: Immunohistochemical staining; IP: Intraperitoneal injections; MCP-1: Monocyte chemoattractant protein-1; PGE2: Prostaglandin E2; RA: Rheumatoid arthritis

Acknowledgements
We are grateful to the Department of Microbiology, School of Basic Medical Science, Wuhan University, for supporting this work. We also thank Quanquan Ding for her help with animal experiments.

Funding
This work was supported by the National Natural Science Foundation of China [grant numbers 81,101,386, 30,901,356] and the Natural Science Foundation of Hubei Province, China [grant number 2014CFB158], also supported by the Wuhan Science and Technology Project, China [grant number 2016060101010045] and Hubei Provincial Science and Technology Support Program [grant number 2015BCA316].

Authors' contributions
Conceived and designed the experiments: D L, L C; Performed the experiments: L C, X W, J Z; Analyzed the data: X W, J Z.; Wrote the paper: D L and X W. All authors have read and approved the manuscript.

Competing interests
We declare no conflicts of interest related to this paper.

Author details
[1]Department of Orthopedics, Renmin Hospital of Wuhan University, 9 Zhangzhidong Street, Wuhan, Hubei 430060, People's Republic of China. [2]Laboratory of Immunology, University of Lorraine, Avenue du Morvan, 54511 Vandoeuvre lès Nancy, Nancy, France. [3]Department of Microbiology, School of Basic Medical Science, Wuhan University, 185 Donghu Road, Wuhan, Hubei 430071, People's Republic of China.

References
1. Sakkas LI, Bogdanos DP, Katsiari C, Platsoucas CD. Anti-citrullinated peptides as autoantigens in rheumatoid arthritis-relevance to treatment. Autoimmun Rev. 2014;13:1114–20.
2. Lee HS, Woo SJ, Koh HW, Ka SO, Zhou L, Jang KY, et al. Regulation of apoptosis and inflammatory responses by insulin-like growth factor binding protein 3 in fibroblast-like synoviocytes and experimental animal models of rheumatoid arthritis. Arthritis Rheumatol. 2014;66:863–73.
3. Bai F, Tian H, Niu Z, Liu M, Ren G, Yu Y, et al. Chimeric anti-IL-17 full-length monoclonal antibody is a novel potential candidate for the treatment of rheumatoid arthritis. Int J Mol Med. 2014;33:711–21.
4. Boyle DL, Kim HR, Topolewski K, Bartok B, Firestein GS. Novel phosphoinositide 3-kinase delta,gamma inhibitor: potent anti-inflammatory effects and joint protection in models of rheumatoid arthritis. J Pharmacol Exp Ther. 2014;348: 271–80.
5. Cribbs AP, Kennedy A, Penn H, Read JE, Amjadi P, Green P, et al. Treg cell function in rheumatoid arthritis is compromised by ctla-4 promoter methylation resulting in a failure to activate the indoleamine 2,3-dioxygenase pathway. Arthritis Rheumatol. 2014;66:2344–54.
6. Sarkar S, Fox DA. Targeting IL-17 and Th17 cells in rheumatoid arthritis. Rheum Dis Clin N Am. 2014;36:345–66.
7. Kosmaczewska A, Ciszak L, Swierkot J, Szteblich A, Kosciow K, Frydecka I. Exogenous IL-2 controls the balance in Th1, Th17, and Treg cell distribution in patients with progressive rheumatoid arthritis treated with TNF-alpha inhibitors. Inflammation. 2015;38:765–74.
8. Luo CT, Li MO. Transcriptional control of regulatory T cell development and function. Trends Immunol. 2013;34:531–9.
9. Kurebayashi Y, Nagai S, Ikejiri A, Koyasu S. Recent advances in understanding the molecular mechanisms of the development and function of Th17 cells. Genes Cells. 2013;18:247–65.
10. Tang EH, Libby P, Vanhoutte PM, Xu A. Anti-inflammation therapy by activation of prostaglandin EP4 receptor in cardiovascular and other inflammatory diseases. J Cardiovasc Pharmacol. 2013;59:116–23.
11. Aida T, Furukawa K, Suzuki D, Shimizu H, Yoshidome H, Ohtsuka M, et al. Preoperative immunonutrition decreases postoperative complications by modulating prostaglandin E2 production and T-cell differentiation in patients undergoing pancreatoduodenectomy. Surgery. 2014;155:124–33.
12. Kowsar R, Hambruch N, Liu J, Shimizu T, Pfarrer C, Miyamoto A. Regulation of innate immune function in bovine oviduct epithelial cells in culture: the homeostatic role of epithelial cells in balancing Th1/Th2 response. J Reprod Dev. 2013;59:470–8.
13. Sheibanie AF, Yen JH, Khayrullina T, Emig F, Zhang M, Tuma R, et al. The proinflammatory effect of prostaglandin E2 in experimental inflammatory bowel disease is mediated through the IL-23/IL-17 axis. J Immunol. 2009;78: 8138–47.
14. McCoy JM, Wicks JR, Audoly LP. The role of prostaglandin E2 receptors in the pathogenesis of rheumatoid arthritis. J Clin Invest. 2002;110:651–8.
15. Inglis JJ, Simelyte E, McCann FE, Criado G, Williams RO. Protocol for the induction of arthritis in C57BL/6 mice. Nat Protoc. 2008;3:612–8.
16. Yanni SE, Barnett JM, Clark ML, Penn JS. The role of PGE2 receptor EP4 in pathologic ocular angiogenesis. Invest Ophthalmol Vis Sci. 2009;50:5479–86.
17. Chen L, Li DQ, Zhong J, XL W, Chen Q, Peng H, et al. IL-17RA aptamer-mediated repression of IL-6 inhibits synovium inflammation in a murine model of osteoarthritis. Osteoarthr Cartil. 2011;19:711–8.
18. Park MJ, Park HS, HJ O, Lim JY, Yoon BY, Kim HY, et al. IL-17-deficient allogeneic bone marrow transplantation prevents the induction of collagen-induced arthritis in DBA/1J mice. Exp Mol Med. 2012;44:694–705.
19. Tang EH, Cai Y, Wong CK, et al. Activation of prostaglandin E2-EP4 signaling reduces chemokine production in adipose tissue. J Lipid Res. 2015;56:358–68.
20. Guo TC, Gamil AA, Koenig M, Evensen O. Sequence analysis and identification of new isoform of EP4 receptors in different atlantic salmon tissues (Salmo Salar L.) and its role in PGE2 induced immunomodulation in vitro. PLoS One. 2015;10:e0120483.
21. Schmidt A, Sinnett-Smith J, Young S, et al. Direct growth-inhibitory effects of prostaglandin E2 in pancreatic cancer cells in vitro through an EP4/PKA-mediated mechanism. Surgery. 2017; doi:10.1016/j.surg.2016.12.037.
22. Nandi P, Girish GV, Majumder M, Xin X, Tutunea-Fatan E, Lala PK. PGE2 promotes breast cancer-associated lymphangiogenesis by activation of EP4 receptor on lymphatic endothelial cells. BMC Cancer. 2017;17:11.
23. Sugita R, Kuwabara H, Kubota K, et al. Simultaneous inhibition of PGE2 and PGI2 signals is necessary to suppress hyperalgesia in rat inflammatory pain models. Mediat Inflamm. 2016;2016:9847840.
24. Bender AT, Spyvee M, Satoh T, et al. Evaluation of a candidate anti-arthritic drug using the mouse collagen antibody induced arthritis model and clinically relevant biomarkers. Am J Transl Res. 2013;5:92–102.
25. Abdel-Magid AF. Selective EP4 Antagonist May Be Useful in Treating Arthritis and Arthritic Pain. ACS Med Chem Lett. 2014;5:104–5.
26. Duffy MM, Pindjakova J, Hanley SA, McCarthy C, Weidhofer GA, Sweeney EM, et al. Mesenchymal stem cell inhibition of T-helper 17 cell- differentiation is triggered by cell-cell contact and mediated by prostaglandin E2 via the EP4 receptor. Eur J Immunol. 2011;41:2840–51.
27. Chuang YC, Yoshimura N, Huang CC, Wu M, Tyagi P, Chancellor MB. Expression of E-series prostaglandin (EP) receptors and urodynamic effects of an EP4 receptor antagonist on cyclophosphamide-induced overactive bladder in rats. BJU Int. 2010;106:1782–7.
28. Wang Y, Da G, Li H, Zheng Y. Avastin exhibits therapeutic effects on collagen-induced arthritis in rat model. Inflammation. 2013;36:1460–7.
29. Ye L, Jiang B, Deng J, Du J, Xiong W, Guan Y, Wen Z, et al. IL-37 alleviates rheumatoid arthritis by suppressing IL-17 and IL-17-triggering cytokine production and limiting Th17 cell proliferation. J Immunol. 2015;194:5110–9.
30. Poloso NJ, Urquhart P, Nicolaou A, Wang J. Woodward DF. PGE2 differentially regulates monocyte-derived dendritic cell cytokine responses depending on receptor usage (EP2/EP4). Mol Immunol. 2013;54:284–95.
31. Lubberts E. The IL-23-IL-17 axis in inflammatory arthritis. Nat Rev Rheumatol. 2015;11:562.
32. Liou LB, Tsai WP, Chang CJ, Chao WJ, Chen MH. Blood monocyte chemotactic protein-1 (MCP-1) and adapted disease activity Score28-MCP-1: favorable indicators for rheumatoid arthritis activity. PLoS One. 2013;8:e55346.
33. He M, Liang X, He L, Wen W, Zhao S, Wen L, et al. Endothelial dysfunction in rheumatoid arthritis: the role of monocyte chemotactic protein-1-induced protein. Arterioscler Thromb Vasc Biol. 2013;33:1384–91.

9

Establishment of rat ankle post-traumatic osteoarthritis model induced by malleolus fracture

Dawei Liang[1], Jian Sun[1], Fangyuan Wei[2], Jianzhong Zhang[2], Pengcui Li[1], Yingke Xu[3], Xianwen Shang[4], Jin Deng[4], Ting Zhao[5] and Lei Wei[1,5*]

Abstract

Background: Malleolar fracture, which is present in 37–53% of human ankle osteoarthritis (OA), is the most common type of fracture in the ankle joint. In spite of this, no rat animal model has been developed for this type of injury to date. Here, we established a rat ankle post-traumatic OA (PTOA) model induced by malleolar fracture; this model will be useful in ankle OA research.

Methods: Two-month-old male Sprague Dawley (SD) rats were randomized into 2 groups ($n = 19$ per group): 1) malleolus articular fracture, dislocation, and immediate reduction on the right joints and 2) malleolus articular fracture on the right ankle. The contralateral ankle joints were used as controls. The fracture and healing processes were confirmed and monitored by radiography. Changes in inflammation were monitored in vivo by fluorescence molecular tomography (FMT). Cartilage damage and changes in expression of OA-related genes were analyzed by histology, immunohistochemistry, Real-time quantitative PCR (qPCR) and enzyme-linked immunosorbent assay (ELISA) at 8 weeks post-surgery.

Results: X-rays showed that all fractures were healed at 8 weeks post-surgery. A reproducible, mild to moderate degree of OA cartilage damage with reduced aggrecan was detected by histology in all animals in both groups but there was no significant difference between the two groups. Decreased Col-II and increased Col-X and MMP-13 levels were detected by qPCR, immunohistochemistry, ELISA and FMT from both groups cartilage.

Conclusions: Malleolus articular fracture alone induces ankle OA with lesions on the central weight bearing area of the tibiotalar joint in rats. This model will provide a reproducible and useful tool for researchers to study ankle OA.

Keywords: Ankle, Post-traumatic osteoarthritis, Animal model, Fracture, Rat

Background

Osteoarthritis (OA) is the most common cause of disability in the elderly [1]. Disability stems from pain and limitations in mobility secondary to the degeneration of articular cartilage, a trademark of the disease. Unfortunately, current pharmacological therapy targeting the mechanism of OA is relatively ineffective, largely because the etiology and pathogenesis of OA remain poorly understood. The complex pathobiological changes that occur in human OA may be influenced by a multitude of genetic and environmental factors. The effort to clarify the molecular events that occur in OA during the onset and the progression of OA has necessitated the use of in vivo models [2]. Researchers tend to utilize knee OA models to investigate these factors, but have neglected the establishment of other types of OA models, such as ankle OA.

A recent study indicates that the biomarker and mechanism of ankle OA may not be the same as those of knee OA [3–5]. Researchers have reported that aggrecan (Acan), bone morphogenetic protein (BMP)-2, BMP-7, and fibronectin-aggrecan complex (FAC) can be used as key markers of OA in the ankle, but not in the knee [6, 7]. In the knee and hip, primary OA accounts for 67% and

* Correspondence: lei_wei@brown.edu
[1]Department of Orthopaedics, The Second Hospital of Shanxi Medical University, Taiyuan, China
[5]Department of Orthopaedics, Warren Alpert Medical School of Brown University and Rhode Island Hospital, Providence, RI, USA
Full list of author information is available at the end of the article

58% of all cases, respectively. Meanwhile, 78% of all cases of ankle OA are post-traumatic (PTOA) [8, 9]. In addition, while the incidence of knee OA in the adult population rises from 6% to 10% after 65 years of age, the incidence of ankle OA remains unchanged with age [10]. Malleolar fractures are the most frequent type of fracture in the ankle, presenting in 37–53% of patients with advanced or end-stage ankle OA [11, 12]. More than 50% of patients with fractures of the distal tibial articular surface develop OA [13]. After intra-articular fracture, the ankle joint sustains increased contact stress; in addition, the inflammatory response is a contributory factor to the progress of OA [14]. Chondrocyte necrosis and apoptosis are observed following trauma in human and porcine knees, and associated with cartilage damage and degeneration [15]. An advantage of PTOA models is that there is temporal control of disease induction (when compared with spontaneous animal OA and with human disease), while mimicking the molecular pathology and histopathology of human disease [2]. Despite the high incidence of ankle trauma and OA, ankle-specific OA research is sparse, with the majority of clinical and basic research pertaining to the knee and hip joints [16]. This will greatly limit the study of ankle OA. Thus, there is a need to develop novel ankle PTOA models to facilitate research of this type of OA. Clinically, some patients with malleolar fracture present only, while others present with fracture and dislocation. Therefore, we developed two rat ankle PTOA models in this study: 1) the malleolus fracture with dislocation and reduction; and 2) the malleolus fracture alone. The contralateral ankles were used as controls. To validate the success of our models, X-ray and Safranin-O were used to observe morphological changes in the subchondral bone, joint space and cartilage. FMT, ELISA and immunohistochemistry were used to detect protein levels of several OA-related biomarkers, and qPCR was used to obtain the mRNA levels of several OA related genes.

Methods

Experimental animals

This study was approved by the Institutional Review Board and the Institutional Animal Care and Use Committee of the Shanxi Medical University (2015LL020). Thirty-eight skeletally mature 2-month-old male Sprague Dawley (SD) rats (220 ± 20 g), which were from Shanxi Medical University Experimental Animal Center, were randomized into 2 groups (n = 19 per group): Group 1 (fracture + dislocation + reduction) underwent fracture of the right medial malleolus, dislocation, and immediate reduction; Group 2 (fracture alone) underwent fracture of the right medial malleolus. The contralateral ankle joints were used as controls. Animals were housed in groups of 2 rats per cage. They had free access to food and water throughout the experiment. Eight weeks after surgery, rats were euthanized with an overdose of pentobarbital sodium (150 mg/kg IV).

Surgical fracture of medial malleolus with or without dislocation

The site of fracture was shown in the schematic diagram of right ankle joint (Fig. 1a). The animals were anesthetized, and the ankles were prepared for aseptic surgery as before [17]. Rats were maintained on supine position with the right hip joint in 90 degree abduction, and the right knee joint bent at 90 degree. A 1-cm longitudinal incision was performed on the medial malleolus with a #11 blade. Subsequently, blunt dissection of the superficial and deep fascia and the tibialis posterior tendon was carried out in order to expose the medial malleolus. Two 1-ml syringes were used as retractors. The osteotome, combined with an angle fixator (37 degree, to create a reproducible and stable fracture located at medial 1/3 tibiotalar joint) was put in the distal tibia and peened into the medial malleolus until there was sudden stop of resistance. Micro-surgery forceps were used to clamp and wobble the fracture fragment and ensure that it was completely fractured (Fig. 1b). The dislocation group was performed by a malleolar varus (attention was paid to not injure the lateral ligament) and reduction was immediately performed. Before closing the incision, the fracture fragment was compressed to achieve anatomical restoration. The incision was closed layer by layer with 4–0 suture. These animals were allowed to move freely after surgery. The post-operative analgesia was maintained using buprenorphine hydrochloride (0.03 mg/kg SQ for three days) to relieve pain and distress. No animal was excluded in this study.

Radiography

X-rays were taken immediately in supine position under anesthesia condition after fracture to make sure the malleolus fracture was successful. Fracture healing and OA changes were confirmed at week 8 after fracture by UltraFocus100 x-ray cabinet (Faxitron, Arizona, USA). The exposure time was 4 s and the kV settings were about 30–40 kV.

Fluorescence molecular tomography (FMT)

FMT is a noninvasive and quantitative fluorescence-based technology with high molecular specificity and sensitivity for 3-dimensional tissue imaging of live animals. Using in vivo FMT imaging methods and probes, real-time and deep tissue imaging information can be gained about biological processes [18, 19]. In this study, FMT was used to monitor the levels of inflammation in vivo 24 h after intra-articular injection of MMPSense 680 (10 μl, 13.3 μM) (PerkinElmer, Massachusetts, USA), which detects MMPs-3, -9, and

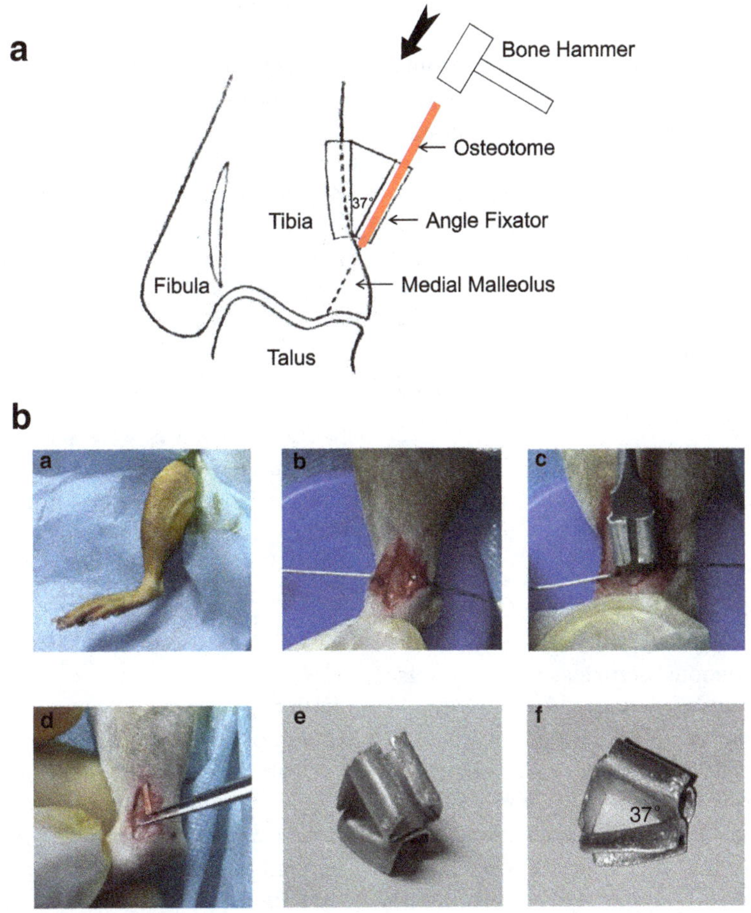

Fig. 1 **a** Schematic illustration of surgical procedure in right ankle joint (anterior view). The dashed line in medial malleolus was the location of fracture. **b** The procedure of ankle surgery-induced OA model. **a** Position of ankle joint. **b** Exposure of medial malleolus. **c** Osteotome and angle fixator placed together on the distal tibia. **d** Micro-surgery forceps were used to make sure fracture was complete. **e-f** Front and lateral views of angle fixator

-13. The picomolar concentrations of probes in the ankle joint were determined using region of interest analysis (ROI), and restricting the area of measurement to the distal-tibia to talus in order to isolate the joint space [20]. Data are reported as means ± SD, $n = 5$/per group.

Enzyme-linked immunosorbent assay (ELISA)

Synovial fluid (SF) lavages were immediately collected from the ankles after euthanasia. Briefly, 100 µl of isotonic saline solution was injected into the ankle joint through the front joint cavity using a 0.3-ml insulin syringe with 31G needle. The joint capsule was visibly distended after injection. Before collection the ankle was manually cycled through flexion and extension 5 times to distribute the fluid. About 70 µl of the injected fluid was recovered. These samples were centrifuged for 20 min at 1000 g and frozen at −80 °C until analysis. MMP-13 content was measured in the SF samples using ELISA Kit (Uscn Life Science, Wuhan, China) according to the instructions of the manufacturer. The samples were diluted at 1:1 in phosphate buffer saline (PBS). Colorimetric density on the developed plates was determined using a Thermo Multskan Mk3 microplate reader (Thermo, Massachusetts, USA) set to 450 nm. Data are reported as means ± SD, $n = 8$/per group.

Histologic evaluation

Rats were humanely sacrificed 8 weeks after surgery. The ankle joints were fixed in 4% formaldehyde for 48 h. Whole joints were decalcified in 20% EDTA for 6 weeks on a shaker. Each ankle joint including the distal tibia and talus was hemisected in the mid-coronal plane, an anterior and a posterior one. The two resulting tissue pieces (anterior and posterior half) were then both embedded in a single paraffin block with the cut planes facing down. Blocks were trimmed to expose cartilage. Ten adjacent sections were collected at intervals of 0 µm, 100 µm, and 200 µm. Two serial 5-µm-thick slides from each interval were stained with Safranin-O and Fast Green. Cartilage degradation was quantified by two independent and blinded observers using a modified Osteoarthritis Research Society International (OARSI) grading system based on OARSI score [21]. The joint surface of the distal tibia and talus was respectively divided into three zones of equal width using an ocular micrometer or a ruler on a photograph. A score of 0 was given to normal cartilage; 1 for samples with 5–10% of the total projected cartilage area affected by Acan, matrix or chondrocyte loss and matrix fibrillation; 2: 11–25% affected; 3: 26–50% affected; 4: 51–75% affected; 5: greater than 75% affected. The maximum cartilage damage score is 30. Data are reported as means ± SD, $n = 11$/per group. Eleven rats were used for histologic analyses; the remaining 8 rats were used for collection of synovial fluid lavage and cartilage for ELISA and qPCR.

Immunohistochemistry

Type II collagen, type X collagen, and MMP-13 were analyzed by immunohistochemistry using an UltraSensitive™ SP IHC Kit (Maixin Biotech, Fuzhou, China). For antigen retrieval, sections were digested with 0.05% trypsin for 20 min at 37 °C. Endogenous peroxidase activity was quenched with endogenous peroxidase block and nonspecific antibody binding was blocked by goat nonimmune serum for 10 min at room temperature. The sections were incubated with primary antibody against either rat type II collagen (Boster, Wuhan, China), type X collagen, or MMP-13 at 4 °C overnight. Thereafter, the sections were incubated with biotinylated secondary antibody and streptavidin-peroxidase conjugate each for 10 min at room temperature, then developed in 3,3′-diaminobenzidine chromogen. Photography was performed with an Olympus BX51 microscope (Olympus, Tokyo, Japan). Counting of positively stained cells was achieved using Image-Pro Plus 6.3 system at ×400 magnification. Five areas of cartilage were counted randomly and results expressed as average mean number of positive cells. Areas near chondrocyte and matrix loss were excluded. Slides were counted by two blinded and independent observers. Data are reported as means ± SD, $n = 3$/per group.

Real-time quantitative PCR (qPCR)

Cartilage samples were scraped with #11 blade and ground with mortar and pestle under liquid nitrogen ($n = 6$). Total RNA was isolated from cartilage using a RNAiso Plus (Takara, Dalian, China). 1 μg total RNA was reverse transcribed to complementary DNA (cDNA) using a Prime Script™ RT Master Mix (Takara, Dalian, China). The resulting cDNA (40 ng/μl) was used as the template to quantify the relative level of messenger RNA (mRNA) using a SYBR Premix Ex Taq™ II (Takara, Dalian, China) with a iQ™5 Optical Module Detection System (Bio-Rad, California, USA). Primer pairs were as follows: for rat Col2a1, AAG-GGA-CAC-CGA-GGT-TTC-ACT-GG (forward) and GGG-CCT-GTT-TCT-CCT-GAG-CGT (reverse); for rat Acan, CAG-TGC-GAT-GCA-GGC-TGG-CT (forward) and CCT-CCG-GCA-CTC-GTT-GGC-TG (reverse); for rat MMP-13, GGA-CCT-TCT-GGT-CTT-CTG-GC (forward) and GGA-TGC-TTA-GGG-TTG-GGG-TC (reverse); and for 18S RNA, CGG-CTA-CCA-CAT-CCA-AGG-AA (forward) and GCT-GGA-ATT-ACC-GCG-GCT (reverse). Relative transcript levels were calculated according to the equation $x = 2^{-\Delta\Delta Ct}$, where $\Delta\Delta Ct = \Delta CtE - \Delta CtC$ ($\Delta CtE = CtE - Ct18S$, $\Delta CtC = CtC - Ct18S$) [17]. Data is reported as means ± SD.

Statistical analysis

Statistical differences were assessed with two-way ANOVA with repeated measures. Follow-up pairwise comparisons were carried out using the Bonferroni post-test. Results were expressed as the mean ± SD, and P values smaller than 0.05 were considered statistically significant. Statistical analysis was performed with GraphPad Prism 5 software.

Results

Radiography

The medial malleolus fracture was confirmed in all rats (Fig. 2c and e). X-ray showed that all fractures were healed completely 8 weeks after surgery (Fig. 2d and f). The joint space in the fracture groups was narrow compared to that on day 0 after surgery and the control groups, and subchondral sclerosis and osteophytes appeared at week 8 after surgery (Fig. 2).

Fluorescence molecular tomography (FMT)

FMT data indicated that MMPs were higher in the operated ankles than in the contralateral sides 8 weeks after fracture. MMPs in the dislocation group vs control were 31.36 ± 18.19 pmol vs 23.05 ± 14.49 pmol (mean ± SD, $n = 5$), $t = 4.382$, $P < 0.05$. Similarly, MMPs in the fracture group vs control were 33.02 ± 19.19 pmol vs 26.70 ± 19.35 pmol, $t = 3.328$, $P < 0.05$ (Fig. 3a and b). Detailed data are shown in Fig. 3c. There was no significant difference in MMPs between the dislocation and fracture-alone animals ($F = 0.056$, $P > 0.05$).

Enzyme-linked immunosorbent assay (ELISA)

The MMP-13 concentration in SF lavages as detected by ELISA was 3.33 ± 1.93 ng/ml in the dislocation group (mean ± SD, $n = 8$) and in the control it was 2.05 ± 1.69 ng/ml ($t = 3.348$, $P < 0.05$). The level of MMP-13 in the fracture group was 2.30 ± 1.07 ng/ml and in the control it was 1.23 ± 0.75 ng/ml ($t = 2.792$, $P < 0.05$) (Fig. 3d). Similarly, no differences were detected by ELISA between the dislocation and fracture-alone animals ($F = 1.928$, $P > 0.05$).

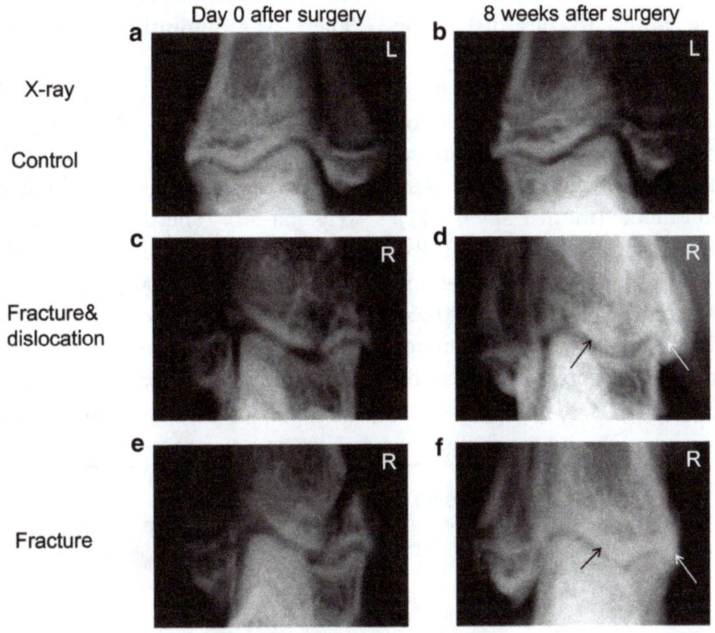

Fig. 2 Radiography demonstrated the OA changes in the ankle joint 8 weeks after surgery (**b, d,** and **f**) when compared with immediately after surgery (**a, c,** and **e**). **d** and **f** suggested that the joint space became narrow. Black arrow shows subchondral sclerosis and white arrow shows osteophytes

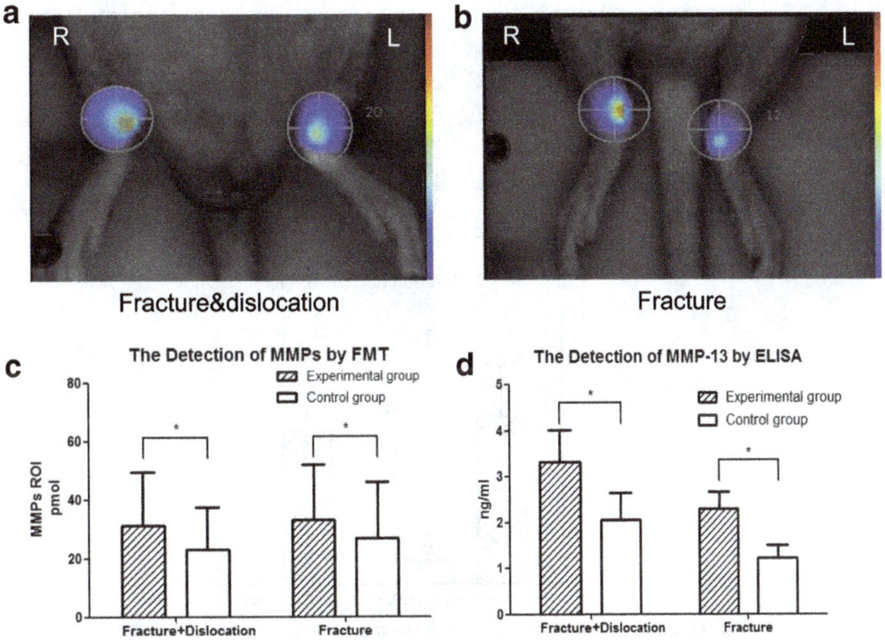

Fig. 3 MMP-13 was detected by FMT and ELISA. FMT indicated that the positive MMPs signals were enhanced in the fractured ankles 8 weeks after surgery. **a** and **b** showed images of FMT signals. **c** showed quantitative FMT data. Values are the mean ± SD, * = $P < 0.05$ versus controls. **d** The concentration of MMP-13 detected by ELISA indicated that MMP-13 levels in the surgical sides were higher than those in the control. Values are the mean ± SD, * = $P < 0.05$ versus controls

Histologic evaluation

Representative sections of the control, fracture/dislocation and fracture-alone rats are shown in Fig. 4a. Cartilage degeneration was detected in the ankle joint, including the distal tibia and talus cartilage. In both models, OA lesion was more severe in the center cartilage than that in the peripheral parts. The summed ankle joint scores were 12.45 ± 4.01 in the dislocation model (mean ± SD, $n = 11$), and 1.73 ± 1.10 in its contralateral controls ($t = 9.512$, $P < 0.05$); while it was 11.45 ± 2.81 in the fracture model and 1.27 ± 0.90 in its contralateral controls ($t = 9.028$, $P < 0.05$). However, there was no significant statistical difference detected in the summed ankle joint scores of dislocation and fracture-alone models ($F = 0.970$, $P > 0.05$, Fig. 4b).

Immunohistochemistry

There was diminished type II collagen staining in the fracture/dislocation and the fracture alone groups than that in their contralateral control ankles. Strong Type X collagen and MMP-13 staining was detected both in the fracture/dislocation and in the fracture alone groups compared with their contralateral control ankle joints (Fig. 5a-5d). There were 27.67 ± 2.52 type X collagen positive cells in the fracture/dislocation group (mean ± SD, $n = 3$) and 5.00 ± 1.00 in its contralateral control group ($t = 8.636$, $P < 0.05$); as well as 29.67 ± 6.66 in fracture alone group and 4.67 ± 0.58 in its contralateral control group ($t = 9.525$, $P < 0.05$). There were 35.00 ± 4.00 MMP-13 positive cells in the fracture/dislocation group

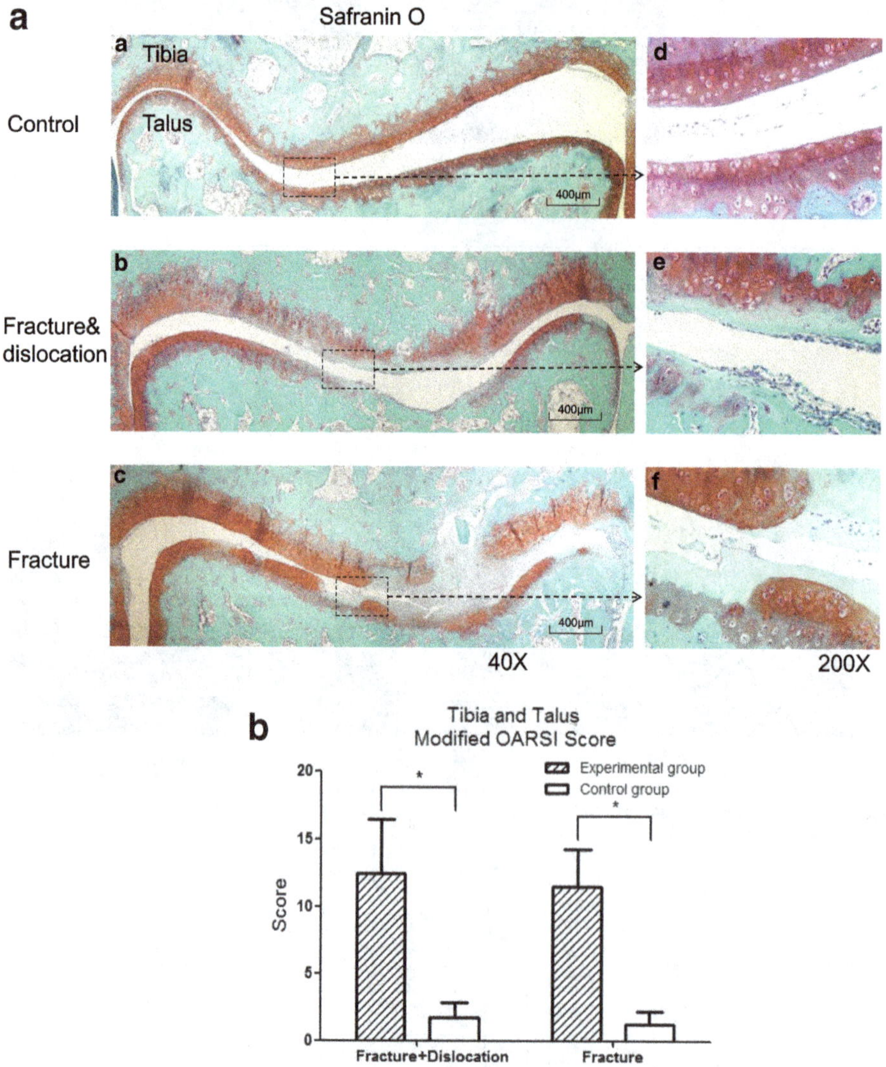

Fig. 4 Safranin-O staining and quantification of the histological results. **a** Unlike the control groups (**a** and **d**), OA changes were observed in fracture groups, including cartilage fibrillation and cranny, rough articular surface, the loss of Acan, matrix and chondrocytes (**b-c** and **e-f**). Particularly, OA lesions were more severe in the central cartilage when compared with the peripheral cartilage. **b** Quantification of the histological results obtained using the modified OARSI score; there was a significant statistical difference between surgical sides and control sides in both models. No difference was observed between the two models. Values are the mean ± SD, * = $P < 0.05$ versus controls

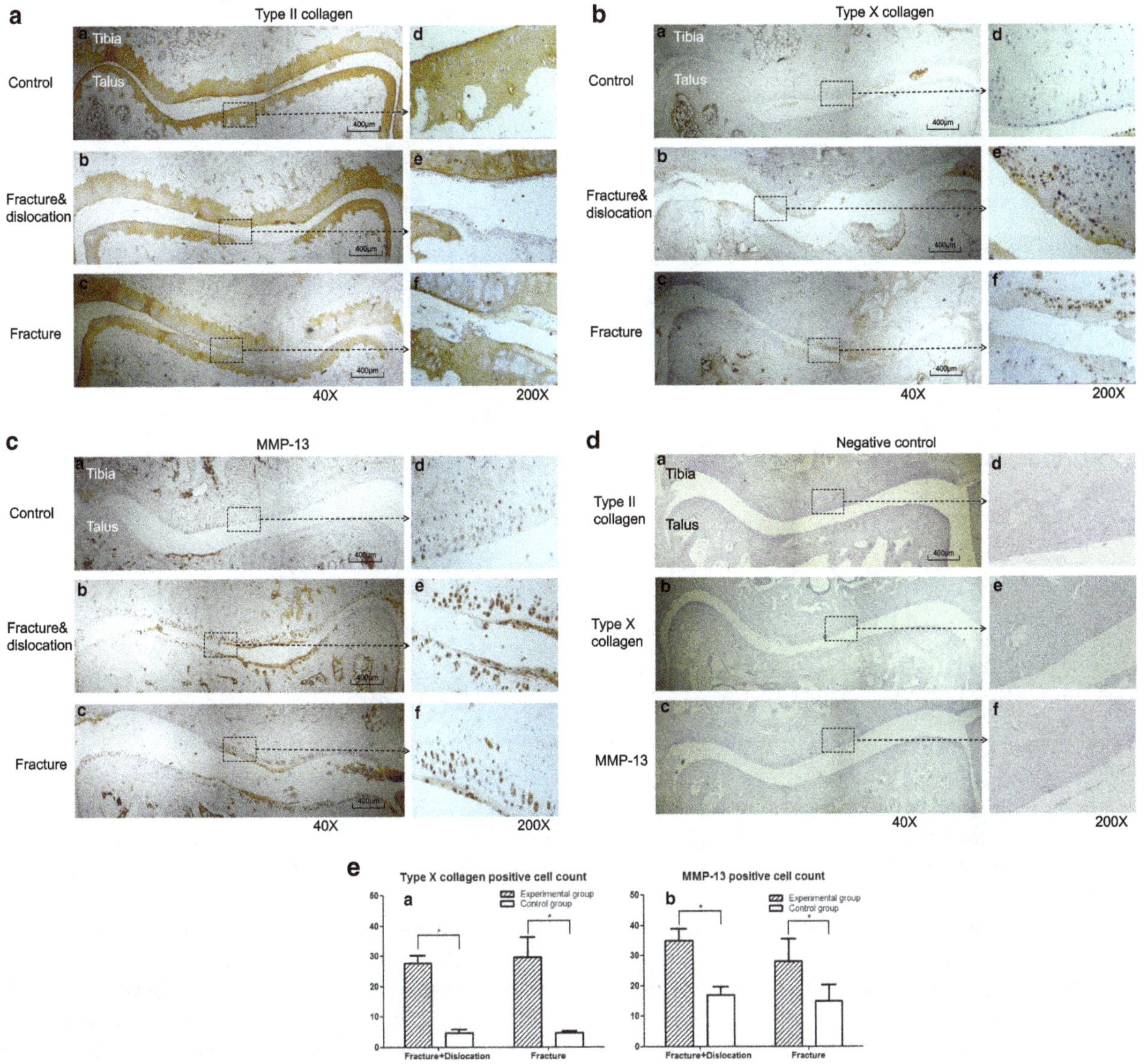

Fig. 5 OA biomarkers were detected by immunohistochemistry. **a** Type II collagen staining was lower in the fracture/dislocation group and in the fracture alone group than in the control group. **b** Strong type X collagen staining was detected in both experimental groups. **c** Strong MMP-13 staining was detected in both experimental groups. **d** Negative control. **e** Cell counting results indicated that the number of type X collagen and MMP-13 positive cells was increased in experimental groups than control groups. Values are the mean ± SD, * = $P < 0.05$ versus controls

and 17.00 ± 2.65 in the contralateral control group (t = 7.152, $P < 0.05$); while there were 28.00 ± 7.55 in the fracture alone group and 15.00 ± 5.29 in the contralateral control group (t = 5.166, $P < 0.05$). However, there were no significant statistical differences detected between the fracture/dislocation and the fracture alone group (F = 0.1330, 1.365 respectively, $P > 0.05$, Fig. 5e).

Real-time quantitative PCR (qPCR)

The qPCR results indicated that both OA models had lower levels of mRNA for Col2a1 ($n = 6$) and Acan ($n = 6$), and higher levels of mRNA for MMP-13 ($n = 6$) compared with their contralateral controls (Fig. 6).

Discussion

Approximately 1% of the world's adult population is affected by joint pain and disability resulting from ankle OA [8]. Although knee OA has been surveyed thoroughly, the diagnosis and treatment of ankle OA may be different from those of knee OA due to the difference of metabolism, articular surface thickness and biomechanical properties [16, 22]. In healthy cadaver joints, ankle chondrocytes had increased proteoglycan (PG) and collagen synthetic rates when compared with knee chondrocytes [23]. When fibrillations and fissuring occur on the cartilage surface during early OA, markers of collagen synthesis and aggrecan turnover are increased in the ankle, but down-regulated in

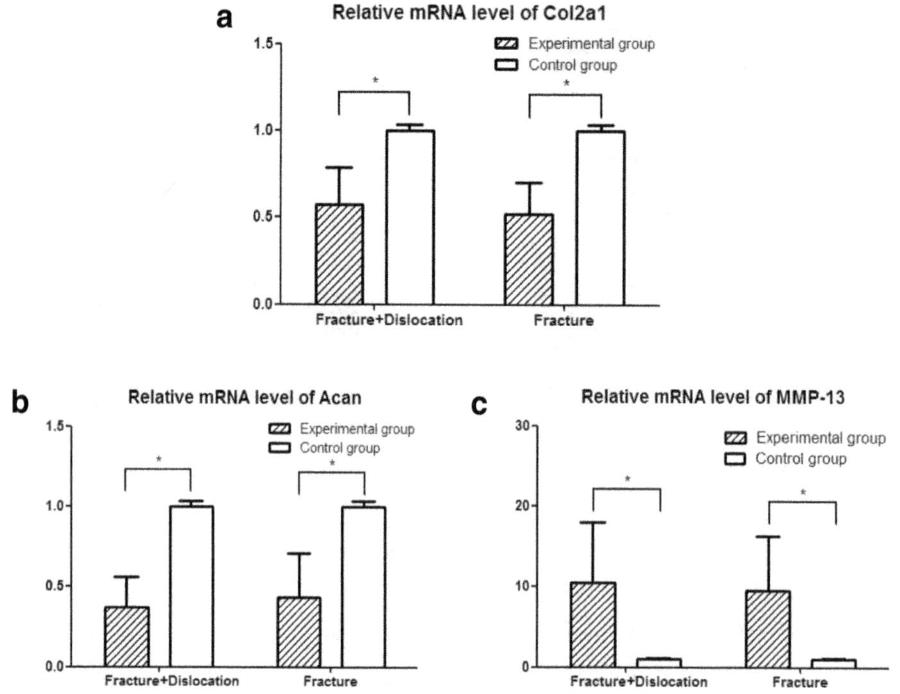

Fig. 6 Enhanced catabolism gene expression from ankle OA cartilage detected by qPCR. The qPCR results revealed that the both experimental groups had low levels of mRNA of Col2a1 (**a**) and Acan (**b**) and increased the level of mRNA of MMP-13 (**c**) compared with the contralateral control. Values are the mean ± SD, * = $P < 0.05$ versus controls

the knee; while markers of collagen degradation are higher in the knee than that in the ankle [24]. Ankle chondrocytes are more resistant to the effects of interleukin-1 or fibronectin fragments than those of knee cartilage, and are able to reverse their effects under the influence of BMP-7 [25]. Furthermore, ankle cartilage is significantly thinner (1–1.45 mm) than knee cartilage (3–6 mm). Joints with higher congruency appear to have thinner cartilage and have a lower incidence of osteoarthritis than noncongruent joints such as the knee [26]. In addition, ankle cartilage has a higher dynamic stiffness and compressive modulus than knee cartilage in compression, that is, ankle cartilage is more resistant to compressive loads [26].

Several OA models are available for knee OA study such as anterior cruciate ligament transection (ACLT) and destabilization of the medial meniscus (DMM), but only two ankle PTOA models have been established recently in mouse (by medial and lateral ligament resection) and mini-pig (by fracture) [27–29]. The ankle joint of mouse ligament resection model is too small to collect SF and cartilage for biomarker studies using ELISA and gene arrays using qPCR. The mini-pig model is expensive for most research groups and is not suitable for drug screen. However, the rat models have the advantages of being low cost and relative large size of joints to collect SF lavage and cartilage, as well as genetically similar within a specific breed strain, and amenable to genetic manipulation [16]. Furthermore, the anatomical and histological features of human and rodent ankle joints are comparable [28]. Therefore, it is necessary to create an innovative ankle fracture OA model for ankle OA research in the field.

Valderrabano and his colleagues showed that ankle PTOA was seen in 78% of 406 ankle OA cases; among these, malleolar ankle fractures accounted for 39% [8]. Moreover, ankle PTOA induced by fracture with dislocation is also common in clinic. Therefore, it is necessary to compare whether there is a difference between the medial malleolus fracture with dislocation injury and the medial malleolus fracture alone. Our results indicated that both the malleolar fracture models with and without dislocation/reduction were healed at 8 weeks post fracture. Based on our pilot study, we found that the 37 degree of the angle fixator created a stable fracture model located at medial 1/3 tibiotalar joint. Our results indicated that these fracture models were stable and no fixation was required. All animal fractures were completely healed without ankle joint deformity at 8 weeks after the fracture. Histology data determined by Safranin-O staining demonstrated that OA changes were similar to changes in human ankle and knee OA, including cartilage fibrillation, rough articular surface, decrease of Acan, matrix and chondrocyte numbers [17, 24, 28, 30, 31]. Increased MMP-13 and type X collagen as well as decreased type II and Acan were further detected by FMT, immunohistochemistry, qPCR and ELISA respectively. Noticeably, the fracture of medial malleolus resulted in mild to moderate OA cartilage lesions. The lesions were primarily located on the central weight-bearing region of the tibiotalar joint with a rare subchondral sclerosis. Compared with our model, the loss of cartilage and subchondral sclerosis are severe and common in the mouse ligament transection ankle OA model [28]. Our model resembles the slowly-progressive human ankle OA and should allow for evaluation of target drugs studies.

There are a few potential limitations to our study. Firstly, we used the contralateral ankle joints as controls instead of sham injured joints and unoperated joints control. The surgically-induced gait alteration may occur in the contralateral side as a result of altered loading. However, our surgical results are significantly more evident than the contralateral limbs. Nevertheless, future studies should add additional sham control groups as an ideal control. Secondly, the growth plates close at skeletal maturity and longitudinal growth ceases in adult human while the rats maintain a growth plate into old age [32]. Although this provides the potential for continued longitudinal growth, in reality bone growth ceases after a certain time (the rate of growth increases before first 5 weeks, then declines at 11.5–13 weeks, ceases until 26 weeks) [32]. Despite of all this, the difference between rodents and human should not affect our results.

The results of this study suggest that the two models can successfully induce OA, but the differences between them are not significant. Compared with the mouse ankle OA models created by transecting several ankle ligaments, our rat fracture OA model is more relevant to human ankle OA and allows for the collection of enough cartilage tissue and SF lavage for gene and inflammation biomarker analyses. Furthermore, compared with the mini-pig model, our model will be beneficial for rapid screening of targets drug with low cost.

Conclusions

We have successfully established two rat ankle PTOA models induced by malleolus fracture. Although the OA changes observed in the two ankle OA models are similar to the changes that occur in human ankle OA cartilage, we recommend the fracture alone model as it is simpler and there is no significant difference between the two models. Thus, our ankle PTOA models will accelerate ankle OA research in the future, especially for ankle OA induced by the fracture injury.

Abbreviations

Acan: aggrecan; ACLT: anterior cruciate ligament transection; BMP: bone morphogenetic protein; DMM: destabilization of the medial meniscus; ELISA: enzyme-linked immunosorbent assay; FAC: fibronectin-aggrecan complex; FMT: fluorescence molecular tomography; MMP-13: matrix metalloproteinase-13; OA: osteoarthritis; OARSI: Osteoarthritis Research Society International; PBS: phosphate buffer saline; PTOA: post-traumatic OA; qPCR: real-time quantitative PCR; ROI: region of interest analysis; SF: synovial fluid

Acknowledgements

The authors gratefully acknowledge Ericka M. Bueno, Ph.D., for help with the paper preparation and editorial services.

Funding

The project was supported by Grant R01AR059142 from NIH/NIAMS, NSFC 81171676, 31271033, 81572098 and 81601949, SXNSF 201308050, 20150313012-6, 201605D211024 and 20161100006. The content is solely the responsibility of the authors and does not necessarily represent the official view of the National Institutes of Health.

Authors' contributions

DL performed the experiments, statistical analysis and drafted the manuscript. DL, FW, JZ, TZ and LW designed the study. JS, PL and LW assisted with the acquisition of data. YX, XS, JD and LW assisted with analysis and interpretation of data. LW revised the manuscript. All authors read and approved the final manuscript.

Competing interests

The authors declare that they have no competing interests.

Author details

[1]Department of Orthopaedics, The Second Hospital of Shanxi Medical University, Taiyuan, China. [2]Foot and Ankle Orthopaedic Surgery Center, Beijing Tongren Hospital, Beijing, China. [3]School of Community Health Science, Nevada Institute of Personalized Medicine, University of Nevada, Las Vegas, Nevada, USA. [4]Department of Orthopaedics, Affiliated Hospital of Guizhou Medical University, Guiyang, China. [5]Department of Orthopaedics, Warren Alpert Medical School of Brown University and Rhode Island Hospital, Providence, RI, USA.

References

1. Thomas AC, Hubbard-Turner T, Wikstrom EA, Palmieri-Smith RM. Epidemiology of posttraumatic osteoarthritis. J Athl Train. 2017;52:491–6.
2. Little CB, Smith MM. Animal models of osteoarthritis. Curr Rheumatol Rev. 2008;4:175–82.
3. Furman BD, Kimmerling KA, Zura RD, Reilly RM, Zlowodzki MP, Huebner JL, et al. Articular ankle fracture results in increased synovitis, synovial macrophage infiltration, and synovial fluid concentrations of inflammatory cytokines and chemokines. Arthritis Rheumatol. 2015;67:1234–9.
4. Dang Y, Cole AA, Homandberg GA. Comparison of the catabolic effects of fibronectin fragments in human knee and ankle cartilages. Osteoarthr Cartil. 2003;11:538–47.
5. Swann AC, Seedhom BB. The stiffness of normal articular cartilage and the predominant acting stress levels: implications for the aetiology of osteoarthrosis. Br J Rheumatol. 1993;32:16–25.
6. Schmal H, Salzmann GM, Langenmair ER, Henkelmann R, Südkamp NP, Niemeyer P. Biochemical characterization of early osteoarthritis in the ankle. ScientificWorldJournal. 2014; doi:10.1155/2014/434802.
7. San Giovanni TP, Golish SR, Palanca A, Hanna LS, Scuderi GJ. Correlation of intra-articular ankle pathology with cytokine biomarkers and matrix degradation products. Foot Ankle Int. 2012;33:627–31.
8. Valderrabano V, Horisberger M, Russell I, Dougall H, Hintermann B. Etiology of ankle osteoarthritis. Clin Orthop Relat Res. 2009;467:1800–6.
9. Günther KP, Stürmer T, Sauerland S, Zeissig I, Sun Y, Kessler S, et al. Prevalence of generalised osteoarthritis in patients with advanced hip and knee osteoarthritis: the Ulm osteoarthritis study. Ann Rheum Dis. 1998;57:717–23.

10. Aurich M, Hofmann GO, Rolauffs B, Gras F. Differences in injury pattern and prevalence of cartilage lesions in knee and ankle joints: a retrospective cohort study. Orthop Rev (Pavia). 2014;6:5611.
11. Lübbeke A, Salvo D, Stern R, Hoffmeyer P, Holzer N, Assal M. Risk factors for post-traumatic osteoarthritis of the ankle: an eighteen year follow-up study. Int Orthop. 2012;36:1403–10.
12. Horisberger M, Valderrabano V, Hintermann B. Posttraumatic ankle osteoarthritis after ankle-related fractures. J Orthop Trauma. 2009;23:60–7.
13. Anderson DD, Chubinskaya S, Guilak F, Martin JA, Oegema TR, Olson SA, et al. Post-traumatic osteoarthritis: improved understanding and opportunities for early intervention. J Orthop Res. 2011;29:802–9.
14. Kraeutler MJ, Kaenkumchorn T, Pascual-Garrido C, Wimmer MA, Chubinskaya S. Peculiarities in ankle cartilage. Cartilage. 2017;8:12–8.
15. Backus JD, Furman BD, Swimmer T, Kent CL, McNulty AL, Defrate LE, et al. Cartilage viability and catabolism in the intact porcine knee following transarticular impact loading with and without articular fracture. J Orthop Res. 2011;29:501–10.
16. Delco ML, Kennedy JG, Bonassar LJ, Fortier LA. Post-traumatic osteoarthritis of the ankle: a distinct clinical entity requiring new research approaches. J Orthop Res. 2017;35:440–53.
17. Wang S, Wei X, Zhou J, Zhang J, Li K, Chen Q, et al. Identification of α2-macroglobulin as a master inhibitor of cartilage-degrading factors that attenuates the progression of posttraumatic osteoarthritis. Arthritis Rheumatol. 2014;66:1843–53.
18. Weissleder R, Ntziachristos V. Shedding light onto live molecular targets. Nat Med. 2003;9:123–8.
19. Ntziachristos V, Bremer C, Weissleder R. Fluorescence imaging with near-infrared light: new technological advances that enable *in vivo* molecular imaging. Eur Radiol. 2003;13:195–208.
20. Thomas NP, Li P, Fleming BC, Chen Q, Wei X, Xiao-Hua P, et al. Attenuation of cartilage pathogenesis in post-traumatic osteoarthritis (PTOA) in mice by blocking the stromal derived factor 1 receptor (CXCR4) with the specific inhibitor, AMD3100. J Orthop Res. 2015;33:1071–8.
21. Gerwin N, Bendele AM, Glasson S, Carlson CS. The OARSI histopathology initiative-recommendations for histological assessments of osteoarthritis in the rat. Osteoarthr Cartil. 2010;18(Suppl 3):24–34.
22. Saltzman CL, Salamon ML, Blanchard GM, Huff T, Hayes A, Buckwalter JA, et al. Epidemiology of ankle arthritis: report of a consecutive series of 639 patients from a tertiary orthopaedic center. Iowa Orthop J. 2005;25:44–6.
23. Huch K. Knee and ankle: human joints with different susceptibility to osteoarthritis reveal different cartilage cellularity and matrix synthesis in vitro. Arch Orthop Trauma Surg. 2001;121:301–6.
24. Aurich M, Squires GR, Reiner A, Mollenhauer JA, Kuettner KE, Poole AR, et al. Differential matrix degradation and turnover in early cartilage lesions of human knee and ankle joints. Arthritis Rheum. 2005;52:112–9.
25. Hendren L, Beeson PA. Review of the differences between normal and osteoarthritis articular cartilage in human knee and ankle joints. Foot (Edinb). 2009;19:171–6.
26. Treppo S, Koepp H, Quan EC, Cole AA, Kuettner KE, Grodzinsky AJ. Comparison of biomechanical and biochemical properties of cartilage from human knee and ankle pairs. J Orthop Res. 2000;18:739–48.
27. Glasson SS, Blanchet TJ, Morris EA. The surgical destabilization of the medial meniscus (DMM) model of osteoarthritis in the 129/SvEv mouse. Osteoarthr Cartil. 2007;15:1061–9.
28. Chang SH, Yasui T, Taketomi S, Matsumoto T, Kim-Kaneyama JR, Omiya T, et al. Comparison of mouse and human ankles and establishment of mouse ankle osteoarthritis models by surgically-induced instability. Osteoarthr Cartil. 2016;24:688–97.
29. Goetz JE, Fredericks D, Petersen E, Rudert MJ, Baer T, Swanson E, et al. A clinically realistic large animal model of intra-articular fracture that progresses to post-traumatic osteoarthritis. Osteoarthr Cartil. 2015;23:1797–805.
30. Eger W, Schumacher BL, Mollenhauer J, Kuettner KE, Cole AA. Human knee and ankle cartilage explants: catabolic differences. J Orthop Res. 2002;20: 526–34.
31. Muehleman C, Li J, Aigner T, Rappoport L, Mattson E, Hirschmugl C, et al. Association between crystals and cartilage degeneration in the ankle. J Rheumatol. 2008;35:1108–17.
32. Roach HI, Mehta G, Oreffo RO, Clarke NM, Cooper C. Temporal analysis of rat growth plates: cessation of growth with age despite presence of a physis. J Histochem Cytochem. 2003;51:373–83.

10

CT-based analysis of muscle volume and degeneration of gluteus medius in patients with unilateral hip osteoarthritis

Takako Momose, Yutaka Inaba*, Hyonmin Choe, Naomi Kobayashi, Taro Tezuka and Tomoyuki Saito

Abstract

Background: The gluteus medius (GMED) affects hip function as an abductor. We evaluated muscle volume and degeneration of the GMED by using CT-based analysis and assessed factors that affect hip abductor strength in patients with unilateral hip osteoarthritis (OA).

Methods: We examined clinical and imaging findings associated with hip abductor strength in consecutive 50 patients with unilateral hip OA. Hip abductor muscle strength and Harris hip score (HHS) were assessed. Leg length discrepancy (LLD) and femoral offset were assessed using X-ray; CT assessment was employed for volumetric and qualitative GMED analysis. Volumetric analysis involved measurement of cross sectional area (CSA) and three-dimensional (3D) muscle volume. CT density was measured for the qualitative assessment of GMED degeneration with or without adjustment using a bone mineral reference phantom.

Results: Hip abductor muscle strength on the affected side was significantly lower than that on the contralateral healthy side and positively correlated with overall score and score for limping of gait of HHS, demonstrating the importance of hip abductor strength for normal hip function. A significant correlation was found between CSA and 3D muscle volume, unadjusted CT density and adjusted CT density, and hip abductor strength and these CT measurements. Multiple linear regression analysis demonstrated that 3D muscle volume, adjusted CT density, and LLD are independent factors affecting hip abduction.

Conclusions: 3D measurement of muscle volume and adjusted CT density more accurately reflect quantity and the GMED quality than do conventional assessments. Increase in muscle volume, recovery of muscle degeneration, and correction of LLD are important for improving limping in patients with hip OA.

Keywords: Gluteus medius, Muscle volume, Fatty degeneration, Cross-sectional area, Hip osteoarthritis

Background

Hip abductor muscles are important determinants for hip function [1]. Abductor function ensures stability of the hip joint and controls pelvic posture in standing and walking [1]. The gluteus medius (GMED) is one of the main muscles in the hip abductor muscle group. The GMED provides stabilization of the pelvis in a single leg stance [1]. Thus, dysfunction of the GMED is responsible for unstable hip and postural imbalance of the pelvis during ambulation. A reduction in the volume of the GMED in patients with hip osteoarthritis (OA) is a major reason for limping gait [2–4]. Therefore, quantification of the GMED can provide vital information for obtaining normal gait in patients with hip OA.

Computed tomography (CT) is one of the commonly used imaging tools for the quantification of muscle volume around the hip [3, 5]. Measurement of cross-sectional area (CSA) has been demonstrated as a method for evaluating muscle volume [3, 5]; however, such measurements in cross-sectional images are widely variable and depend on the place of section. Since the GMED transverses from the pelvis to the femur and is widely variable in each patient [6], three-dimensional (3D) analysis can more precisely quantify GMED muscle volume. In addition to muscle volume, muscle quality is also responsible for muscle

* Correspondence: yute0131@med.yokohama-cu.ac.jp
Department of Orthopaedic Surgery, Yokohama City University, 3-9 Fukuura, Kanazawa-ku, Yokohama, Japan

weakness [7, 8]. However, few studies have assessed the relationship between muscle quality and muscle strength around the hip, although measurement of CT density can be used to assess muscle degeneration [9]. CT density can be affected by CT scan settings; as demonstrated in measurements of bone mineral density, adjustment of CT density using a bone mineral reference phantom may improve the evaluation of muscle degeneration [10].

The purposes of our study were to evaluate muscle volume and muscle degeneration of GMED using CT based analysis, and to assess the effect of hip abductor muscle strength on hip function and factors affecting hip abductor strength in patients with unilateral hip OA. For this purpose, we quantified clinical parameters, X-ray findings, and CT measurements of the GMED. CT measurements involved muscle volume quantified by CSA and 3D reconstruction and muscle degeneration by CT density with or without adjustment using bone mineral reference phantom.

Methods

Patients

This prospective study was approved by our institutional review board. We enrolled 50 consecutive patients with unilateral hip OA between April 2012 and May 2014 with informed consent. Those patients suffered from symptomatic hip for an average of 9 years (range, 0.5-45 years) before initial presentation to our hospital. For clinical assessment, the Harris hip score (HHS) was recorded. To assess hip abductor strength, isometric hip abductor strength measurements were performed on all patients using a manual isokinetic/isometric dynamometer (microFET; Hoggan Health Industries, Inc., Draper, UT, USA). During the test, the participants lay on their side with the test leg up and with the dynamometer secured on the lateral side of their thigh. The pad on the dynamometer was centered over the distal lateral femur at a standardized point of 80% of the length between the greater trochanter and the lateral femoral condyle. The testing leg was positioned straight (0° of hip and knee flexion and 0° of hip rotation), whereas the non-testing leg was positioned in approximately 30° of hip flexion and 30° of knee flexion against the table for comfort and stability. During the hip abduction testing, a careful causation was given on the reproducibility of lower leg motion, especially in patients with severe hip pain. The participant was asked to perform three maximal isometric contractions for 5 s with 30 s of rest between the repetitions on each side. The peak force from the 3 trials was used for statistical analysis. Abductor muscle strength was measured by hip surgeons in our institution.

Imaging tests

All patients were scanned with a plain anterior-posterior X-ray of the hip in a standing position and computed tomography (CT) using transaxial CT scans (Sensation16; Siemens AG, Erlangen, Germany). Scanner settings were approximately 120 kV and 300 mA, with a slice thickness of 1.5 mm. The 50 patients were examined in the supine position using a spiral CT-scanner with their pelvis in the neutral position and the lower limb placed in patient's natural rotation. Natural rotation meant the lower leg position in relax position. Since stretch of muscle might affect the muscle volumes, we did not enforce lower legs to patella median position. Transverse images were obtained from the iliac crest to the condyles of the femur in each patient.

Leg length discrepancy [11] and femoral offset [12] and Kellgren and Lawrence (KL) grade [13] were measured using a plain anterior-posterior X-ray of the hip in a standing position. CSA was measured by locating the mid-point of the anterior superior iliac spine and greater trochanter using cross-sectional images obtained by CT (Fig. 1). Muscle volume was measured using dedicated software (Synapse Vincent®: Fujifilm Medical Systems, Japan). The software provided tools for measuring distances, areas, volumes, and radiological density. 3D muscle volume of the GMED was calculated in free-hand-draw fashion by tracking the margins of the GMED (Fig. 2). The margin of the GMED was drawn from proximal to distal slices, where the GMED was visible and on every third slice in between these start- and end-point slices. The decision to use every third slice was based on the minimum number of slices that the software required to trace the muscle margins and to calculate muscle volume. Whole muscle was carefully detected by excluding the surrounding fat or connective tissue and partial volume artifacts. The software reconstructed the GMED and output data included volume and CT density of the muscle (Fig. 2).

Muscle degeneration was quantified by calculating the mean CT density, which was measured as hounsfield units (HU). CT density was adjusted by calculating the equivalent hydroxyapatite amount in muscle area and a calibration phantom (B-MAS 200; Kyoto-Kagaku, Kyoto, Japan) using dedicated software that calculates adjusted HU of the muscle in the CT image based upon reference values measured in bone mineral reference phantom (Fig. 1) [14].

Statistics

Pearson's test was used for correlation analyses. Statistical significance of differences was determined by Student t-test or non-parametric Mann-Whitney test of data sets that were not normally distributed. To assess intra-observer and inter-observer reliabilities in measuring muscle volume of the GMED, intra-class correlation coefficients were calculated. For this purpose, 3D muscle volumes of the GMED in 12 patients were measured twice by the author with

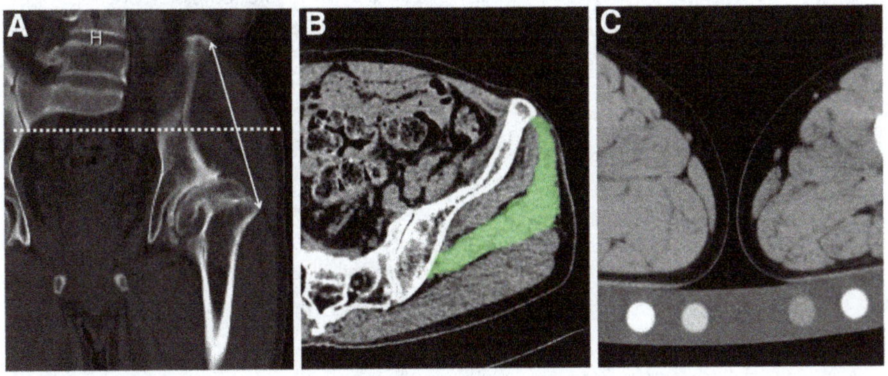

Fig. 1 Cross-sectional analysis of the gluteus medius and bone mineral reference phantom for adjustment of CT density. **a** and **b** Cross sectional area (colored area in panel **b**) was measured using the mid-point of the anterior superior iliac spine and greater trochanter, which were visualized using cross-sectional images obtained by CT (dot line in panel **a**). **c** A calibration phantom (B-MAS 200; Kyoto-Kagaku, Kyoto, Japan) is placed in a CT scanner and an equivalent amount of hydroxyapatite in the bone mineral reference phantom was utilized to adjust CT density by using dedicated software

6 months of interval period (TM) to determine intra-observer reliability, and those values in the same patients were also measured by another blinded orthopedic surgeon (HC) to determine inter-observer reliability. Multiple linear regression analysis was performed to identify the factors affecting abductor muscle strength. At first, a univariate regression analysis was performed with the following factors as explaining variables: muscle volume of the GMED, adjusted CT density, CSA of the GMED, CT density of the GMED, age, sex, BMI, LLD, femoral offset and KL grade. Secondly, all the variables were analyzed by multiple linear regression analysis (forced entry method). Thereafter, a backward selection method of multiple linear regression analysis was done with selected variables with p values less than 0.2 in forced entry method (final model). A p-value of <0.05 was considered significant.

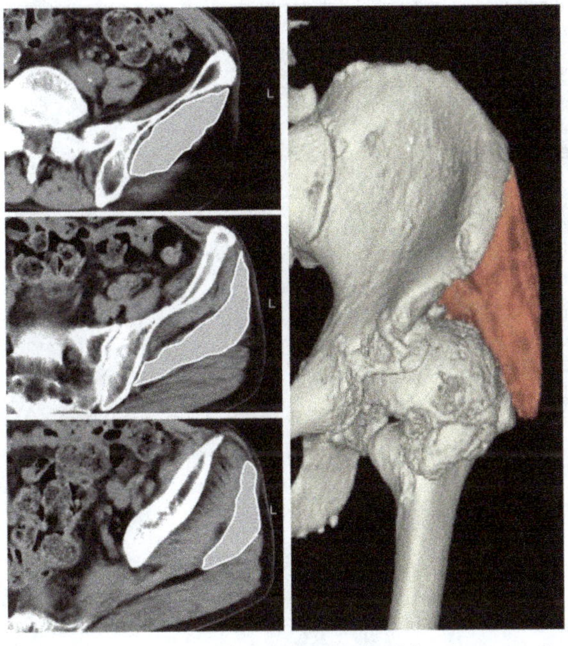

Fig. 2 Muscle volume and fatty degeneration of the gluteus medius (GM). By tracing the cross-sectional areas of the GM on every third slice of the CT images using three-dimensional (3D) image analysis software (stripe area), GM muscle was reconstructed three-dimensionally (colored area). Muscle volume and fatty degeneration of the reconstructed GM were quantified using dedicated software

Results

Fifty patients (12 males and 38 females) with an average body mass index of 23.3 kg/m^2 (standard deviation, ±4.1) and a mean age of 62 years (range, 30-82 years) were enrolled. Mean femoral offset on the affected hip was significantly lower than that on the healthy hip (34.6 mm and 38.3 mm, $p < 0.01$). Mean LLD was −10.9 mm (range, −55–0 mm) on the affected side and 4, 8 and 38 patients had a hip OA with KL grade 2, 3, and 4, respectively. The muscle strength of the hip abductor on the affected side was significantly lower than that on the contralateral healthy side (Table 1). The average ratio of the muscle strength of the hip abductor on the affected side to the healthy side was 69.9%. CSA and 3D muscle volume of the GMED on the affected side measured on CT images were significantly smaller than those on the contralateral healthy side in all patients (Table 1). The average ratios of the CSA and muscle volume on the affected side to those on the healthy side were 83.7% and 79.4%, respectively. CT density and adjusted CT density of the GMED on the affected side were significantly lower than those on the contralateral healthy side (Table 1). The average ratios of CT density and adjusted CT density of the GMED on the affected side to the healthy side were 78.2% and 76.5%, respectively. Hip abductor muscle strength had a positive correlation with overall HHS score and significantly correlated with the limping score, but not with

Table 1 Comparison of hip abductor strength and radiological measurements of the GMED between the affected side and healthy side

	Affected side (mean ± SD)	Healthy side (mean ± SD)	*P* value
Strength of hip abduction (N)	67.8 ± 31.0	94.5 ± 26.1	<0.001
Cross-sectional area of GMED (mm^2)	1838 ± 494	2260 ± 503	<0.001
Muscle volume of GMED (cm^3)	206 ± 57	260 ± 61	<0.001
CT density of the GMED (HU)	35.6 ± 10.6	45.5 ± 6.7	<0.001
Adjusted CT density of the GMED (mg/cm^3)	29.1 ± 10.8	37.3 ± 7.2	<0.001

GMED gluteus medius, *HU* Hounsfield unit

the scores of hip joint pain, requirement of gait support, or walking distance in HHS (Table 2). Intra-observer reliability and inter-observer reliability for 3D muscle volume of the GMED were 0.998 (95% CI, 0.996–0.999) and 0.948 (95% CI, 0.887–0.977), respectively.

To assess the factors that affect hip abductor muscle strength among clinical and radiological findings, univariate and multiple linear regression analysis were performed. Univariate linear regression analysis determined that CSA, 3D muscle volume, CT density, adjusted CT density, sex, and BMI, were factors that affected hip abductor muscle strength on the affected side. With further investigation using multiple linear regression analysis, 3D muscle volume, adjusted CT density, and LLD were found to be the factors that affected hip abductor strength on the affected side (Tables 3 and 4). Similar factors were found upon univariate analysis on the healthy side, but LLD was excluded from the factors affecting hip abductor strength in multivariate analysis.

Cross-sectional and 3D muscle volume of the GMED showed a strong positive correlation (Fig. 3), and these measurements were both correlated with muscle strength of the hip abductor (Fig. 3). CT density and adjusted CT density showed a significant correlation (Fig. 4). Hip abductor strength correlated with CT density and adjusted CT density (Fig. 4). There was also a significant correlation between LLD and GMED

Table 2 Correlation of hip abductor muscle on the affected side with Harris hip score (HHS)

HHS score (points)	r	*P* value
Overall	0.42	0.002
Pain	0.25	0.09
limping	0.51	<0.001
Required support for walking	0.11	0.45
Walking distance	0.22	0.13

Table 3 Univariate regression analysis for evaluating the association between hip abductor strength and clinical and radiological parameters on the affected side

	Regression coefficient	Standardized regression coefficient	*P* value
Muscle volume of the GMED	0.34	0.62	<0.001
Adjusted CT density of the GMED	1.36	0.47	0.001
CSA of the GMED	0.04	0.56	<0.001
CT density of the GMED	1.46	0.50	<0.001
Age	−0.04	−0.02	0.91
Sex	29.8	0.42	0.003
BMI	2.31	0.31	0.03
LLD	−0.17	−0.07	0.65
Femoral offset	0.32	0.06	0.68
KL grade	−0.01	0.02	0.31

GMED gluteus medius, *CSA* cross-sectional area, *RD* radiological density, *BMI* body mass index, *LLD* leg length discrepancy, *KL* Kellgren and Lawrence

Table 4 Multilinear regression analysis for evaluating the association between hip abductor strength and clinical and radiological parameters on the affected side

		Regression coefficient	Standardized regression coefficient	*P* value	Variance inflation factor
Forced Entry Method	Muscle volume of the GMED	0.28	0.52	0.07	6.63
	Adjusted CT density of the GMED	0.93	0.32	0.18	4.95
	CSA of the GMED	−0.003	−0.05	0.85	5.96
	CT density of the GMED	0.37	0.13	0.59	4.8
	Age	0.37	0.14	0.24	1.16
	Sex	−11.1	−0.15	0.35	2.44
	BMI	0.95	0.13	0.34	1.48
	LLD	0.71	0.28	0.09	2.31
	Femoral offset	0.42	0.08	0.55	1.49
	KL grade	−1.91	−0.04	0.77	1.46
Final model	Muscle volume of the GMED	0.3	.54	<0.001	1.29
	Adjusted CT density of the GMED	1.13	.39	0.005	1.65
	LLD	0.81	.32	0.014	1.43

GMED gluteus medius, *CSA* cross-sectional area, *RD* radiological density, *BMI* body mass index, *LLD* leg length discrepancy, *KL* Kellgren and Lawrence

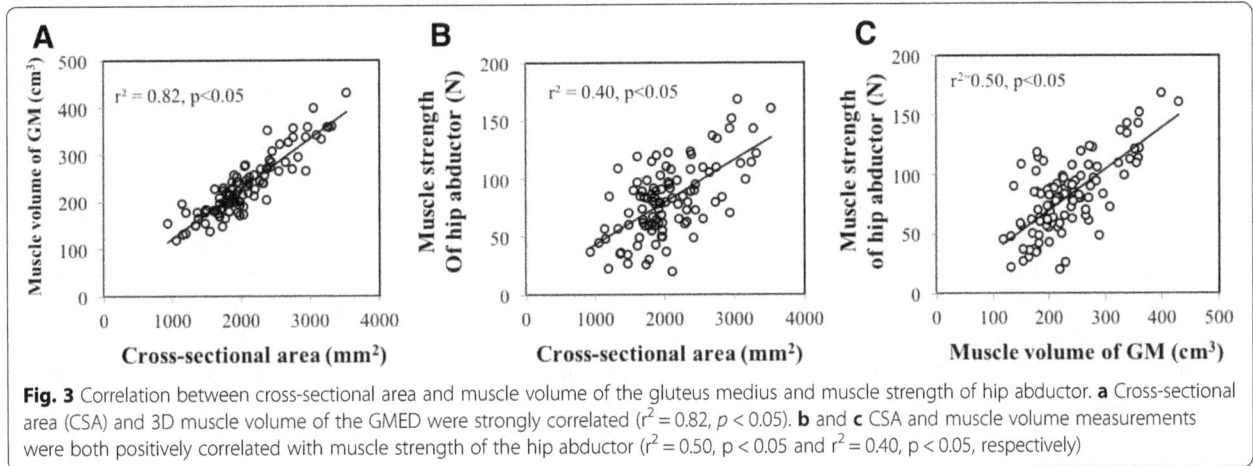

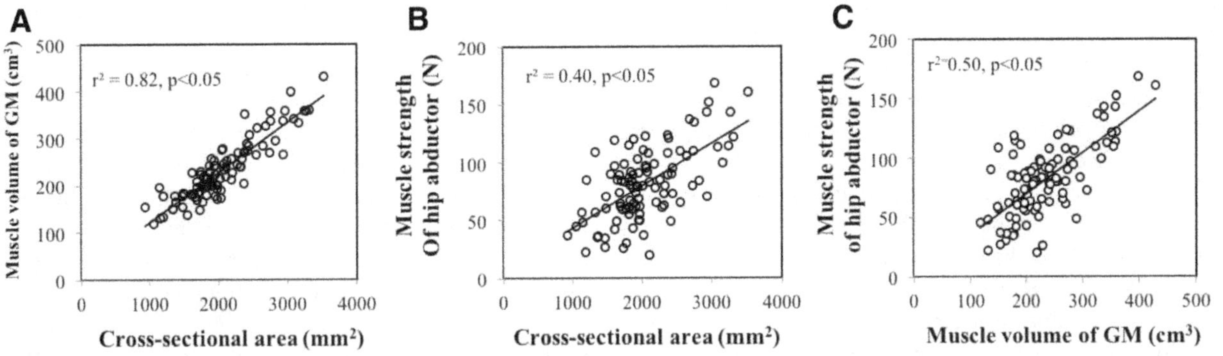

Fig. 3 Correlation between cross-sectional area and muscle volume of the gluteus medius and muscle strength of hip abductor. **a** Cross-sectional area (CSA) and 3D muscle volume of the GMED were strongly correlated ($r^2 = 0.82$, $p < 0.05$). **b** and **c** CSA and muscle volume measurements were both positively correlated with muscle strength of the hip abductor ($r^2 = 0.50$, $p < 0.05$ and $r^2 = 0.40$, $p < 0.05$, respectively)

volume ($r = -0.19$, $p = 0.024$) or LLD and adjusted CT density ($r = -0.545$, $p < 0.001$).

Discussion

The purposes of our study were to evaluate the effect of hip abductor muscle strength on hip function, to validate the utility of our CT-based analysis for the quantification of muscle volume and muscle degeneration of GMED, and to assess factors that affect hip abductor strength in patients with unilateral hip OA. Reduction of muscle volume and degeneration of the GMED were evident in the present study, which agrees with findings of previous reports [2–4]. Correlation of hip abductor strength with limping score of HHS, rather than hip pain or walking distance, indicated the importance of hip abductor muscle strength for normal gait in patients with unilateral hip OA.

Previous studies have demonstrated an association between two-dimensional area of the GMED and hip abductor muscle strength [2–4]; however, few studies have focused on the 3D volume of the GMED. Measurements of the muscle CSA using MRI or CT imaging is a simple and easy way to determine muscle volume [2, 3, 5]. However, the shape of the muscle is widely variable, while cross-sectional analysis affects the place of the measurement section, particularly in patients with severe hip deformity. Because most patients with hip OA in Japan have acetabular dysplasia or femoral deformity, 3D quantification is attractive to assess muscle volume precisely. Therefore, in the present study, we performed 3D quantification of muscle volume and explored whether the 3D quantification is more likely associated with muscle strength. Although CSA has a strong correlation with 3D quantification of muscle volume, the results of multilinear regression analysis indicate that 3D measurement of muscle volume is a better method that accurately reflects muscle strength. The limitation of 3D quantification of muscle volume is that it requires the scanning of the entire muscle and additional time for 3D analysis. Assessment for muscle volume by cross-sectional images may be an alternative method for the quantification of muscle volume with minimal effort. However, intra-observer and inter-observer reliability analysis have demonstrated the good reproducibility of 3D measurement of muscle volume

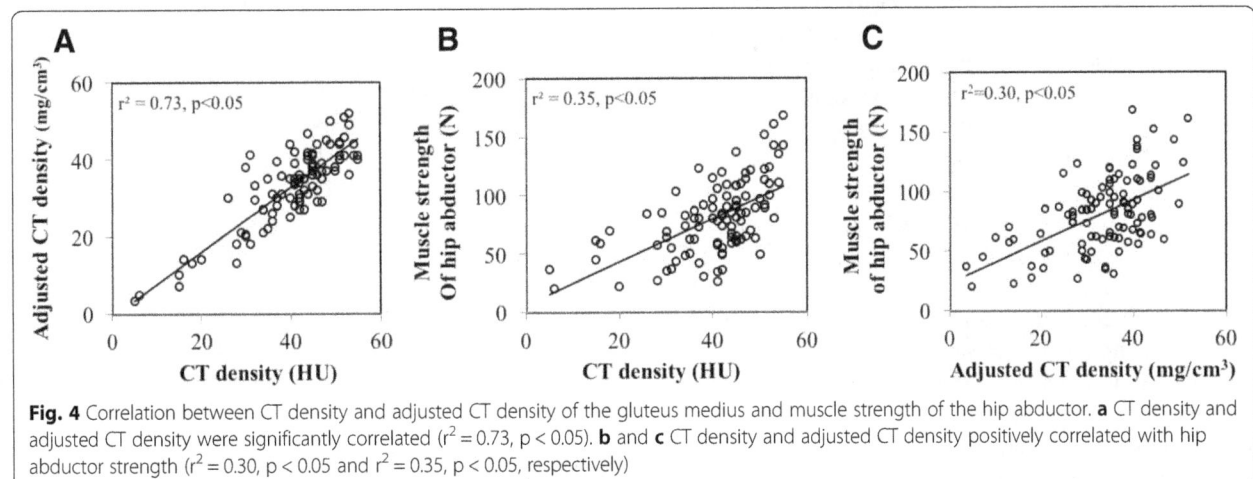

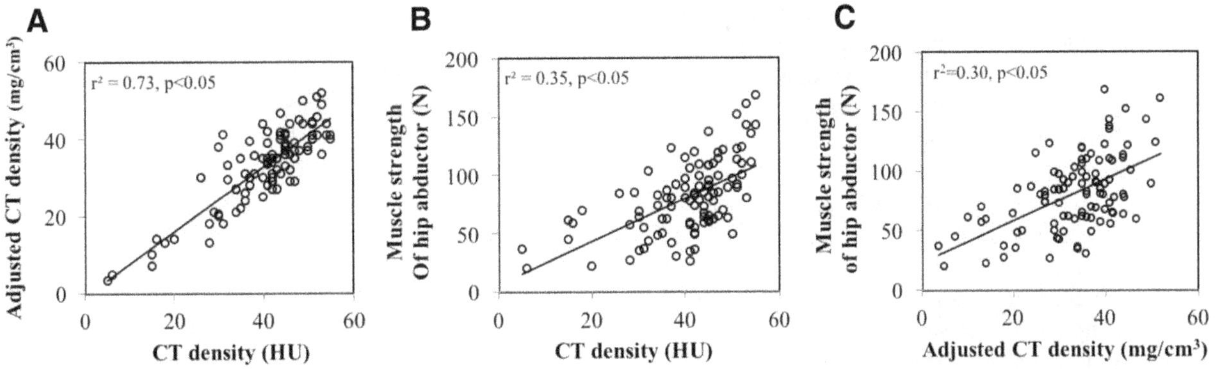

Fig. 4 Correlation between CT density and adjusted CT density of the gluteus medius and muscle strength of the hip abductor. **a** CT density and adjusted CT density were significantly correlated ($r^2 = 0.73$, $p < 0.05$). **b** and **c** CT density and adjusted CT density positively correlated with hip abductor strength ($r^2 = 0.30$, $p < 0.05$ and $r^2 = 0.35$, $p < 0.05$, respectively)

and we believe that 3D measurement is better to evaluate the accurate muscle volume of GMED in CT analysis.

Atrophic changes in muscle property may also be responsible for muscle weakness in patients with gait disorder. Nevertheless, quantification of muscle degeneration has not received sufficient attention. Upon CT assessment, several studies have measured radiological density to evaluate muscle degeneration [3, 5, 15]. However, radiological density can be affected by the different settings used during CT scanning. Hence, in the current study, we corrected CT values using bone mineral reference phantom for a more accurate assessment of muscle degeneration. Adjustment with bone mineral reference phantom is a widely used method to quantify bone mineral density using CT [14]. We applied this method to measure CT density in muscle area and investigated whether adjustment with bone mineral reference phantom improves the quantification of muscle properties in the GMED. In the current study, multilinear regression analysis indicated that adjusted radiological density of the GMED was a more important factor affecting hip abductor muscle strength compared to unadjusted CT density. The use of a bone mineral reference phantom eliminates the effect of different CT settings and ensures greater accuracy in assessing muscle degeneration using CT data.

No study yet has comprehensively demonstrated the effect of related factors on hip abductor muscle strength by using multilinear regression analysis. Few studies have evaluated the relevance of implant orientations, including hip center and femoral offset for hip abductor strength in total hip arthroplasty patients [12]. Patients with Hip OA have severe pain on the affected limbs, thereby disuse of abductor muscle caused muscle atrophy and reduction of volume in our patients. In addition to the 3D measurement of muscle volume and adjusted CT density, LLD, rather than femoral offset or KL grade, was found to be an important independent factor that affects abductor muscle strength in patients with unilateral hip OA. This finding indicates that LLD affects muscle strength in a different manner from muscle atrophic change, possibly because a superior shift in the hip center and greater trochanter may result in mechanical incompatibility of the hip abductor muscles on the affected side. Thus, correction of LLD can lead to improvement in hip abductor muscle properties and gait limping, as often observed in patients after total hip arthroplasty. The severity of OA quantified by KL grade on the affected side had no correlation to GMED strength, although the affected hip (KL grade 2-4) has significantly lower GMED strength than the healthy hip (KL grade 0) in this study. Because some patients in our series suffered from severe hip pain regardless of their KL grade, the severe pain of the affected hip likely eliminated the effect of the difference in KL grade on GMED strength.

One of the limitations in this study was that we only assessed the gluteus medius. Since hip motion requires complicated coordination of several muscles, assessment of other muscles is necessary for a practical understanding of functional disability in patients with hip OA. However, our volumetric and qualitative CT analysis may be useful in the assessment of other muscles and provides better information compared to CSA-based conventional analysis. The second limitation of this study was that we used a bone mineral reference phantom to adjust muscle density. The reference system, which was specifically prepared for muscle assessment, should be assessed in future CT-based studies. The third limitation was that discrepancies in strength testing may be related to hip pain, rather than true muscle weakness. During the testing, a careful causation was given on the reproducibility of lower leg motion, especially in patients with severe hip pain. However, although we tried to exclude the effect of hip pain on the testing, the severe hip pain might affect the measurement of muscle strength.

Conclusions

In conclusion, we investigated factors that affected hip abductor muscle strength in patients with unilateral hip OA by using a novel volumetric and qualitative CT-based analysis of GMED. 3D measurement of muscle volume rather than CSA, adjusted CT density rather than unadjusted CT density, and LLD rather than femoral offset were found to be important factors that affect abductor muscle strength in patients with unilateral OA. An increase in muscle volume, recovery of muscle degeneration, and correction of LLD are important for improving gait limping in patients with hip OA.

Abbreviations

3D: Three-dimensional; CSA: Cross sectional area; CT: Computed tomography; GMED: Gluteus medius; HHS: Harris hip score; HU: Hounsfield units; KL: Kellgren and Lawrence; LLD: Leg length discrepancy; OA: Osteoarthritis

Acknowledgements

Not applicable.

Funding

No funding was obtained for this study.

Authors' contributions

TM, YI, and TS designed this study. TM, YI, HC, TT, and NK contributed to execution of the study and collection of data. TM, YI, HC prepared the manuscript. YI, HC, NK and TS edited the manuscript. All authors have read and approved the submission of this manuscript.

Competing interests

The authors declare that they have no competing interests.

References

1. Preininger B, Schmorl K, von Roth P, Winkler T, Schlattmann P, Matziolis G, Perka C, Tohtz S. A formula to predict patients' gluteus medius muscle volume from hip joint geometry. Man Ther. 2011;16(5):447–51.
2. Arokoski MH, Arokoski JP, Haara M, Kankaanpaa M, Vesterinen M, Niemitukia LH, Helminen HJ. Hip muscle strength and muscle cross sectional area in men with and without hip osteoarthritis. J Rheumatol. 2002;29(10):2185–95.
3. Rasch A, Bystrom AH, Dalen N, Berg HE. Reduced muscle radiological density, cross-sectional area, and strength of major hip and knee muscles in 22 patients with hip osteoarthritis. Acta Orthop. 2007;78(4):505–10.
4. Preininger B, Schmorl K, von Roth P, Winkler T, Matziolis G, Perka C, Tohtz S. The sex specificity of hip-joint muscles offers an explanation for better results in men after total hip arthroplasty. Int Orthop. 2012;36(6):1143–8.
5. Liu R, Wen X, Tong Z, Wang K, Wang C. Changes of gluteus medius muscle in the adult patients with unilateral developmental dysplasia of the hip. BMC Musculoskelet Disord. 2012;13:101.
6. Grimaldi A. Assessing lateral stability of the hip and pelvis. Man Ther. 2011;16(1):26–32.
7. Miozzari HH, Dora C, Clark JM, Notzli HP. Late repair of abductor avulsion after the transgluteal approach for hip arthroplasty. J Arthroplast. 2010;25(3): 450–457 e451.
8. Seo JB, Yoo JS, Jang HS, Kim JS. Correlation of clinical symptoms and function with fatty degeneration of infraspinatus in rotator cuff tear. Knee Surg Sports Traumatol Arthrosc. 2015;23(5):1481–8.
9. van de Sande MA, Stoel BC, Obermann WR, Tjong a Lieng JG, Rozing PM. Quantitative assessment of fatty degeneration in rotator cuff muscles determined with computed tomography. Investig Radiol. 2005;40(5):313–9.
10. Cann CE, Genant HK. Precise measurement of vertebral mineral content using computed tomography. J Comput Assist Tomogr. 1980;4(4):493–500.
11. Kjellberg M, Al-Amiry B, Englund E, Sjoden GO, Sayed-Noor AS. Measurement of leg length discrepancy after total hip arthroplasty. The reliability of a plain radiographic method compared to CT-scanogram. Skelet Radiol. 2012;41(2):187–91.
12. McGrory BJ, Morrey BF, Cahalan TD, An KN, Cabanela ME. Effect of femoral offset on range of motion and abductor muscle strength after total hip arthroplasty. J Bone Joint Surg Br. 1995;77(6):865–9.
13. Kellgren JH, Lawrence JS. Radiological assessment of osteo-arthrosis. Ann Rheum Dis. 1957;16(4):494–502.
14. Maeda Y, Sugano N, Saito M, Yonenobu K. Comparison of femoral morphology and bone mineral density between femoral neck fractures and trochanteric fractures. Clin Orthop Relat Res. 2011;469(3):884–9.
15. Daguet E, Jolivet E, Bousson V, Boutron C, Dahmen N, Bergot C, Vicaut E, Laredo JD. Fat content of hip muscles: an anteroposterior gradient. J Bone Joint Surg Am. 2011;93(20):1897–905.

Structural effects of intra-articular TGF-β1in moderate to advanced knee osteoarthritis: MRI-based assessment in a randomized controlled trial

A. Guermazi[1*], G. Kalsi[2], J. Niu[3], M. D. Crema[1], R. O. Copeland[2], A. Orlando[2], M. J. Noh[2] and F. W. Roemer[1]

Abstract

Background: To determine effects of allogeneic human chondrocytes expressing TGF-β1 (TG-C) on structural progression of MRI features of knee osteoarthritis over a 1 year period.

Methods: This phase II randomized controlled trial of TG-C included patients with moderate to advanced osteoarthritis. Patients were randomized to receive an intraarticular 3:1 mixture of non-transduced allogeneic human chondrocytes and TG-C or placebo. 3 T MRI was acquired for all patients at baseline and follow-up (3, 6 and 12 months). MRIs were assessed using the WORMS system including cartilage damage, bone marrow lesions (BMLs), meniscal damage/extrusion, Hoffa-, effusion-synovitis, and osteophytes. Analyses were performed on a whole knee level, compartmental level, and subregional level. Binary logistic regression with Generalized Estimating Equation was used to compare risks of progression, adjusting for baseline age and gender. Mann – Whitney – Wilcoxon tests were used to assess differences for continuous variables.

Results: Fifty-seven Patients were included in the TG-C group and 29 in the placebo group. At 12 months, knees in the TG-C group showed less progression of cartilage damage compared to placebo on a whole knee level (34.6% vs. 47.9%; adjusted RR 0.7, 95%CI [0.5–1.1], $p = 0.077$). Less progression of Hoffa-synovitis and effusion-synovitis was observed in the TG-C group compared to placebo (9.6% vs. 21.1%, adjusted RR 0.5, 95%CI [0.2,1.2], $p = 0.115$). No statistically significant differences were seen for BMLs, meniscal damage and osteophytes.

Conclusions: Intraarticular treatment with TG-C showed fewer patients in the treated group with progression in structural OA features and other MRI-defined inflammatory markers such as Hoffa-synovitis and effusion-synovitis. However, no differences were observed in regard to progression of BMLs and meniscal damage, or hypertrophic osteophyte formation.

Trial registration: NCT01221441.Registered 13th October, 2010

Keywords: Tgf-β1, Osteoarthritis, MRI, Randomized controlled trial

* Correspondence: guermazi@bu.edu
[1]Department of Radiology, Quantitative Imaging Center, Boston University School of Medicine, 820 Harrison Avenue, FGH Building, 3rd Floor, Boston, MA, USA
Full list of author information is available at the end of the article

Background

TGF-β proteins induce osteogenesis and chondrogenesis, and play a role in cell growth, differentiation, and extracellular matrix protein synthesis [1]. TGF-β stimulates proteoglycan synthesis and chondrocyte proliferation, and may also have anti-inflammatory and immunosuppressive characteristics [1]. A new treatment approach for knee osteoarthritis (OA) involves intraarticular administration of human chondrocytes transduced with a viral vector containing the gene for TGF-β1 transcription. Recently, a preliminary evaluation of the efficacy of non-transduced allogeneic human chondrocytes and allogeneic human chondrocytes virally transduced to express TGF-β1 (TG-C) was done. TG-C is made of human chondrocytes which has immunosuppressive effect and is grown from tissue obtained from a polydactyly finger of a single infant donor [2]. TG-C represents a cell-mediated cytokine gene therapy approach for local intra-articular administration in patients with OA. TG-C showed positive effects on pain levels in patients with moderate to advanced knee OA, as demonstrated by the visual analogue scale (VAS) and International Knee Documentation Committee (IKDC) scores at 1 year follow-up compared to the control cohort [3]. Patients receiving TG-C had less knee pain, and they were less likely to need analgesics compared to placebo. However, effects of TG-C on MRI-assessed structural changes in knee joint tissues have only been assessed in a single study demonstrating mixed results after 12 months, i.e. those who received low-dose TG-C showed worsening mean MRI score of cartilage signal intensity, while those who had high-dose TG-C showed worsening mean MRI scores in bone surface osteophytes and periarticular inflammation [4].

Our study aimed to assess effects of intraarticular TG-C on structural progression of knee OA features based on semi-quantitative MRI evaluation compared with placebo during 12-months of follow-up period.

Method

Subject inclusion and exclusion

Our study was a multi-center double-blind placebo-controlled phase II randomized clinical trial (ClinicalTrials.gov identifier: NCT01221441.Registered 13th October, 2010). It was conducted in accordance with the International Conference on Harmonization Tripartite Guideline, Guideline for Good Clinical Practice, ethical principles with origin in the Declaration of Helsinki, as well as the USA Code of Federal Regulations. Patient recruitment started in May 2011 and ended in October 2013. Institutional review board ethical approval was obtained from all five recruitment sites – Center for Joint Preservation and Reconstruction, Baltimore, MD); Commonwealth Orthopedics, Arlington, PA; Advent Orthopaedics and Rehabilitation LLC, Pinellas Park, FL; University Orthopedics Center, State College, PA; and The Rothman Institute, Philadelphia, PA. We included both male and female subjects aged between 18 and 70 years; body mass index (BMI) between 18.5 and 45.5 kg/m^2; grade 3 radiographic knee OA as determined by the criteria of Kellgren and Lawrence [5] and pain symptoms for more than four consecutive months with an intensity of ≥ 40 and ≤ 90 on the 100-mm VAS. Subjects were generally healthy based on physical examination, normal blood work including hematology and serum chemistry, and urinalysis. All laboratory values were within 20% of normal ranges. All patients had negative history of significant organ system disorders. Written informed consent was obtained from all subjects after the nature of the study was fully explained and understood by them.

Exclusion criteria included: Patients taking non-steroidal anti-inflammatory medications within 14 days of baseline visit unless washed out; Patients taking steroidal anti-inflammatory medications within 2 months of baseline visit; Patients with a recent (within 1 year) history of drug abuse and/or a positive urine drug test at the time of screening; Patients receiving injections to the treated knee within 2 months prior to study entry; Patients who had contraindications for 3 T MRI; Patients who were pregnant or currently breast-feeding; Patients with a history of systemic, rheumatic or inflammatory disease or chondrocalcinosis, hemochromatosis, inflammatory arthritis, necrosis of the femoral condyle, arthropathy of the knee associated with juxta-articular Paget's disease of the femur or tibia, ochronosis, hemophilic arthropathy, infectious arthritis, Charcot's knee joint, villonodular synovitis, synovial chondromatosis, and/or history of inflammatory arthropathy; Patients with ongoing infectious disease, including HIV and hepatitis B or C; Patients with clinically significant cardiovascular, renal, hepatic, endocrine disease, cancer, or Type I diabetes; Patients participating in a study of an experimental drug or medical device within 30 days of study entry; Patients that were unable to comply with the requisite study follow-up and not able to complete all of the follow-up office visits and 3 T MRI exams.

Treatment

Patients were randomized to receive a 3:1 mixture of non-transduced allogeneic human chondrocytes and allogeneic human chondrocytes virally transduced to express TGF-β1 (TG-C) (TissueGene-C; TissueGene Inc., Rockville, Maryland, USA) or placebo (2 ml normal saline 0.9%). Details of the randomization procedure and determination of the sample size have been published previously [3]. TG-C was derived from a single human donor, grown from cartilage tissue from an infant polydactyly finger. Absence of viruses and other adventitious donor agents and the cell line were tested. Prior to TG-C or placebo administration, synovial fluid was aspirated from the patients' knee joints. TG-C or placebo was then injected intra-articularly using an 18 gauge needle with an inferolateral or inferomedial approach while the knee was flexed to 90-degrees. Injection was performed over about 10 s to avoid shearing of cells. Both patients and physicians were blinded to drug/placebo status.

Magnetic resonance imaging acquisition and interpretation

All patients underwent 3 T MRI at baseline and follow-up visits (3, 6 and 12 months) using a dedicated knee coil and the following protocol (triplanar intermediate-weighted fat suppressed sequences: TE 30–40 msec, TR 3600–4000 msec, 14 cm field of view, slice thickness 3 mm, 1 excitation, no phase wrap). MRIs were read by one expert musculoskeletal radiologist (AG, 18 years of experience in semiquantitative MRI assessment of OA) in sequential order - unblinded to the time sequence of MRI but blinded to all clinical information including treatment - using the modified semi-quantitative Whole Organ MRI Scoring (WORMS) system [6] including assessment of cartilage morphology (grade 0 = normal thickness and signal; grade 1 = normal thickness but increased signal on T2-weighted images; grade 2.0 = partial-thickness focal defect < 1 cm in greatest width; grade 2.5 = full-thickness focal defect < 1 cm in greatest width; grade 3 = multiple areas of partial-thickness (Grade 2.0) defects intermixed with areas of normal thickness, or a Grade 2.0 defect wider than 1 cm but < 75% of the region; grade 4 = diffuse (≥ 75% of the region) partial-thickness loss; grade 5 = multiple areas of full thickness loss (grade 2.5) or a grade 2.5 lesion wider than 1 cm but < 75% of the region; grade 6 = diffuse (≥ 75% of the region) full-thickness loss.), bone marrow lesions (BMLs – grade 0 = none;grade 1 = < 25% of the region; grade 2 = 25% to 50% of the region; grade 3 = > 50% of the region.), meniscal damage (grade 0 = intact; grade 1 = minor radial tear or parrot-beak tear; grade 2 = nondisplaced tear or prior surgical repair; grade 3 = displaced tear or partial resection; grade 4 = complete maceration/destruction or complete resection) and meniscal extrusion (grade 0 = < 2 mm; Grade 1 = 2–2.9 mm; grade 2 = 3–4.9 mm; grade 3 = > 5 mm), and inflammatory markers of disease (Hoffa-synovitis, grade 0 = normal; grade 1 = mild; grade 2 = moderate; grade 3 = severe, and effusion-synovitis, grade 0 = normal; grade 1 = < 33% of maximum potential distention; grade 2 = 33%–66% of maximum potential distention; grade 3 = > 66% of maximum potential distention.). Longitudinal changes were recorded including within-grade changes.

As TGF-β1 is considerd to be an anabolic agent, osteophyte presence and severity (grade 0–7) and change over time were additionally evaluated to compare rates of progression of osteophyte formation between groups.

Analytic approach

Data analyses were carried out in three ways using the data at baseline and at 12-month follow-up only: First, using 'delta-subregional' approach, the number of subregions showing progression (score increase at 12-month follow-up), no change, or improvement (score decrease at 12-month follow-up), respectively, were added to give a single score for each knee. There were a total of 14 subregions in the knee by WORMS definition (5 subregions each for the medial and lateral tibiofemoral [MTF, LTF] and 4 subregions for the patello-femoral [PF] compartment). For example, if 4 subregions show progression (delta [+1] × 4 = [+4]), 8 subregions show improvement (delta [−1] × 8 = [−8]) and 2 subregions show no change (delta 0), the 'delta-subregion change' for this knee would be '-4' (4 + [−8] = [−4]). Second, using 'delta-sum' approach, the absolute scores of all subregions were added within each compartment or within the whole knee. For these two approaches, progression was defined as overall delta > 0. Third, progression was defined as an increase in score in any of the subregions.

Binary logistic regression with Generalizing Estimating Equations was performed to assess relative risks of progression comparing data at baseline and 12-month follow-up, adjusting for baseline age and gender. Moreover, Mann – Whitney – Wilcoxon tests were used to evaluate differences of the continuous variables between treatment and placebo groups. All statistical analyses were carried out using SAS for Windows, version 9.1. Statistical significance was defined at $p < 0.05$.

Results

TG-C group had 57 patients and placebo group had 29 patients. Baseline demographic characteristics of the TG-C and placebo groups were comparable without statistically significant differences regading age (55.9 ± 7.9 vs. 56.6 ± 9.4 years) and gender (37 [64.9%] vs. 17 [58.6%] female). There was no statistically significant difference between two groups regarding baseline summary score.

Regarding change in cartilage morphology from baseline to 12 months, a lower proportion of knees showed progression of cartilage damage (progression in any subregion) in the treatment group on a whole knee level with a trend towards statistical significance (34.6% vs. 47.9%; adjusted RR 0.7, 95% CI [0.5–1.1], $p = 0.077$). The delta-sum approach or delta-subregional approach showed no statistically significant differences between two groups on a whole knee or compartmental level (Table 1).

A lower proportion of knees showed progression of Hoffa-synovitis and/or effusion synovitis (TG-C 9.6% vs.

Table 1 Presence and relative risk of progression of cartilage damage, Hoffa-synovitis and effusion-synovitis in different knee compartments for all visits combined from baseline to 12 months

		Number of subjects who had follow-up visits and included in analysis		Number of subjects with MRI progression		Analysis adjusted for age and gender	
Compartment	*Definition*	*T*[a]	*P*	*T*	*P*	*RR (95% CI)*	*p-value*
Knee	Progression in any subregion	133	71	46 (34.6%)	34 (47.9%)	0.7 (0.5,1.1)	0.077
	Delta Subregion > 0	123	71	43 (35.0%)	32 (45.1%)	0.8 (0.5,1.2)	0.207
	Delta Sum > 0	123	71	26 (21.1%)	23 (32.4%)	0.6 (0.3,1.2)	0.176
Lateral TFJ	Progression in any subregion	133	71	20 (15.0%)	12 (16.9%)	0.8 (0.3,1.9)	0.617
	Delta Subregion > 0	128	71	20 (15.6%)	12 (16.9%)	0.8 (0.4,1.9)	0.680
	Delta Sum > 0	128	71	13 (10.2%)	10 (14.1%)	0.7 (0.2,1.9)	0.434
Medial TFJ	Progression in any subregion	133	71	23 (17.3%)	12 (16.9%)	1.1 (0.5,2.5)	0.767
	Delta Subregion > 0	133	71	23 (17.3%)	12 (16.9%)	1.1(0.5,2.5)	0.767
	Delta Sum > 0	133	71	16 (12.0%)	5 (7.0%)	1.9(0.5,7.2)	0.345
PF	Progression in any subregion	131	71	18(13.7%)	16(22.5%)	0.6(0.3,1.3)	0.176
	Delta Subregion > 0	128	71	17(13.3%)	15(21.1%)	0.6(0.3,1.3)	0.210
	Delta Sum > 0	128	71	10(7.8%)	10(14.1%)	0.5(0.2,1.9)	0.327
MRI feature	*Definition*	*T*	*P*	*T*	*P*	*RR (95% CI)*	*p-value*
Hoffa-synovitis/ Effusion-synovitis combined	Any worsening	136	71	13 (9.6%)	15 (21.1%)	0.5 (0.2,1.2)	0.115
Hoffa-synovitis	Any worsening	133	71	4 (3.0%)	5 (7.0%)	0.3 (0.1,1.8)	0.200
Effusion-synovitis	Any worsening	136	71	12 (8.8%)	11 (15.5%)	0.6 (0.2,2.0)	0.428

T treatment group, *P* placebo group, *TFJ* tibiofemoral joint, *RR* relative risk

[a]Note: We excluded knees with MRI score missing in any subregion at either baseline or follow-up visit when defining delta subregion and delta sum, but did not exclude these knees when defining progression in any subregion. So N used for progressoin in any subregion was equal to or larger than N used in the two delta approaches

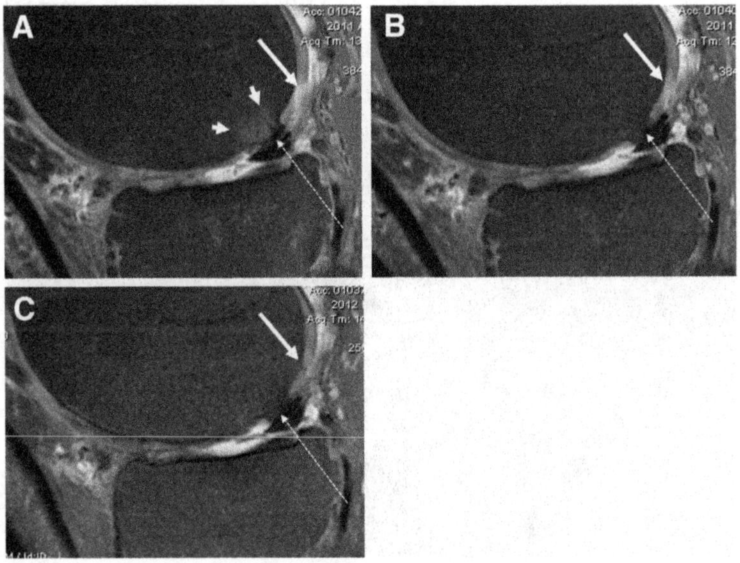

Fig. 1 Sagittal intermediate-weighted fat suppressed MRI in treated patient at baseline (**a**), 3 months (**b**) and 6 months (**c**) follow up show improvement of cartilage focal defect of the posterior medial femoral condyle with almost perfect filling at 6 months (long arrows). Also note the grade 1 BML at the central weight-bearing medial femoral condyle disappears at 3 months (**a**, short arrows). There is a Hoffa-synovitis grade 1 and moderate size tibial osteophytes. There is a femoral intrachondral osteophyte that seems to be slightly increasing in size (dotted arrows)

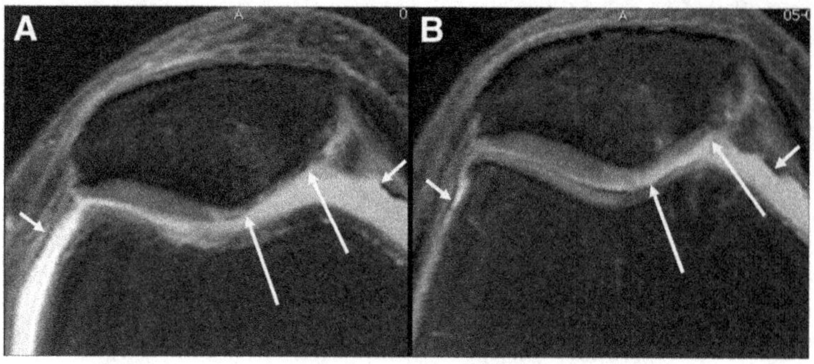

Fig. 2 Axial intermediate-weighted fat-suppressed MRI in treated patient at baseline (**a**) and 12 months (**b**) follow up show improvement of cartilage focal defect and thickness of the medial patella (long arrows). Also note the decrease in volume of the joint effusion (small arrows)

placebo 21.1%, $p = 0.115$), although the difference was not statistically significant.

Regarding change in BMLs and meniscal damage from baseline to 12 months, there was no significant difference using any of the three analytic approaches with similar rates of progression in both groups (TG-C vs. placebo: any BML progression 66.2% vs. 60.6%, $p = 0.612$; any meniscal damage progression, 31.6% vs. 32.4%, $p = 0.993$).

The Least Squared Mean Difference (95% CI) between the two groups in the osteophytes sum scores at the 12-month visit was 0.65 (−2.07 to 3.36), which was not statistically significant.

Table 1 summarizes the details of the baseline to 12 months analyses for cartilage and inflammatory markers. Figures 1, 2 and 3 show examples of cases with positive effect of TG-C on MRI-depicted structural changes, as well as a case which did not show positive effect of TG-C.

Discussion

In our phase II trial of allogeneic human chondrocytes expressing TGF-β1 (TG-C) vs. placebo in patients with moderate to advanced OA, a lower proportion of knees showed progression of cartilage damage on a knee level as well as less progression of MRI-based inflammatory markers for the treatment group compared to placebo. No preventive effect in regard to potential hypertrophic osteophyte formation was observed for the treatment group compared to placebo. Likewise, no significant differences between treatment and placebo were seen for change in BML and meniscal damage.

Previously, safety and tolerability of TG-C was demonstrated in a phase I human study [7]. More recently, positive effects of TG-C on knee function and pain in patients with moderate to advanced knee osteoarthritis were reported, showing some improvement in knee pain, function, and physical ability [3, 8, 9]. In these studies, however, MRI-based –structural assessment was not included.

MRI has become an essential research tool for knee OA studies thanks to its ability to non-invasively visualize the morphology of different knee joint tissues relevant to the disease process, and especially hyaline cartilage [10, 11]. Potential beneficial effects of TG-C on

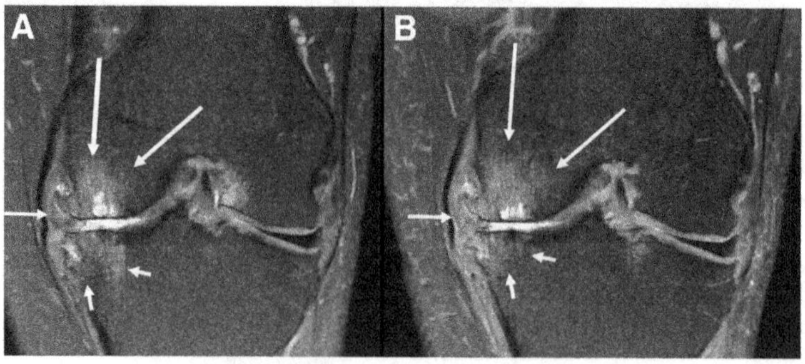

Fig. 3 Coronal intermediate-weighted fat-suppressed MRI in treated patient at baseline (**a**) and 3 months (**b**) follow up show no improvement of cartilage damage in the medial tibiofemoral compartment (WORMS grade 6 at central medial femur; WORMS grade 5 at central medial tibia). There is a medial meniscal maceration/extrusion (arrow). There is a slight improvement of the subchondral bone marrow lesion/cysts at the central medial tibia (small arrows) and slight worsening of the subchondral bone marrow lesion/cysts at the central medial femur (long arrows). Note large medial osteophytes

cartilage formation/growth for treatment of articular cartilage defects was first reported by Noh and colleagues in preclinical studies using mice, rabbits and goats [12]. In these animal studies, cartilage status after treatment was evaluated histologically at autopsy. Such an outcome measure is not appropriate in a phase II human study and therefore we deployed MRI which is a non-invasive imaging method.

Cho and colleagues reported a Korean phase IIa clinical trial in which MRI was used to evaluate effects of TG-C on structural changes including BMLs, cartilage damage, osteophytes, meniscal damage, effusion and periarticular inflammation 6-months and 12-months after TG-C injection [4]. In this study, effects of TG-C on MRI-based structural outcomes (assessed using the WORMS) were variable depending on TG-C dosage (low vs. high) and length of observation (6 months vs. 12 months). At 6 months, the low-dose cohort demonstrated worsening in mean MRI scores in one parameter (osteophytes), while the high-dose cohort demonstrated no worsening in mean scores. At 12 months, the low-dose cohort had worsening in the mean score in a subset of one parameter of unknown clinical significance, i.e. cartilage signal intensity, and the high-dose cohort demonstrated worsening in mean scores in two parameters (osteophytes and periarticular inflammation). This study was limited by a small number of subjects ($n = 27$), relatively short follow-up time and lack of a placebo group. The US phase II study described herein had more than double the sample size, had a placebo group, and deployed a more detailed outcome analyses.

Despite the fact that TGF-β1 is understood to be an anabolic agent, our study did not show any preventive effect of TG-C on progression of osteophyte formation in kneeOA. In fact, failing to reach statistical significance in all of our analyses may partly be due to sample size and low rates of progression overall. Also, since OA is a slowly progressing disease, a follow-up period of 12 months may have been too short to observe statistically significant effects of the TGF-β1 on structural progression of knee OA. Therefore, a future study with a larger number of subjects and a longer period of follow-up is necessary to confirm our preliminary observation regarding the effects of TGF-β1 on structural progression of knee OA. However, based on our results and thus far available literature evidence from animal and human studies, continued research efforts utilizing MRI-based structural outcomes to assess clinical efficacy of TG-C seem justifiable, especially focusing on cartilage regeneration.

Conclusion

In conclusion, intraarticular treatment with TG-C may potentially show benefits on delayed progression of cartilage damage and MRI markers of inflammation in osteoarthritis with fewer patients in the treated group showing progression of these structural OA features. However, TG-C showed no preventive effect for progression of BMLs and meniscal damage, or hypertrophic osteophyte formation within 12 month follow-up.

Abbreviations

BMI: Body mass index; BML: Bone marrow lesion; HIV: Human immunodeficiency virus; IKDC: International Knee Documentation Committee; MRI: Magnetic resonance imaging; OA: Osteoarthritis; TE: Time to echo; TG-C: Allogeneic human chondrocytes expressing TGF-β1; TGF: Transforming growth factor beta 1; TR: Time to repetition; VAS: Visual analogue scale; WORMS: Whole Organ Magnetic Resonance Imaging Score

Acknowledgements

We would like to thank the participants and staff of our clinical trial especially all principal investigators from:
Michael Mont, MD.
Rubin Institute for Advanced Orthopedics.
Center for Joint Preservation and Reconstruction, Baltimore, MD.
David Romness, MD.
Commonwealth Orthopedics, Arlington, VA.
Javad Parvizi, MD.
The Rothman Institute, Philadelphia, PA.
Dale Bramlet, MD.
Advent Orthopaedics and Rehabilitation LLC, Pinellas Park, FL.
Kenneth Cherry, MD.
University Orthopedics Center, State College, PA.

Funding

There were no research grants for this study. No funds were provided for this manuscript preparation.

Authors' contributions

All authors made the following contribution in preparation of this paper. Made substantial contributions to conception and design, or acquisition of data, or analysis and interpretation of data; AG, GK, JN, MDC, ROC, AO, MJN, FWR. Been involved in drafting the manuscript or revising it critically for important intellectual content; AG, GK, JN, MDC, ROC, AO, MJN, FWR. Given final approval of the version to be published. Each author should have participated sufficiently in the work to take public responsibility for appropriate portions of the content; AG, GK, JN, MDC, ROC, AO, MJN, FWR. Agreed to be accountable for all aspects of the work in ensuring that questions related to the accuracy or integrity of any part of the work are appropriately investigated and resolved; AG, GK, JN, MDC, ROC, AO, MJN, FWR. All authors read and approved the final manuscript.

Competing interests

AG received consulting fees from TissueGene, AstraZeneca, Merck Serono, GE Healthcare, Pfizer, SanofiAventis and OrthoTrophix. He is the President of Boston Imaging Core Lab (BICL), LLC. FWR is the CMO of BICL and received consulting fees from Merck Serono and National Institute of Health. MDC is a shareholder of BICL. GK, OC, MN and AO are employees of TissueGene, Inc. JN has nothing to disclose.

Author details

[1]Department of Radiology, Quantitative Imaging Center, Boston University School of Medicine, 820 Harrison Avenue, FGH Building, 3rd Floor, Boston, MA, USA. [2]TissueGene, Rockville, MD, USA. [3]Baylor College of Medicine, Houston, TX, USA.

References

1. MacFarlane EG, Haupt J, Dietz HC, Shore EM. TGF- β family signaling in connective tissue and skeletal diseases. Cold Spring Harb Perspect Biol. 2017. doi: 10.1101/cshperspect.a022269. [Epub ahead of print].
2. Lim CL, Lee YJ, Cho JH, Choi H, Lee B, Lee MC, et al. Immunogenicity and immunomodulatory effects of the human chondrocytes, hChonJ. BMC Musculoskelet Disord. 2017;18:199.
3. Cherian JJ, Parvizi J, Bramlet D, Lee KH, Romness DW, Mont MA. Preliminary results of a phase II randomized study to determine the efficacy and safety of genetically engineered allogeneic human chondrocytes expressing TGF-β1 in patients with grade 3 chronic degenerative joint disease of the knee. Osteoarthr Cartil. 2015;23:2109–18.
4. Cho JJ, Totterman S, Elmallah RK, Kim TW, Lee B, Mont MA. An MRI evaluation of patients who underwent treatment with a cell-mediated gene therapy for degenerative knee arthritis: a phase IIa clinical trial. J Knee Surg. 2016; doi: 10.1055/s-0036-1597275 [Epub ahead of print].
5. Kellgren JH, Lawrence JS. Radiological assessment of osteo-arthrosis. Ann Rheum Dis. 1957;16:494–502.
6. Peterfy CG, Guermazi A, Zaim S, Tirman PF, Miaux Y, White D, et al. Whole-organ magnetic resonance imaging score (WORMS) of the knee in osteoarthritis. Osteoarthr Cartil. 2004;12:177–90.
7. Ha CW, Noh MJ, Choi KB, Lee KH. Initial phase I safety of retrovirally transduced human chondrocytes expressing transforming growth factor-beta-1 in degenerative arthritis patients. Cytotherapy. 2012;14:247.
8. Ha CW, Cho JJ, Elmallah RK, Cherian JJ, Kim TW, Lee MC, et al. A multicenter, single-blind, phase IIa clinical trial to evaluate the efficacy and safety of a cell-mediated gene therapy in degenerative knee arthritis patients. Hum Gene Ther Clin Dev. 2015;26:125–30.
9. Lee MC, Ha CW, Elmallah RK, Cherian JJ, Cho JJ, Kim TW, et al. A placebo-controlled randomized trial to assess the effect of TGF-β1-expressing chondrocytes in patients with arthritis of the knee. Bone Joint J. 2015;97-B(7):924–32.
10. Alizai H, Roemer FW, Hayashi D, Crema MD, Felson DT, Guermazi A. An update on risk factors for cartilage loss in knee osteoarthritis assessed using MRI-based semiquantitative grading methods. Eur Radiol. 2015;25:883–93.
11. Hayashi D, Roemer FW, Guermazi A. Imaging for osteoarthritis. Ann Phys Rehabil Med. 2016;59:161–9.
12. Noh MJ, Copeland RO, Yi Y, Choi KB, Meschter C, Hwang S, et al. Pre-clinical studies of retrovirally transduced human chondrocytes expressing transforming growth factor-beta-1 (TG-C). Cytotherapy. 2010;12:384.

12

Functional midterm follow-up comparison of stemless total shoulder prostheses versus conventional stemmed anatomic shoulder prostheses using a 3D-motion-analysis

David M. Spranz, Hendrik Bruttel, Sebastian I. Wolf, Felix Zeifang and Michael W. Maier*

Abstract

Background: The aim of this study is to compare the functional midterm outcome of stemless shoulder prostheses with standard anatomical stemmed shoulder prostheses and to show that the STEMLESS results are comparable to the STEMMED with respect to active maximum range of shoulder motion (ROM) and Constant score (CS).

Methods: Seventeen patients underwent total shoulder arthroplasty (TSA) in 25 shoulder joints. Stemless TSA was performed in 12 shoulder joints (group STEMLESS), third-generation stemmed TSA in 13 shoulder joints (group STEMMED). Functional results were documented using the CS. 3D-motion-analysis using the Heidelberg upper extremity model (HUX) was conducted to measure active maximum (ROM).

Results: The group STEMLESS achieved a CS of 67.9 (SD 12.0) points and the group STEMMED of 70.2 (SD 5.8 points) without significant difference between the groups ($p = 0.925$). The maximum ROM of the group STEMLESS, ascertained by 3-D-motion-analysis, was in forward flexion 125.5° (SD 17.2°), in extension 49.4° (SD 13.8°), in abduction 126.2° (SD 28.5°) and in external rotation 40.3° (SD 13.9°). The maximum ROM of the group STEMMED, also ascertained by 3-D-motion analysis, was in forward flexion 135.0° (SD 16.8°), in extension 47.2° (SD 11.5°), in abduction 136.3° (SD 24.2°) and in external rotation 40.1° (SD 12.2°). The maximum ROM of the STEMLESS group was lower in forward flexion and abduction, higher in extension and almost identical in external rotation. But there was no significant difference (forward flexion $p = 0.174$, extension $p = 0.470$, abduction $p = 0.345$, external rotation $p = 0.978$).

Conclusion: Both types of shoulder prostheses achieve a similar and good active ROM and similar results in CS.

Trial registration: DRKS00013166, retrospectively registered, 11.10.2017

Keywords: Shoulder arthroplasty, Stemless shoulder arthroplasty, Osteoarthritis, 3D motion analysis, HUX Model

Background

As the anatomical TSA has shown quite successful results in reducing pain and improving function when performed in patients with glenohumeral osteoarthritis (OA) and an intact rotator cuff it is the golden standard in surgical treatment. [1, 2]. However, stem-related complications, which include such as bone stock loss, stress shielding, intraoperative and postoperative periprosthetic fractures, mal-positioning of the humeral head component relative to the metaphysis, and in situations of infection difficulty with stem and cement extraction [3–6], have been described in several studies. Therefore, stemless shoulder prostheses, such as the Total Evolution Shoulder System (TESS®; Biomed, France) have been developed to reduce these stem-related complications [3]. Today, different models of stemless TSA are available and increasingly used, but studies about their clinical results are rare [2, 7–11]. The aim of this study is to investigate the clinical

* Correspondence: Michael.Maier@med.uni-heidelberg.de
Clinic for Orthopedics and Trauma Surgery, Heidelberg University Hospital, Schlierbacher Landstraße 200a, D-69118 Heidelberg, Germany

midterm outcome of stemless TSA in comparison with a standard anatomical TSA.

Methods

Seventeen patients (10 female, 7 male) with mean age 72.0 (SD 5.3, range 64-79) years participated in a prospective case series. All patients received a minimum of 3 months of physical therapy (strengthening of the rotator cuff and instruction for self-training) but in the end they suffered from persistent pain.

All participants underwent anatomical TSA. A total of 25 shoulder joints was treated. Two patients were left-handed, 15 patients were right-handed. In 9 cases, only the dominant side was treated, 8 cases were treated bilaterally. Eleven of the participants (5 female, 4 male) with mean age 71.0 (SD 5.4, range 64 - 79) received third-generation stemmed TSA in 13 shoulders (Aequalis Shoulder, Tornier, Lyon, France) with a mean follow-up of 6.3 (SD 2.4, range 3.0 – 11.1) years (group STEMMED). Nine participants (6 female, 5 male) with mean age 74.0 (SD 5.7, range 64-79) received stemless TSA in 12 shoulders (Biomet T.E.S.S., Biomet, Warsaw, USA) with a mean follow-up of 4.3 (SD 1.1, range 2.7 – 6.1) years (group STEMLESS). Inclusion criteria were the diagnosis with primary glenohumeral osteoarthritis with an intact rotator cuff. Exclusion criteria were previous operations at the shoulder and rotator cuff tears. Patients were recruited over a time period of 3.5 months. All patients were operated on by a single surgeon (FZ). By using a deltopectoral approach the subscapularis tendon was detached, the capsular was released and the joint was exposed. In no case a rotator cuff tear was found. A biceps tendon tenodesis was conducted. After the placement of the implants, the subscapularis tendon was reconstructed by using non-absorbable tendon-to-tendon sutures.

To protect the reconstructed subscapularis tendon postoperatively, the operated arm was placed in internal rotation in a shoulder abduction pillow for 4 weeks. The operated shoulder joint was mobilized passively by a physiotherapist with the limitation to 60° of flexion and abduction over a time period of 6 weeks. Patients were requested to support these movements actively. External rotation was strictly prohibited. Free range of motion was allowed 6 weeks postoperatively.

In accordance with the World Medical Association Declaration, the ethics committee of the Heidelberg medical school approved the study protocol. Informed consent was obtained from all individual participants included in the study. All patients were clinically examined to exclude further shoulder pathologies such as shoulder impingement, rotator cuff tear and shoulder instability. Constant Score [12, 13] was obtained for both sides. The Constant Score was used to grade pain (with 0 points indicating severe pain and 15 points indicating no pain), activity of daily living (ADL) (with 0 points indicating no mobility and 20 points indicating full mobility), power (with 0 points indicating 0 kp [0 N] and 25 points indicating 25 kp [110.4 N] and ROM (max. 40 points). Shoulder flexion and abduction were recorded in degrees with a goniometer, whereas external and internal rotation were graded according to landmarks that could be reached by hand. For internal rotation the landmarks were gluteal region, lumbosacral region, 3rd lumbal vertebra, 12th thoracic vertebra and reaching between the scapulas. For external rotation five different positions were tested: Ability to reach over the head, hand on top of the head and hand on the neck both with elbows pointing forward and pointing lateral. The Mann-Whitney-U test was used to search for significant differences.

Afterwards all shoulders were examined via 3D-motion-analysis with an optoelectronic system consisting of 12 infrared cameras (T40-S, Vicon Motion Systems Ltd., Oxford, United Kingdom). All trials were recorded using Vicon Nexus 2 software (Vicon Motion System Ltd., Oxford, United Kingdom). The Heidelberg Upper Extremity Model (HUX) by Rettig et al. [14] was used as a biomechanical model. It used a least-squares method by Gamage and Lasenby [15] to calculate the glenohumeral center of rotation and elbow axis of rotation. Forward flexion/extension and abduction were calculated as projection angles in sagittal and frontal plane respectively. External rotation was calculated as "conjunct rotation" as proposed by Wolf et al. [16]. For reference a coordinate system for the thorax was defined by incisura jugularis, processus xiphoideus, processus spinosus of 7th cervical and 10th thoracic vertebra [14] essentially following the recommendations of the International Society of Biomechanics, which propose using the 8th thoracic vertebra [17]. All angles were calculated by using customized Java software. Subjects were asked to move their arm back and forth between maximum forward flexion and maximum extension with elbow fully extended to assess ROM in sagittal plane. Movements from neutral position to maximum abduction were used to assess ROM in frontal plane. Adduction was not accounted for, as visibility of thorax markers would have been restricted by the upper arm. Rotation was tested by moving arm back and forth between maximum external rotation and hand-to-belly position with elbow flexed by 90°. As it did not resemble maximum internal rotation only external rotation was evaluated. Between one to four repetitions could be evaluated and the maximum achieved position was used. Minimum and maximum values were calculated using Matlab R2015a (The MathWorks Inc., Natick, USA). The Shapiro-Wilk test was used to test for normal distribution. The Levene's test was used to assess equality of variance. The

Mann-Whitney-U test was used for non-normally distributed data. Normally distributed data were analyzed using Student's t-test. *P*-values < 0.05 were considered significant. All statistical analysis was performed in SPSS 23 (International Business Machines Corporation, Armonk, USA).

Results

The group STEMLESS achieved a Constant Score of 67.9 (SD 12.0) points and the group STEMMED of 70.2 (SD 5.8) points without significant difference between the groups ($p = 0.925$) (see Fig. 1). The categories pain, ADL, ROM and power did not show any significant differences either (see Fig. 2 and Table 1).

The maximum ROM of the group STEMLESS, ascertained by 3-D-motion-analysis, was in forward flexion 125.5° (SD 17.2°), in extension 49.4° (SD 13.8°), in abduction 126.2° (SD 28.5°) and in external rotation 40.3° (SD 13.9°) (see Fig. 3 and Table 2).

The maximum ROM of the group STEMMED, also ascertained by 3-D-motion analysis, was in forward flexion 135.0° (SD 16.8°), in extension 47.2° (SD 11.5°), in abduction 136.3° (SD 24.2°) and in external rotation 40.1° (SD 12.2°) (see Fig. 3 and Table 2).

The maximum ROM of the group STEMLESS compared with the group STEMMED was lower in forward flexion and abduction, higher in extension and almost identical in external rotation. But there was no significant difference (forward flexion $p = 0.174$, extension $p = 0.470$, abduction $p = 0.345$, external rotation $p = 0.978$) (see Table 2).

Discussion

It has been shown that the prosthetic anatomic stemmed TSA produces quite successful results in reducing pain and improving function when performed in patients with OA and an intact rotator cuff in the long-term follow up and is therefore the golden standard in the surgical treatment [18]. The Aequalis TSA is an unconstrained third-generation prosthesis with variable medial and posterior offset which replicates the complex shape of the proximal humerus. This type of stemmed TSA has shown excellent results in long-term follow up studies [18, 19].

The restoration of the individual anatomy of the glenohumeral joint with superior reconstruction of the humeral head geometry is an essential factor for postoperative functional results [9]. Possibilities to adjust the position of the head component are limited in stemmed TSA. In case of the stemmed Aequalis prosthesis the inclination can only be modified in steps and the offset of the center of rotation can only be set along a simple eccentric track. Stemless TSA has been performed since 2004 in Europe [11]. The stemless system enables the individual anatomic reconstruction of the center of rotation of the humeral head without any external restraints, e.g. the shaft axis [11]. Moreover stemless TSA might reduce the risk of perioperative bleeding, and the operative time seems to be lower [3, 7, 9, 20]. Furthermore, in case of revision, the integrity of the humeral shaft and neck more easily allows further implants [20].

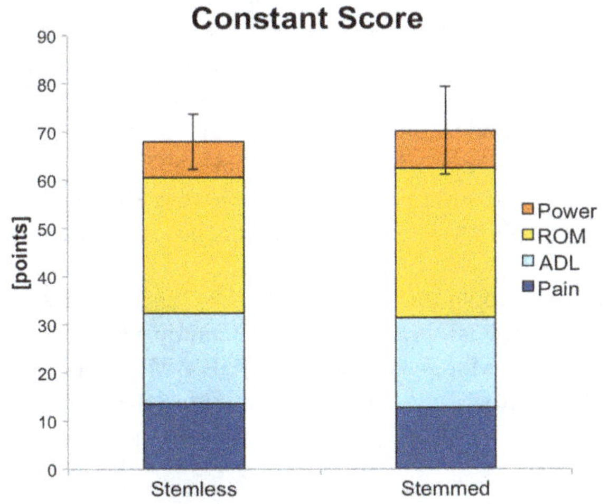

Fig. 1 Postoperative Constant Score of the group STEMLESS and the group STEMMED

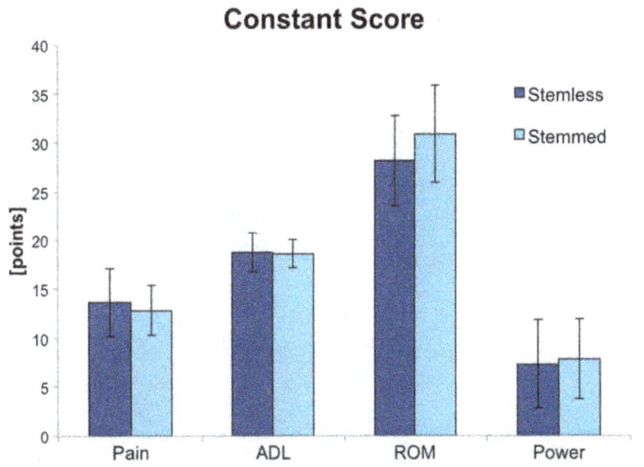

Fig. 2 Postoperative Constant Score categories pain, ADL, ROM, and power of the group STEMLESS and the group STEMMED

Table 1 Postoperative Constant Score of the group STEMLESS and the group STEMMED

	STEMLESS	STEMMED	*p*-value
Pain (/15)	13.7 ± 3.5	12.8 ± 2.5	0.167
ADL (/20)	18.8 ± 2.0	18.6 ± 1.4	0.535
ROM (/40)	28.2 ± 4.6	30.9 ± 4.9	0.283
Power (/25)	7.3 ± 4.5	7.8 ± 4.1	0.543
Total (/100)	67.9 ± 12.0	70.2 ± 5.8	0.925

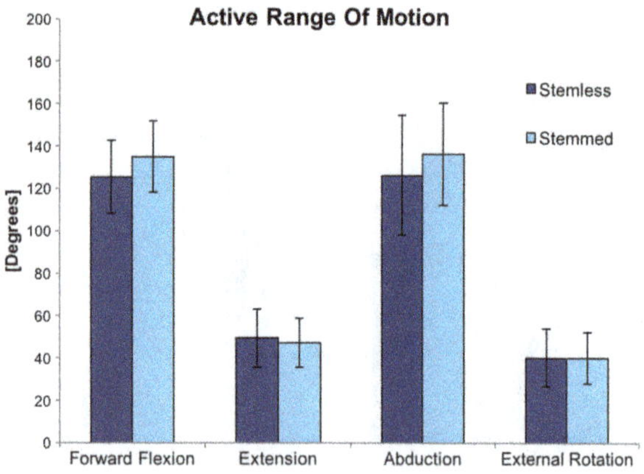

Fig. 3 Postoperative maximum active ROM of the group STEMLESS and the group STEMMED in forward flexion, extension, abduction, and external rotation

The results provided by stemless TSA must be compared with the very good results achieved by using the existing anatomic stemmed TSA concept.

In this study, we have compared the clinical results of patients with primary OA of the shoulder who had been surgically treated with either a standard stemmed TSA or an anatomical stemless TSA.

The aim of this study has been to investigate the clinical midterm outcome of stemless TSA in comparison with a standard anatomical TSA related to the CS and the active ROM.

In our study we have used the HUX-Model, described previously by Rettig et al. [14] and applied in some studies [21–23] to evaluate the maximum range of motion. It promises high objectivity and high intra- and interrater reliability.

Only few studies have reported the clinical results of stemless shoulder arthroplasty in the short-term follow-up. All these studies have used a goniometer.

Schoch et al. [24] once reported early results of 96 stemless TSA with primary OA with a mean follow-up of 13.2 month (± 3.5). The patients achieved significant improvement of the absolute Constant Score from 44 points preoperatively to 66 points at follow up. ROM improved significantly with forward flexion of 145°, abduction of 105° and external rotation of 41° [24]. Huguet et al. [9] reported results of stemless TSA with a mean follow-up of 45 months in 63 patients. The Constant Score increased significantly from 29.6 points preoperatively to 75 points postoperatively. Active forward flexion improved to 145° and external rotation improved to 40°. The author concluded that the early results of stemless TSA improved functional results similar to those of third-generation and fourth-generation stemmed implants [9].

Habermeyer et al. [11] reported results of stemless TSA in midterm follow-up with a mean follow up of 72.9 months. The constant score improved significantly from 38.1 to 75.3 points. Active range of motion, ascertained by using a goniometer, improved significantly for forward flexion (from 114° to 141°), abduction (from 74° to 130°) and external rotation (from 25° to 44°). The author concluded that the functional results of stemless TSA were comparable to third and fourth generation of standard stemmed TSA in midterm follow-up [11].

In accordance with this study we have detected no significant difference in the maximum ROM or in the Constant Score in the midterm follow-up between stemless and stemmed shoulder arthroplasty.

Thus we can compress that the stemless shoulder prosthesis provides very good clinical results in patients with primary OA without the need of a humeral stem.

One limitation of our study was the short duration of our follow-up. Our assessment with a mean follow-up of 4.3 years in the TESS group was too short to detect possible differences in the survivorship of stemless TSA. Further investigations would be necessary to determine the long-term performance of this kind of prosthesis. Another limitation was that some patients included in this study were treated and examined on both sides while others only were treated unilaterally. Although the results can be regarded as the results of independent surgical treatments, patient factors such as postoperative training motivation and compliance, pain perception, handedness and others possibly have an impact on the overall outcome that may influence both shoulders and thus violate the assumption of independence of statistical testing.

But we would like to record the fact that, to our knowledge, there is currently no other study with a longer follow-up. Moreover, using the HUX-Model promises high objectivity and high intra- and interrater reliability.

Table 2 Postoperative maximum active ROM of the group STEMLESS and the group STEMMED in forward flexion, extension, abduction and external rotation

	STEMLESS	STEMMED	*p*
Forward Flexion	125.5 ± 17.2	135.0 ± 16.8	0.174
Extension	49.4 ± 13.8	47.2 ± 11.5	0.470*
Abduction	126.2 ± 28.5	136.3 ± 24.2	0.345
External Rotation	40.3 ± 13.9	40.1 ± 12.2	0.978

*Mann-Whitney-U test was used to assess Extension as Shapiro-Wilk test indicated that data was not normally distributed

Conclusion

Both types of shoulder prostheses achieve similar results for active ROM and CS in the midterm follow-up.

Abbreviations
ADL: Activity of daily living; CS: Constant score; HUX: Heidelberg Upper Extremity Model; OA: Glenohumeral osteoarthritis; ROM: Range of shoulder motion; TSA: Total shoulder arthroplasty

Acknowledgements
We thank the research fund of the Deutsche Arthrose-Hilfe e.V.

Funding
There is no funding source.

Authors' contributions
DS conceived the study and drafted the manuscript. HB performed the statistical analysis. SW participated in the sequence alignment. FZ participated in the sequence alignment. MM participated in the design of the study and ist coordination and helped to draft the manuscript. All authors read and approved the final manuscript.

Competing interests
The authors declare that they have no competing interests.

References

1. Bell SN, Coghlan JA. Short stem shoulder replacement. Int J Shoulder Surg. 2014;8:72–5. doi:10.4103/0973-6042.140113.
2. Maier MW, Lauer S, Klotz MC, Bulhoff M, Spranz D, Zeifang F. Are there differences between stemless and conventional stemmed shoulder prostheses in the treatment of glenohumeral osteoarthritis? BMC Musculoskelet Disord. 2015;16:275. doi:10.1186/s12891-015-0723-y.
3. Churchill RS. Stemless shoulder arthroplasty: current status. J Shoulder Elb Surg. 2014;23:1409–14. doi:10.1016/j.jse.2014.05.005.
4. Bohsali KI, Wirth MA, Rockwood CA Jr. Complications of total shoulder arthroplasty. J Bone Joint Surg Am. 2006;88:2279–92. doi:10.2106/JBJS.F.00125.
5. Chin PY, Sperling JW, Cofield RH, Schleck C. Complications of total shoulder arthroplasty: are they fewer or different? J Shoulder Elb Surg. 2006;15:19–22. doi:10.1016/j.jse.2005.05.005.
6. Farng E, Zingmond D, Krenek L, Soohoo NF. Factors predicting complication rates after primary shoulder arthroplasty. J Shoulder Elb Surg. 2011;20:557–63. doi:10.1016/j.jse.2010.11.005.
7. Berth A, Pap G. Stemless shoulder prosthesis versus conventional anatomic shoulder prosthesis in patients with osteoarthritis: a comparison of the functional outcome after a minimum of two years follow-up. J Orthop Traumatol. 2013;14:31–7. doi:10.1007/s10195-012-0216-9.
8. Geurts GF, van Riet RP, Jansen N, Declercq G. Placement of the stemless humeral component in the Total Evolutive Shoulder System (TESS). Tech Hand Up Extrem Surg. 2010;14:214–7. doi:10.1097/BTH.0b013e3181e397c5.
9. Huguet D, DeClercq G, Rio B, Teissier J, Zipoli B, Group T. Results of a new stemless shoulder prosthesis: radiologic proof of maintained fixation and stability after a minimum of three years' follow-up. J Shoulder Elb Surg. 2010;19:847–52. doi:10.1016/j.jse.2009.12.009.
10. Kadum B, Mafi N, Norberg S, Sayed-Noor AS. Results of the Total Evolutive Shoulder System (TESS): a single-centre study of 56 consecutive patients. Arch Orthop Trauma Surg. 2011;131:1623–9. doi:10.1007/s00402-011-1368-4.
11. Habermeyer P, Lichtenberg S, Tauber M, Magosch P. Midterm results of stemless shoulder arthroplasty: a prospective study. J Shoulder Elb Surg. 2015;24:1463–72. doi:10.1016/j.jse.2015.02.023.
12. Constant CR, Murley AH. A clinical method of functional assessment of the shoulder. Clin Orthop Relat Res. 1987;214:160–4.
13. Constant CR, Gerber C, Emery RJ, Sojbjerg JO, Gohlke F, Boileau P. A review of the constant score: modifications and guidelines for its use. J Shoulder Elb Surg. 2008;17:355–61. doi:10.1016/j.jse.2007.06.022.
14. Rettig O, Fradet L, Kasten P, Raiss P, Wolf SI. A new kinematic model of the upper extremity based on functional joint parameter determination for shoulder and elbow. Gait Posture. 2009;30:469–76. doi:10.1016/j.gaitpost.2009.07.111.
15. Gamage SS, Lasenby J. New least squares solutions for estimating the average centre of rotation and the axis of rotation. J Biomech. 2002;35:87–93.
16. Wolf SI, Fradet L, Rettig O. Conjunct rotation: Codman's paradox revisited. Med Biol Eng Comput. 2009;47:551–6. doi:10.1007/s11517-009-0484-6.
17. Wu G, van der Helm FC, Veeger HE, Makhsous M, Van Roy P, Anglin C, Nagels J, Karduna AR, McQuade K, Wang X, Werner FW, Buchholz B, International Society of B. ISB recommendation on definitions of joint coordinate systems of various joints for the reporting of human joint motion–part II: shoulder, elbow, wrist and hand. J Biomech. 2005;38:981–92.
18. Raiss P, Schmitt M, Bruckner T, Kasten P, Pape G, Loew M, Zeifang F. Results of cemented total shoulder replacement with a minimum follow-up of ten years. J Bone Joint Surg Am. 2012;94:e1711–0. doi:10.2106/JBJS.K.00580.
19. Khan A, Bunker TD, Kitson JB. Clinical and radiological follow-up of the Aequalis third-generation cemented total shoulder replacement: a minimum ten-year study. J Bone Joint Surg Br. 2009;91:1594–600. doi:10.1302/0301-620X.91B12.22139.
20. Mariotti U, Motta P, Stucchi A, Ponti di Sant'Angelo F. Stemmed versus stemless total shoulder arthroplasty: a preliminary report and short-term results. Musculoskelet Surg. 2014;98:195–200. doi:10.1007/s12306-014-0312-5.
21. Kasten P, Maier M, Wendy P, Rettig O, Raiss P, Wolf S, Loew M. Can shoulder arthroplasty restore the range of motion in activities of daily living? A prospective 3D video motion analysis study. J Shoulder Elb Surg. 2010;19:59–65. doi:10.1016/j.jse.2009.10.012.
22. Rettig O, Maier MW, Gantz S, Raiss P, Zeifang F, Wolf SI. Does the reverse shoulder prosthesis medialize the center of rotation in the glenohumeral joint? Gait Posture. 2013;37:29–31. doi:10.1016/j.gaitpost.2012.04.019.
23. Maier MW, Niklasch M, Dreher T, Wolf SI, Zeifang F, Loew M, Kasten P. Proprioception 3 years after shoulder arthroplasty in 3D motion analysis: a prospective study. Arch Orthop Trauma Surg. 2012;132:1003–10. doi:10.1007/s00402-012-1495-6.
24. Schoch CHJ, Aghajev E, Bauer G, Mauch F. Die metaphysär verankerte Prothese beimposttraumatischer und primärer Omarthrose. Obere Extremität. 2011;4:275–81.

13

The effectiveness of interventions aimed at increasing physical activity in adults with persistent musculoskeletal pain

Joanne Marley[1,4], Mark A. Tully[2,3*], Alison Porter-Armstrong[1], Brendan Bunting[1], John O'Hanlon[4], Lou Atkins[5], Sarah Howes[1] and Suzanne M. McDonough[1,3,6]

Abstract

Background: Individuals with persistent musculoskeletal pain (PMP) have an increased risk of developing co-morbid health conditions and for early-mortality compared to those without pain. Despite irrefutable evidence supporting the role of physical activity in reducing these risks; there has been limited synthesis of the evidence, potentially impacting the optimisation of these forms of interventions. This review examines the effectiveness of interventions in improving levels of physical activity and the components of these interventions.

Methods: Randomised and quasi-randomised controlled trials were included in this review. The following databases were searched from inception to March 2016: CENTRAL in the Cochrane Library, Cochrane Database of Systematic Reviews (CDSR), MEDLINE, Embase, CINAHL, PsycINFO and AMED. Two reviewers independently screened citations, assessed eligibility, extracted data, assessed risk of bias and coded intervention content using the behaviour change taxonomy (BCTTv1) of 93 hierarchically clustered techniques. GRADE was used to rate the quality of the evidence.

Results: The full text of 276 articles were assessed for eligibility, twenty studies involving 3441 participants were included in the review. Across the studies the mean number of BCTs coded was eight (range 0–16); with 'goal setting' and 'instruction on how to perform the behaviour' most frequently coded. For measures of subjective physical activity: interventions were ineffective in the short term, based on very low quality evidence; had a small effect in the medium term based on low quality evidence (SMD 0.25, 95% CI 0.01 to 0.48) and had a small effect in the longer term (SMD 0.21 95% CI 0.08 to 0.33) based on moderate quality evidence. For measures of objective physical activity: interventions were ineffective - based on very low to low quality evidence.

Conclusions: There is some evidence supporting the effectiveness of interventions in improving subjectively measured physical activity however, the evidence is mostly based on low quality studies and the effects are small. Given the quality of the evidence, further research is likely/very likely to have an important impact on our confidence in effect estimates and is likely to change the estimates. Future studies should provide details on intervention components and incorporate objective measures of physical activity.

Keywords: Physical activity, Low back pain, Osteoarthritis, Musculoskeletal pain, Chronic pain, Persistent pain, Behaviour change techniques, Systematic review

* Correspondence: m.tully@qub.ac.uk; http://go.qub.ac.uk
[2]Centre for Public Health, Queens University Belfast, Royal Victoria Hospital, Grosvenor Road, Belfast BT12 6BA, UK
[3]UKCRC Centre of Excellence for Public Health (Northern Ireland), Centre for Public Health, School of Medicine, Dentistry and Biomedical Sciences, Queens University Belfast Room 02020, Institute of Clinical Science B, Royal Victoria Hospital, Grosvenor Road, Belfast, BT 12 6BJ, UK
Full list of author information is available at the end of the article

Background

Epidemiological studies suggest one in five people across Europe suffer from persistent pain [1, 2]. Most persistent pain arises from musculoskeletal disorders, such as low back pain and osteoarthritis; both of which are considered leading causes of disability, worldwide [3]. It can be expected that with aging populations, the health, economic, and social problems associated with these conditions are likely to rise [1, 2, 4]. In addition to causing considerable disability, persistent musculoskeletal pain (PMP) also increases an individual's risk of developing other health conditions including; depression, obesity, heart disease [5–7], cancer [8] and indeed early mortality [7–9]. Despite this, efforts to address these broader health implications of PMP are somewhat lacking.

Description of the intervention

Clinical guidelines widely endorse exercise and/or physical activity (PA) in the management of PMP [10–17]. This is largely due to the positive impact these interventions can have on reducing pain and disability. However, improving levels of PA can lead to broader health benefits: with even small changes in PA levels leading to substantial health gains [18, 19].

PA can be defined as any movement produced by skeletal muscles resulting in energy expenditure, it occurs across several domains including: social and domestic activities, commuting, recreational and leisure activities [20]. PA may or may not include exercise: exercise is a subset of PA tending to be planned, structured or repetitive [20] with a specific purpose such as improving strength, it has been recommended that the terms PA and exercise are not confused [21].

How the intervention might work

Improving levels of PA requires behaviour change. Behaviour change interventions are coordinated sets of activities designed to change specified patterns of behaviour [22]. Behaviour change techniques (BCTs) are the components of interventions that effect change [23]. Taxonomies of BCTs have been used to describe intervention content in a number of PA behaviour change interventions [24–28]. Across these interventions and in line with NICE recommendations for individual level behaviour change [29], some consistent techniques appear to be associated with effective interventions e.g. self-monitoring behaviour, providing feedback, and goal setting.

Why it is important to do this review

PA and exercise interventions are often recommended in the management of PMP as they can have a positive effect on pain and disability levels. However, the extent to which these interventions actually result in changes to behaviour and consequently increased levels of physical activity is less clear. Although individual studies have demonstrated it is possible to increase PA levels in those with back pain [30] or osteoarthritis [31, 32], the results of systematic reviews are conflicting and limited. In adults with osteoarthritis a systematic review concluded that self-management programmes achieve small improvements in subjectively measured PA in the short-term [32]: whereas, a review of PA interventions in adults with PMP reported no improvements in objectively measured PA [33]. Furthermore, the BCTs used within these forms of interventions and the relationship if any, to outcomes has not yet been systematically explored.

Objectives

This systematic review investigated the effectiveness of any form of intervention with a clear aim of increasing PA in adults with PMP. Possible associations between BCTs or intervention characteristics and intervention effects were also investigated.

The objectives of this review are to:

1. Determine the effectiveness of interventions in increasing PA levels in adults with PMP.
2. Identify BCTs used within interventions.
3. Determine if particular BCTs or other intervention characteristics (intensity, recruitment route, type of PA, etc.) are associated with greater effect sizes.

Methods

The full protocol for this review has been published [34].

Population

Randomised and quasi-randomised controlled trials in adults (≥18) with PMP (pain lasting ≥3 months), in the axial skeleton or large peripheral joints were included. We excluded studies focusing on fibromyalgia, inflammatory and/or autoimmune disorders and perioperative patients, which may require a different management strategy.

Types of interventions

All interventions that had a clear aim of increasing PA in adults with PMP were eligible for inclusion. We excluded site specific rehabilitative exercise interventions unless it was clear the intervention also addressed habitual PA. We included trials with a comparative control group and trials with multiple intervention arms. We did not include population or community-wide interventions.

Types of outcome measures

The primary outcome of interest was PA measured by self-reported or objective measures; questionnaires, recall diaries, pedometers or actigraphy. Measurements of adherence or attendance at classes alone, were not sufficient. The secondary outcome of interest was adverse incidents.

Search methods for identification of studies

Search strategies were developed for each electronic database and were based on the initial Medical Literature Analysis and Retrieval System Online (MEDLINE) strategy (Additional file 1). We searched the Cochrane Central Register of Controlled Trials (CENTRAL) in the Cochrane Library, the Cochrane Database of Systematic Reviews (CDSR) in the Cochrane Library, Ovid MEDLINE(R) Daily Update, Ovid MEDLINE(R), Ovid MEDLINE (R) - includes new records, not yet fully indexed, Ovid Embase, EBSCO Cumulative Index to Nursing and Allied Health Literature (CINAHL), Ovid PsycINFO, AMED (Allied and Complementary Medicine). All databases were searched from inception to March 2016.

Reference lists of systematic reviews and articles retrieved from the search were scanned for additional references.

Data collection and analysis

Selection of studies

Results from the searches were imported into EndNote (X7) bibliographic software (Thomson Reuters, Philadelphia, PA, USA) and duplicates removed. Titles and abstracts obtained from the search were independently screened by two authors (JM 100%, MAT 70% and SMcD 30%). Articles not meeting the inclusion criteria and outside the scope of the review were removed. Full text reports of the remaining publications were retrieved. Two review authors (JM, SMcD) used a standardised form tested prior to use, to select trials eligible for inclusion. Non-English papers were assessed and, where necessary, translated in part or in full.

Data extraction and management

Data was extracted independently by two reviewers (JM, SMcD) using a customised form tested prior to use. Relevant data was extracted for methodological issues, intervention characteristics, study design, study characteristics and adverse events. Intervention content was coded according to the BCTTv1 [35]. Two coders (JM, SH) independently coded BCTs, inter-rater reliability was assessed using the prevalence-adjusted bias-adjusted Kappa (PABAK) statistic [36]. PABAK adjusted for the high frequency of agreement on absent BCTs. Values of 0.60–0.79 indicated 'substantial' reliability and 0.80 and above 'outstanding' reliability [37].

Assessment of risk of bias in included studies

Two reviewers (JM, SMcD) independently assessed studies for risk of bias (ROB), using the Cochrane risk of bias tool [38]. An additional domain was added to determine if studies were adequately powered. For cluster randomised controlled trials, five additional domains were assessed, as recommended by Cochrane (16.3.2) [38].

Quality of the evidence

The Grading of Recommendations, Assessment, Development and Evaluation (GRADE) approach was used to interpret and evaluate the quality of the evidence [39, 40]. The methods and recommendations described in the Cochrane handbook [38] and by the GRADE working group [33] were used to assess the quality of a body of evidence using five domains: risk of bias, inconsistency, indirectness of evidence, imprecision of effect estimates and potential publication bias. Data for each outcome was entered into GRADEpro to create 'Summary of Findings' table and footnotes were used to justify all decisions on the downgrading of the quality of the evidence.

The definitions described by the GRADE working group were used to grade the quality of evidence as follows:

- High – Further research is very unlikely to change our confidence in the estimate of effect.
- Moderate – Further research is likely to have an important impace on our confidence in the estimate of effect and may change the estimate.
- Low – Further research is very likely to have an important impact on our confidence in the estimate of effect and is likely to change the estimate.
- Very low – Any estimate of effect is very uncertain.

Measures of treatment effect

Continuous outcomes were analysed using post intervention measures, we reported effect sizes using the standardised mean difference (SMD) as outcomes were reported across different scales. For comparisons of the results we categorised studies into effect sizes according to Cohen's classification; SMD; $0.2 < 0.3$ as small, 0.3–0.8 as moderate, >0.8 as large [41]. *P*-values of <0.05 and confidence intervals that excluded null values were considered statistically significant.

Unit of analysis issues

Where studies involved multiple intervention groups we followed recommendations suggested by the Cochrane collaboration (16.5.4) [38] by combining similar intervention groups to perform a single pairwise comparison.

Where studies reported PA domains separately or reported more than one PA outcome, data were extracted for each, however, for the effect size analysis, measures of overall PA were given preference, if these were not available leisure time PA was given preference'.

To facilitate exploration of results not suitable for quantitative synthesis we grouped studies by effect size using an aggregate of subjective and objective measures (objective measures given preference to subjective where available) at the post intervention time point.

Dealing with missing data

Attempts were made to contact original investigators to request missing data.

The frequency and duration of the intervention was used to calculate an estimated overall intervention contact time 'intensity'. The calculation was based on the full intervention being delivered as planned. If the duration of a session was not reported or the data was unobtainable from authors, we allocated 20 min for telephone follow up and 45 min for face to face interventions.

Assessment of heterogeneity

Diversity across the studies was qualitatively assessed in terms of the intervention, participant demographics, outcome measures and follow-up. Data was assessed for statistical heterogeneity using RevMan version 5.3 using the I^2 statistic, values of I^2 ranging from 30% to 60% were considered to represent moderate heterogeneity and 50% to 90% substantial heterogeneity [38].

Data synthesis

Separate meta-analyses were completed for subjective and objective outcome data at three time points; short term (not longer than 12 weeks' post-randomisation), medium term (not longer than 6 months' post randomisation) and long term (greater than 6 months post randomisation). Outcomes were analysed using the SMD, with the inverse variance method to calculate the overall effect and standard error, a random effects model was applied to incorporate heterogeneity.

Subgroup analysis and investigation of heterogeneity

We performed the following pre-specified subgroup analysis:

- Clinical subgroups: classified as 'persistent low back pain' and 'osteoarthritis'
- Frequency and duration of intervention (intensity) classified as 'higher' or 'lower' relative to the median number of contact hours across the studies

The following subgroups were planned but not conducted as the data generated was deemed insufficient.

- BCTs
- Recruitment routes

Descriptive statistics were therefore used to explore possible associations between these factors and other intervention characteristics and intervention effects.

Sensitivity analysis

A sensitivity analysis was performed to check if excluding studies with a higher ROB affected results. The threshold for sensitivity analysis was set for studies meeting at least 50% of the criteria of the ROB assessment, excluding blinding of participants and providers.

Results

Results of the search

The electronic searches returned 18,953 records, (Fig. 1) after de-duplication in the referencing software, 11,323 title and abstracts were screened against the inclusion criteria. In total 276 records were identified as potentially relevant, and the full text reports were retrieved. Twenty-six studies were initially agreed for inclusion; six studies were subsequently found to contain unusable

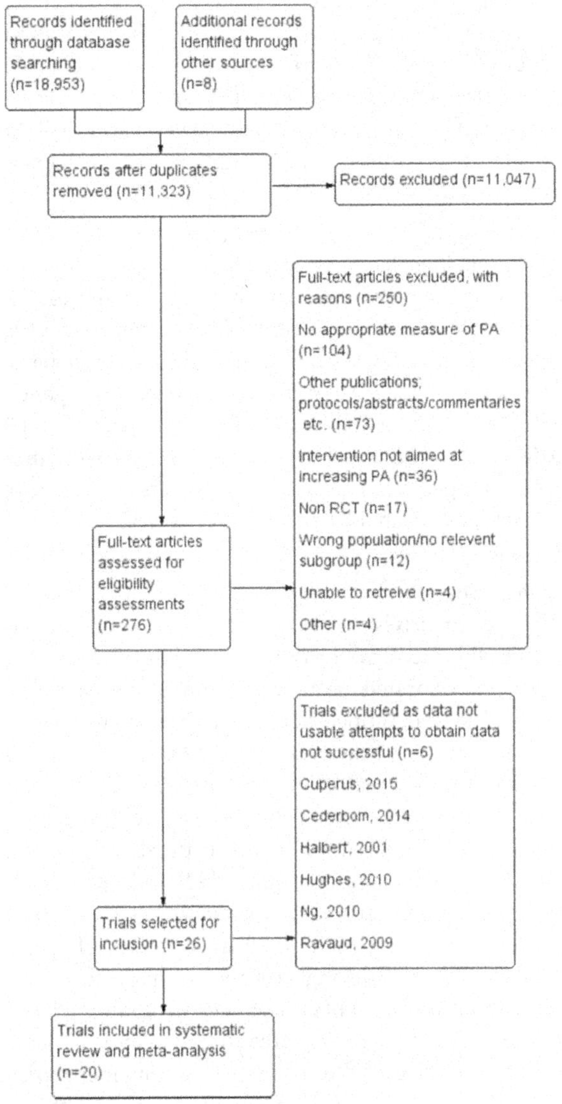

Fig. 1 Study Flow Diagram

outcome data, requests to obtain the data were not successful (Fig. 1). Twenty studies had sufficient data to be included in a meta-analysis [30–32, 42–58]. Nine authors were contacted regarding studies that were deemed to have potentially usable data; six replied, four authors provided the information needed to include their study [43, 44, 52, 58].

Eight non-English language studies were translated but none were eligible for inclusion.

Excluded studies

A total of ($n = 250$) studies were excluded from the review. Exclusions were most often due to no or unacceptable measures of PA and studies having no clear aim of increasing PA (Fig. 1).

Characteristics of included studies

Ten studies were described as randomised controlled trials (RCTs), three were cluster RCTs [43, 44, 55], five feasibility or pilot RCTs [30, 32, 48, 51, 56] and one was a controlled clinical trial [42]. Sullivan et al. [57] reported a one year follow-up of patients who had participated in an RCT [59]. The maximum number of groups within studies was three, [44, 46, 47, 52].

Participants in included studies

The studies involved 3441 suitable participants (4875 in total) (Table 1), over half were female (approx. 59.2%). Thirteen studies focused on osteoarthritis (1874 participants; $n = 7$ knee, $n = 5$ hip and/or knee, $n = 1$ generalised) and seven on persistent low back pain ($n = 1567$ participants). The mean age of participants with osteoarthritis ranged from 61 to 73.8 years, and for persistent low back pain from 40.4 years to 51.9 years.

Interventions

Table 2 summarises modes of delivery, intervention content, provider and intensity for each intervention. Most studies incorporated more than one mode of delivery but have been described according to what was considered the 'primary' delivery mode. Most interventions were provided by healthcare professionals (12/20), other providers included exercise and fitness professionals and a counsellor. Intervention contact times ranged from <1 h for a educational pamphlet [32] to approximately 200 h of contact time [46] occurring over a twelve month intervention. The median number of contact hours was 8.3 h. Walking was the most common form of PA, followed by multicomponent programmes utilising a mixture of aerobic, strengthening and/or general flexibility exercises. All of the interventions incorporated some form of educative component relating to the role of PA in managing PMP.

A total of 160 BCTs (mean per study 8, range 0–16) were coded across the 20 studies (Table 2). The most frequently coded techniques were 'goal setting (behaviour)' and 'instruction on how to perform the behaviour' (65%) followed by 'behavioural practice/rehearsal' and 'self-monitoring of the behaviour' (55%). A mean PABAK score of (0.9) indicated outstanding agreement on identification of BCTs.

Control groups

The content of control groups varied (Table 1); seven studies referred to control groups as 'treatment as usual' or some form of 'standard care' [30, 43, 49, 52, 55–57]. Two studies [45, 58] used waiting list control groups. A clinical guideline posted to GP's was used as a control in the study by Becker et al. [44]. Pamphlets were used as a control in the study by Brosseau et al. [46] and a copy of the 'Arthritis Help book' was given to controls in the study by Hughes et al. [50]. Two studies used self-management programmes in their intervention, but provided it as a stand-alone intervention for controls; [31, 47]. Two studies directly compared two forms of back rehabilitation programmes of varying intensity and content [42, 54]. In the study by Williams et al. [32] the control booklet content differed to the intervention booklet. Krein et al. [53] provided controls with an uploading pedometer and reminder emails to upload data but not access to the web-based intervention, available to the intervention group. In two studies [48, 51] in addition to exercise classes, intervention groups received additional intervention components.

Outcome measures

Across the 20 studies 13 scales or tools for measuring PA were identified (Table 1) twelve studies reported subjective PA; five objective PA and three reported both. Self-reported measures of PA included estimates of total PA and estimates of frequency, intensity and time in different domains of activity. Only two tools were used in more than one study; the International Physical Activity Questionnaire, [32, 51, 52], and the Freiburg Questionnaire of PA, [44, 54]. Objective measures of PA included steps per day or total PA and/or time in different intensities of PA, measured by accelerometers and/or pedometers.

Follow-up (post randomisation) (Table 1)

The longest follow up was 18 months [46] six months after a twelve month intervention. Eleven studies reported outcomes at 12 months [42–45, 48, 50, 52–54, 56, 57] however, the latter two studies involved interventions that lasted the 12 months. Four studies reported outcomes at 6 months [30, 31, 51, 58] and one at 3 months [32]. One study had only post-intervention

Table 1 Characteristics of included studies ($n = 20$)

Author/Year	Study Design	No of Participants	Gender	Age Range	Condition	Intervention	Control Condition	Recruitment Route	PA Outcome	Longest follow-up
Alaranta, 1994 [42]	Controlled Clinical Trial	293	F160 M133	40.4 (4.8) Control 40.5 (4.6) Intervention	PLBP	Home training programme + Inpatient rehabilitation with education	Inpatient rehabilitation 40–50% less strenuous	Finnish Social Security Insurance Institution	Subjective - Leisure time PA (strenuousness)	12 months
Allen, 2016 [43];	Cluster RCT	300 (patients) 30 (providers)	F28 M272	61.6 (9.2)	OA hip/knee	Patients - Physical activity and weight management counselling Healthcare providers received treatment recommendations	Usual care	Medical records veterans affairs	CHAMPS	12 months (12 month intervention)
Becker, 2008 [44];	Cluster RCT	1378 (chronic pain subgroup 332)	F801 M577 (entire group no figures for subgroup)	49.1 (13.3) guideline group 47.4 (13.5) guideline + MC 50.2 (14.3) Control	LBP (mixed)	Practitioner education – guideline implementation Practitioner education – guideline implementation + MI	Guideline delivered via post	Primary Care GP's	Freiburg Questionnaire	12 months
Bossen, 2013 [45];	RCT	199	F129 M70	64 (6.6) All 61 (5.9) Intervention 63 (5.4) Control	OA hip/knee	Web based intervention to increase PA using behavioural graded activity	Waiting list	Volunteers from newspapers and websites	PASE and Subgroup ACTi graph	12 months
Brosseau, 2012; [46];	RCT	222	153F 69M	63.9 (103) Walking 63.9 (8.2) Walking + Booklet 62.3 (6.8) Control	OA Knee	Walking group Walking and behavioural education	Self-directed received educational pamphlet	Unclear	7 day Par (recall)	18 months
Farr, 2010;[47];	RCT	293	F218 M75	55.5 (7.3) Resistance training 55.8 (6.1) Self-Management 54.2 (7.3) Combined	OA Knee	Resistance training + self-management	Self-management	General community mass mailings, media ads and local physicians	ACTi graph 7 days	9 months
Focht, 2014;[48];	RCT (pilot)	80	F67 M13	63.5 (6.86)	OA Knee	Group mediated cognitive behavioural exercise intervention	Traditional centre based exercise	Direct referral State Medical Centre Rheumatologists, ads Arthritis Foundation groups	Accelerometer (PA Lifecorder plus) 7 days	12 months
Hiyama, 2012;[49];	RCT	40	32F 19M	71.9 (5.2) Walking 73.8 (5.7) Control	OA Knee	Instructed to increase number of steps, physical therapy + programme of walking	Physical therapy + advice re walking	Unclear - community dwelling females	Pedometer (steps per day)	4 weeks
Hughes, 2006;[50]	RCT (block randomisation)	215	363F 56M	71.1 (59 -91 yrs)	OA hip/knee	Education, exercise and fitness walking	Arthritis self-help book and information on exercise programmes in community	Senior centres, newsletters, local media, presentations to senior groups	Total minutes exercised	12 months

Table 1 Characteristics of included studies ($n = 20$) *(Continued)*

Author/Year	Study Design	No of Participants	Gender	Age Range	Condition	Intervention	Control Condition	Recruitment Route	PA Outcome	Longest follow-up
Hunter, 2012;[51];	RCT (feasibility)	51	167F M79	43.2 (13.5) Exercise 42.4 (11.3) Exercise Auricular Acupuncture	PLBP	Exercise and acupuncture	Exercise	Primary Care GP's, Physiotherapy waiting list and University population	IPAQ (ActivPal - steps per day)	6 months
Hurley, 2015:[52]:	RCT	246	40F	45.4 (11.4)	PLBP	Walking programme Exercise class	Usual physiotherapy	Physiotherapy departments	IPAQ	12 months
Krien, 2013;[53];	RCT	229	29F 200M	51.2 (12.5) Walking 51.9 (12.8) Enhanced Usual Care	PLBP	Walking group	Enhanced usual care	Individuals referred for back class and medical record system	Pedometer (steps per day)	12 months
McDonough, 2013; [30];	RCT (feasibility)	56	31F 25M	51 (42 – 60 yrs) Exercise 48 (43 – 55 yrs) Exercise Walking Programme	PLBP	Education and advice and walking group	Usual care	Physiotherapy waiting lists primary care	MGROC PA (ActivPal - steps per day)	6 months
Meng, 2011;[54];	RCT	360	231F 129M	50.2 (7.6) Intervention 49.5 (7.7) Control	PLBP	Biopsychosocial back school programme (inpatient)	Traditional back school (setting unclear)	Orthopaedic hospital - patients had applied for inpatient rehabilitation	Freiburger Questionnaire	12 months
Pisters, 2010 [55]	RCT Cluster (analysis of secondary outcomes)	200	F154 M46	64.8 (7.9)	OA Hip or Knee	Behavioural graded activity and operant conditioning and exercise therapy	Usual physiotherapy (per clinical guidelines)	Physiotherapists and press releases in local newspapers	PA SQUASH - Converted using METs total hrs. Per week in health enhancing PA	65 weeks (14.9 months)
Schlenk, 2011;[56];	RCT (feasibility)	26	F25 M1	63.2 (9.8)	OA Knee (overweight)	Counselling, exercise, fitness walking programme	Usual care	Rheumatology practices, arthritis disease network registry, self-referral	Diary - Minutes walked per week and other aerobic PA minutes	12 months
Sullivan, 1998;[57];	RCT (follow-up)	102 (52 in this follow-up)	F85 M17 (f44 m8)	70.38 (9.11) Intervention 68.48 (11.32) Control	OA Knee	Supervised fitness walking and supportive education	Standard medical care, weekly interviews about function and daily activity	Community clinics, private clinics - rheumatology	Recall - Average distance walked per week	12 months
Talbot, 2003;[31];	RCT	34	F26 M8	69.59 (6.74) Pedometer 70.76 (4.71) Education	OA Knee	Arthritis self-management programme + walking programme	Arthritis self-management programme	Senior Centres and ads in local papers	Pedometer (steps per day) + Accelerometer	6 months
Trudeau, 2015;[58];	RCT	228 (Subgroup 94)	F72 M156	49.9 (11.6)	Arthritis (all – subgroup data OA spine, large	Web-based painAction programme, informative articles, self-check assessments etc.	Waiting list control	Flyers in surgeries, Pain association members, google adwords,	Aerobic exercise minutes (all)	6 months

Table 1 Characteristics of included studies ($n = 20$) *(Continued)*

Author/Year	Study Design	No of Participants	Gender	Age Range	Condition	Intervention	Control Condition	Recruitment Route	PA Outcome	Longest follow-up
					peripheral joints via author)			ClinicalTrials.gov. PainEDU.org health professionals		
Williams, 2011 [32]	RCT (feasibility)	119	F76 M43	68.2 (8.1) Intervention 68.6 (8.5) control	OA Hip or Knee	'New' Advice booklet – emphasis on addressing exercise related beliefs	Arthritis UK booklet	GP Practices	IPAQ	3 months

PA Physical Activity, *MI* Motivational Interviewing, *IPAQ* International physical activity questionnaire, *MGROC* Modified global rating of change (physical activity), *SQUASH* Short questionnaire to assess health enhancing physical activity, *PASE* Physical activity scale for elderly, *7 day PAR* 7-day physical activity recall, *CHAMPS* Community healthy activities model programme for seniors, *OA* Osteoarthritis, *LBP* Low back pain, *PLBP* Persistent low back pain, *RCT* Randomised controlled trial

Table 2 Interventions, quality assessment, BCTs - studies grouped post intervention using aggregated outcome measures

Author, Year	Hiyama, 2012;	Hughes, 2006;	Alaranta, 1994;	Focht, 2014;	Pisters, 2010;	Farr, 2010;	Allen, 2016;	Meng, 2011;	Becker, 2008;	Sullivan, 1998;
Effect Size SMD 95% CI	1.96 [1.19, 2.73]	0.87 [0.58, 1.15]	0.77 [0.53, 1.01]	0.56 [0.07, 1.06]	0.51 [0.21, 0.80]	0.29 [−0.03, 0.61]	0.28 [0.04, 0.53]	0.25 [0.02, 0.48]	0.17 [−0.07, 0.41]	0.12 [−0.50, 0.74]
ROB assessment	Lower	Higher	Higher	Lower	Lower	Higher	Lower	Lower	Higher	Higher
Mode of delivery										
Automated Web-based										
Inpatient Programme			x					x		
Centre-based	x	x		x	x	x				x
Home-based		+	+	x	x					
Community-based										
Other							x		x	
Session structure										
Individual	?	+	+		x	x	x	x	x	+
Group based		x	x	x		x		x		x
Type of PA										
Multicomponent Exercise Programme		x	x	x		x		x		
Walking	x	x		x						x
User Selected					x		x		x	
Other/Unclear							x		x	
Provider										
Physiotherapist	x	x			x					x
Nurse									x	
Doctor									x	
Fitness Professional				x		x				
Multidisciplinary			x					x		
Other						? SM	?			
Estimated Intervention Contact Time (hrs)	3	36	111	36	11.5	134	6	50	1.5	24
No. of BCT's coded	3	12	3	16	9	5	16	1	0	6

+ to a lesser extent, ? unclear from study description,/not explicit, *SM* self-management, *WP* walking programme, *EC* exercise class., *SMD* standardised mean difference, *CI* confidence intervals, *ROB* risk of bias (meeting at least 50% of domains assessed, excluding blinding participants and providers)

Table 2 Interventions, quality assessment, BCTs - studies grouped post intervention using aggregated outcome measures *(Continued)*

Author, Year	Williams, 2011;	Brosseau, 2012;	Trudeau, 2015;	Hunter, 2012;	Bossen, 2013;	Schlenk, 2011;	McDonough, 2013;	Krien, 2013;	Hurley, 2015;	Talbot, 2003;
Effect Size SMD 95% CI	0.11 [−0.31, 0.53]	0.10 [−0.27, 0.48]	0.07 [−0.35, 0.49]	0.06 [−0.60, 0.72]	0.02 [−0.50, 0.54]	−0.00 [−0.77, 0.77]	−0.00 [−0.74, 0.73]	−0.03 [−0.35, 0.30]	−0.29 [−0.59, 0.01]	−0.32 [−1.0, 0.35]
ROB assessment	Lower	Lower	Lower	Lower	Lower	Lower	Lower	Lower	Lower	Higher
Mode of delivery										
Automated Web-based			x		x			x		
Inpatient Programme										
Centre-based				x		x			x	
Home-based							x		x	x
Community-based		x								
Other	x									
Session structure										
Individual		x				x	x		x (WP)	x
Group based		x		x					x (EC)	x
Type of PA										
Multicomponent Exercise Programme				x		x			x (EC)	
Walking		x				x	x	x	x (WP)	x
User Selected	x				x					
Other/Unclear	x		x							
Provider										
Physiotherapist				x		x	x	+	x	
Nurse						x				x
Doctor										
Fitness Professional		x								
Multidisciplinary										
Other	x		x		x			x		
Estimated Intervention Contact Time (hrs)	0.5	200.5	4.3	8	1.166	7.5	3.5	8.6	8	12.15
No. of BCT's coded	2	14	5	7	12	10	11	8	15	5

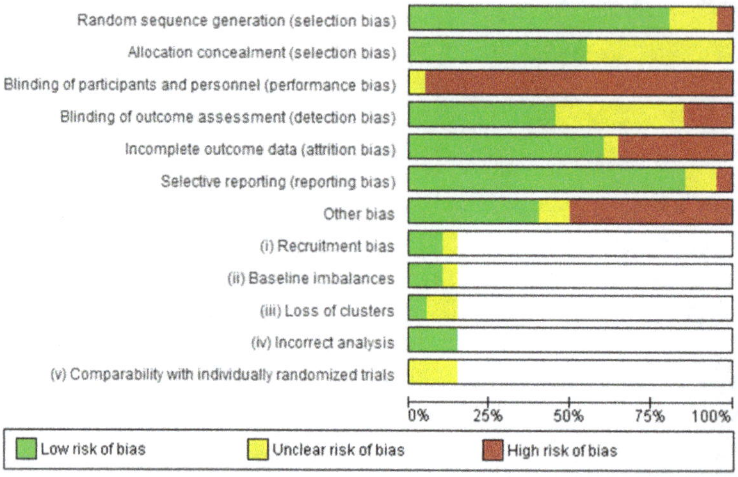

Fig. 2 Risk of bias summary of all studies assessed using Cochrane risk of bias tool

outcomes at four weeks [49] and one study reported outcomes at nine months [47]. Pisters et al. [55] reported outcomes at 65 weeks, the intervention duration was described as 12 weeks however booster sessions were provided to participants up until week 55.

Risk of bias in included studies (Figs. 2 and 3)

The ROB in the included studies is summarised in Figs. 2 and 3. Blinding, inadequately powered studies and attrition bias were considered the greatest ROB in the included studies. Due to the difficultly in blinding participants and providers in PA interventions, the risk of performance bias was considered high in all but one study which involved posting an intervention or control pamphlet to participants [32], the review authors felt there was insufficient information in the report to support a judgement of high or low ROB for this study. The majority of studies included in the review were not sufficiently powered, only nine reported conducting a power calculation for their primary outcome [32, 43–45, 48, 52–55]. Only two studies [45, 55] conducted power calculations for PA outcomes. Attrition bias was considered high in just over one third of the included studies (35%).

Risk of bias in cluster randomised controlled trials

Three studies utilised cluster RCTs [43, 44, 55], summarised in (Figs. 2 and 3). Two studies [43, 55] were judged to be of unclear ROB in relation to loss of clusters, this was due to the loss of clusters not being reported or discussed in the analysis or results. ROB on comparability with individually randomised trials was unclear in all three studies, this was largely due to a lack of reporting of comparability or the influence of clustering on intervention effects.

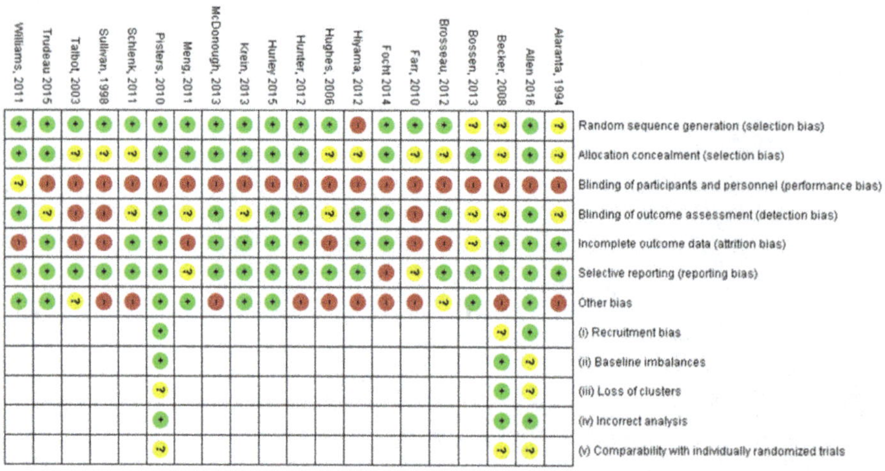

Fig. 3 Risk of bias in individual studies

Effects of interventions: Meta-analysis

Meta-Analysis 1: Effects of Intervention versus control on subjectively measured PA.

Fifteen studies reported continuous measures of subjective self-reported PA [30, 32, 42–46, 50–52, 54–58].

Short term: no longer than 12 weeks post randomisation.

Nine studies (1096 participants) reported short term subjective PA outcomes (Fig. 4) [30, 32, 42, 45, 50–52, 57, 58]. Based on very low quality evidence the pooled effects of the interventions showed no demonstrable effect (SMD 0.24, 95% CI -0.07, 0.55). The quality of the evidence was downgraded from high to very low quality due to substantial statistical heterogeneity ($I^2 = 83\%$), wide confidence intervals around the effect estimate and ROB (Table 3).

Medium term: greater than 3 months, not more than 6 months post randomisation.

Nine studies (1309 participants) reported medium term measures (Fig. 4) [30, 44, 50–52, 54–56, 58]. Based on low quality evidence the pooled effects of the studies at the medium term was significant with a small effect size (SMD 0.25, 95% CI 0.01, 0.48). The quality of the evidence was downgraded from high due to the substantial heterogeneity in the observed effects ($I^2 = 72\%$) and weighting of studies at high ROB included in the analysis (Table 3).

Long term: greater than 6 months post randomisation.

Eleven studies (1872 participants) reported long term follow-up measures (Fig. 4) [42–46, 50, 52, 54–57]. Based on moderate quality evidence the pooled effects were small and statistically significant (SMD 0.21, 95% CI 0.08, 0.33) heterogeneity was moderate in the observed effects ($I^2 = 40\%$). The quality of the evidence was downgraded from high to moderate due to the

Study or Subgroup	Experimental Mean	Experimental SD	Experimental Total	Control Mean	Control SD	Control Total	Weight	Std. Mean Difference IV, Random, 95% CI
1.1.1 Short-term								
Alaranta, 1994	6.744	1.098	149	5.768	1.417	138	13.0%	0.77 [0.53, 1.01]
Bossen, 2013	162	157.63	85	163	120.5423	79	12.4%	-0.01 [-0.31, 0.30]
Hughes, 2006	248.89	150.45	83	126.67	128.66	55	11.9%	0.85 [0.50, 1.21]
Hunter, 2012	3,638.571	4,542.823	21	2,608.46	3,439.95	25	9.4%	0.25 [-0.33, 0.84]
Hurley 2015	1,799.81	1,968.47	126	2,369.89	1,961.46	65	12.4%	-0.29 [-0.59, 0.01]
McDonough, 2013	1.92	3.0849	39	0.94	2.509	17	9.5%	0.33 [-0.24, 0.90]
Sullivan, 1998	6.97	11.87	21	5.83	5.08	19	9.0%	0.12 [-0.50, 0.74]
Trudeau 2015	124.43	95.285	44	131.86	118.904	43	11.2%	-0.07 [-0.49, 0.35]
Williams, 2011	4,859	6,763	43	3,904	4,285	44	11.2%	0.17 [-0.25, 0.59]
Subtotal (95% CI)			**611**			**485**	**100.0%**	**0.24 [-0.07, 0.55]**
Heterogeneity: Tau² = 0.18; Chi² = 46.41, df = 8 (P < 0.00001); I² = 83%								
Test for overall effect: Z = 1.53 (P = 0.12)								
1.1.2 Medium-term								
Becker, 2008	35.87	28.15	205	30.98	27.978	100	14.5%	0.17 [-0.07, 0.41]
Hughes, 2006	214.46	174.11	74	104.66	117.33	44	11.7%	0.70 [0.32, 1.09]
Hunter, 2012	2,952.171	3,367.502	19	2,042.04	2,537.59	24	7.9%	0.30 [-0.30, 0.91]
Hurley 2015	1,534.32	2,259.46	126	2,403.87	2,242.38	65	13.3%	-0.38 [-0.69, -0.08]
McDonough, 2013	1.95	3.1774	39	0	3.3064	17	8.3%	0.60 [0.02, 1.18]
Meng, 2011	10.77	6.57	151	9.21	6.04	145	14.7%	0.25 [0.02, 0.48]
Pisters, 2010	5.6	2.2	90	4.2	2.8	102	13.5%	0.55 [0.26, 0.84]
Schlenk, 2011	99.5	125.2	11	99.9	229.2	10	5.2%	-0.00 [-0.86, 0.85]
Trudeau 2015	153.21	141.317	42	144	119.932	45	11.0%	0.07 [-0.35, 0.49]
Subtotal (95% CI)			**757**			**552**	**100.0%**	**0.25 [0.01, 0.48]**
Heterogeneity: Tau² = 0.08; Chi² = 29.07, df = 8 (P = 0.0003); I² = 72%								
Test for overall effect: Z = 2.08 (P = 0.04)								
1.1.3 Long-term								
Alaranta, 1994	5.955	1.595	149	5.529	1.546	138	13.4%	0.27 [0.04, 0.50]
Allen 2016	16.11	11.36	132	13.1	9.79	131	12.9%	0.28 [0.04, 0.53]
Becker, 2008	48.64	43.832	196	42.009	34.417	97	12.8%	0.16 [-0.08, 0.41]
Bossen, 2013	174	103.59	74	153	118.2951	71	9.3%	0.19 [-0.14, 0.51]
Brosseau, 2012	19.08	17.453	76	24.18	25.59	33	6.8%	-0.25 [-0.66, 0.16]
Hughes, 2006	210.52	153.18	58	115.65	122.67	32	6.1%	0.66 [0.21, 1.10]
Hurley 2015	2,306.28	2,754.85	117	1,972.15	2,742.11	59	9.8%	0.12 [-0.19, 0.43]
Meng, 2011	8.88	5.95	147	8.73	5.7	122	13.0%	0.03 [-0.21, 0.27]
Pisters, 2010	5	2.6	87	3.6	2.9	92	10.4%	0.51 [0.21, 0.80]
Schlenk, 2011	141.3	131.4	11	96.4	152	10	2.0%	0.30 [-0.56, 1.17]
Sullivan, 1998	4.06	6.34	21	4.29	3.6	19	3.5%	-0.04 [-0.66, 0.58]
Subtotal (95% CI)			**1068**			**804**	**100.0%**	**0.21 [0.08, 0.33]**
Heterogeneity: Tau² = 0.02; Chi² = 16.57, df = 10 (P = 0.08); I² = 40%								
Test for overall effect: Z = 3.20 (P = 0.001)								

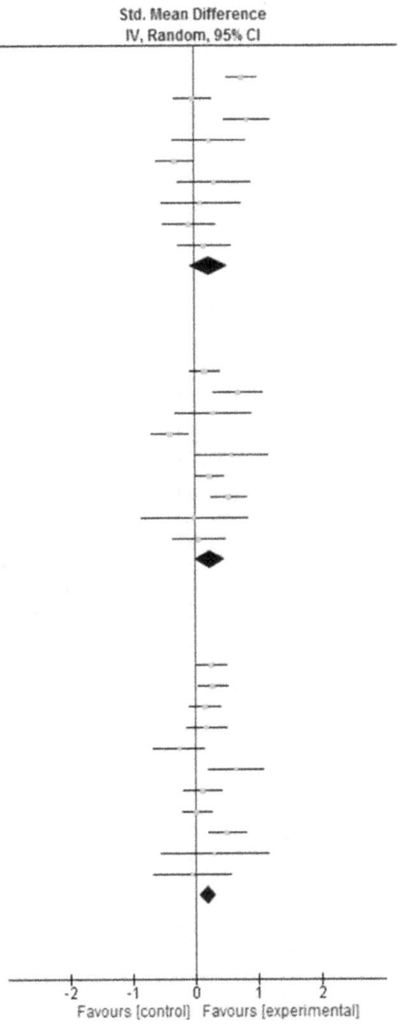

Fig. 4 Forest plot of comparison: 1 Effects of intervention versus control on subjectively measured physical activity: short-term, medium-term and long-term

Table 3 Summary of quality of evidence using the GRADE approach

Quality assessment							№ of patients		Effect	Quality
№ of studies	Study design	Risk of bias (a)	Inconsistency (b)	Indirectness (c)	Imprecision (d)	Other considerations (e)	Interventions	control	Absolute(95% CI)	
Short-term Subjective Physical Activity										
9	randomised trials	serious	serious	not serious	serious	none	611	485	SMD 0.24 SD higher (−0.07 lower to 0.55 higher)	⊕○○○VERY LOW
Medium-Term Subjective Physical Activity (follow up: range 12 weeks to 6 months)										
9	randomised trials	serious	serious	not serious	not serious	none	757	552	SMD 0.25 SD higher (0.01 higher to 0.48 higher)	⊕⊕○○LOW
Long-Term Subjective Physical Activity (follow up: >6 months)										
11	randomised trials	serious	not serious	not serious	not serious	none	1068	804	SMD 0.21 SD higher (0.08 higher to 0.33 higher)	⊕⊕⊕○MODERATE
Short-Term Objective Physical Activity										
7	randomised trials	serious	serious	not serious	serious	none	255	186	SMD 0.31 SD higher (−0.11 lower to 0.74 higher)	⊕○○○VERY LOW
Medium-Term Objective Physical Activity (follow up: range 12 weeks to 6 months)										
4	randomised trials	not serious	not serious	not serious	very serious	none	135	110	SMD −0.02 SD lower (−0.40 lower to 0.36 higher)	⊕⊕○○LOW
Long-Term Objective Physical Activity (follow up: range 6+ months)										
4	randomised trials	serious	not serious	not serious	serious	none	251	184	SMD 0.22 SD higher (−0.02 lower to 0.46 higher)	⊕⊕○○LOW

CI Confidence interval, *SMD* Standardised mean difference

a. Risk of Bias – Using weighting shown in RevMan analysis a serious downgrade is applied where 25% or more of the results are derived from studies judged to be at high risk of bias (see methods for details), a very serious downgrade is applied where 50% of weighting is derived from studies at high risk of bias

b. Inconsistency – a serious downgrade was applied if there is substantial statistical heterogeneity indicated by an (I^2) of 50 to 90%. A very serious downgrade is applied if there was substantial heterogeneity and there was inconsistency arising from the populations, interventions or outcomes

c. Indirectness – a serious downgrade is applied if there was indirectness in one of population, intervention, comparator or outcome. A very serious downgrade was applied if there was indirectness in more than one area

d. Imprecision –a serious downgrade is applied when the total population size is less than 400 (provided there is more than one study). Or, if the 95% CI includes 0 (no effect) or the upper and lower confidence interval cross an effect size (SMD) of 0.5 in either direction. A very serious downgrade is applied where there is a small population and imprecision of the effect estimate

e. Where there was sufficient papers (10) a funnel plot was prepared and inspected, a serious downgrade was applied if this suggested a publication bias

weighting applied to studies judged as high ROB in the analysis (Table 3).

Meta-analysis 2: Effects of intervention versus control on objectively measured PA

Eight studies reported objective measures of PA [30, 31, 45, 47–49, 51, 53].

Short term: no longer than 12 weeks post randomisation.

Seven studies (441 participants) reported short term measures (Fig. 5, Table 3) [30, 31, 45, 47–49, 51]. Based on very low quality evidence, the pooled effect was positive but not significant (SMD 0.31, 95% CI -0.11, 0.74) with substantial heterogeneity ($I^2 = 76\%$). The quality of the evidence was downgraded from high to very low due to wide confidence intervals in the effect estimates and the weighting applied to studies judged as high ROB in the analysis (Table 3).

Medium term: greater than 3 months, not more than 6 months' post randomisation.

Four studies (245 participants) reported medium term measures (Fig. 5) [30, 31, 51, 53]. Based on low quality evidence, the pooled effect was negative (SMD -0.02, 95% CI -0.40, 0.36) with moderate heterogeneity in the observed effects ($I^2 = 41\%$). The quality of the evidence was downgraded due to the small number of participants included in the analysis and wide confidence intervals that included no effect.

Long term: greater than 6 months post randomisation.

Four studies (435 participants) reported long term follow-up measures (Fig. 5) [45, 47, 48, 53]. Based on low quality evidence, the pooled effect was positive but not significant (SMD 0.22, 95% CI -0.02, 0.46) with low heterogeneity in the observed effects ($I^2 = 29\%$). The quality of the evidence was downgraded from high to low due to imprecision of the effect estimates as evidenced by the confidence intervals included no effect and the weighting applied in the analysis to studies at high ROB.

Sensitivity analysis

We examined the pooled effects for the two types of outcomes (subjective and objective) at each time point by an assessment of the ROB. When limited to studies with a lower ROB, effect sizes were not significant at any timepoint.

Subgroup Analyses: To increase statistical power for the planned subgroup analysis we used subjective measures of PA ($n = 16$ studies).

Subgroup analysis 1: Clinical conditions osteoarthritis and low back pain:

Effects were demonstrated for the osteoarthritis subgroup only, effects sizes were moderate in the medium-term (SMD 0.41, 95% CI 0.10, 0.72) and small in the longer term (SMD 0.29, 95%CI 0.08, 0.49).

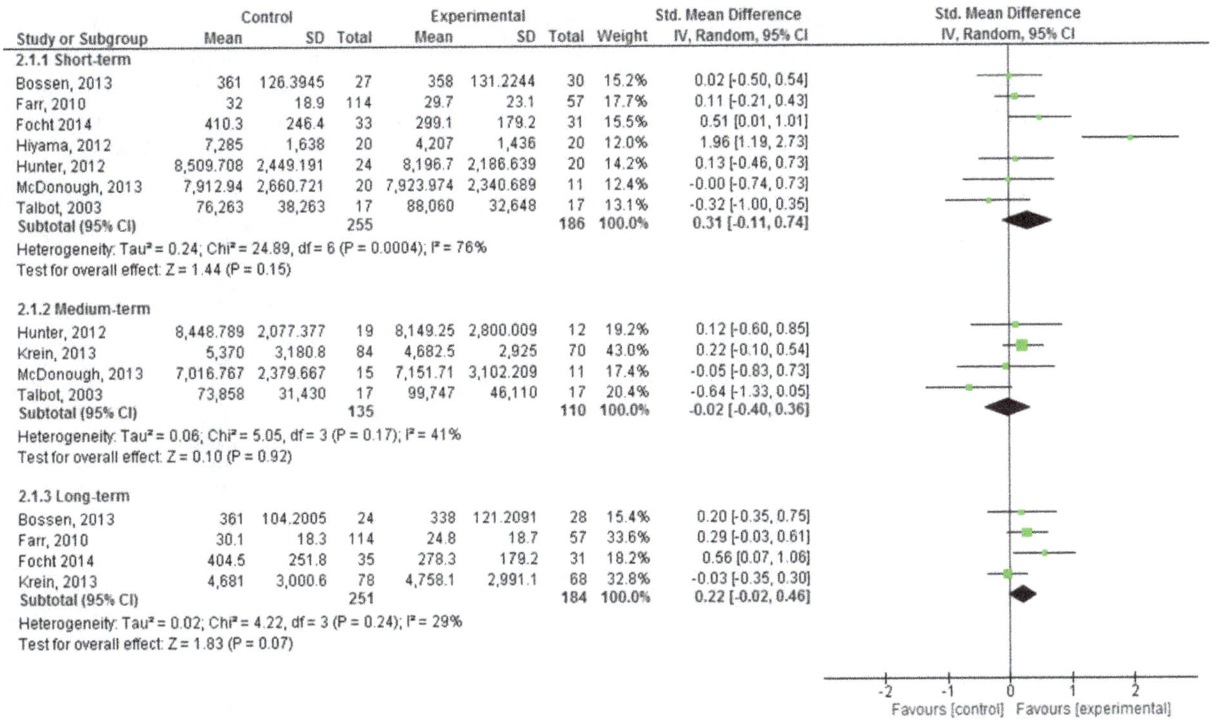

Fig. 5 Forest plot of comparison: 2 Effects of intervention versus control on objectively measured physical activity: short-term, medium term and long-term

Subgroup analysis 2: Intervention Intensity:

Only interventions that were of higher intensity, relative to the median calculated contact hours of the interventions (8.3 h) reached important effect sizes (seven studies). Higher intensity interventions resulted in moderate effect sizes for short term (SMD 0.66 95% CI 0.41, 0.91) and medium term (SMD 0.47 95% CI 0.20, 0.74) outcomes, and small effect sizes for longer term outcomes (SMD 0.25 95% CI 0.02, 0.48).

Influence of BCTS and recruitment route

It was not possible to conduct the quantitative subgroup analysis of BCTs and recruitment routes as the data generated from the review was not sufficient to permit valid comparisons. Descriptive statistics were used to describe possible associations between these factors and other intervention characteristics. To facilitate this exploration, all studies were grouped by effect size, post intervention (Fig. 6).

Behaviour change techniques

Seven studies demonstrated statistically significant small to large effect sizes on post intervention PA (Table 2). Across these studies, 60 BCTs were coded with a mean of 8.57 per study, range (1–16). In total 28 unique BCTs were identified, the most commonly coded were 'goal setting behaviour', and 'instruction on how to perform the behaviour' featuring in 71.4% of studies. 'Self-monitoring behaviour', 'social support (unspecified)', and 'framing/reframing' were also coded frequently and were present in over half of the included studies (57%).

Thirteen studies demonstrated no effect, or negligible effects (<0.2) post intervention (Table 2). Across these studies 100 BCTs were coded with a mean of 7.7 per study, range (0–15) with 31 unique BCTs present. The most commonly coded BCTs were; 'goal setting behaviour', 'information on health consequences' 'instruction on how to perform the behaviour' and 'behavioural practice/rehearsal' which featured in 61.5% of the studies.

Recruitment route and other intervention characteristics: (Tables 1and 2)

No notable differences were observed with regards to the influence of recruitment route, type of PA, mode of delivery and post-intervention effect sizes.

In seven studies demonstrating positive effects, five (71.4%) were delivered by healthcare professionals (2 multidisciplinary and 3 by physiotherapists). In comparison, studies with no effect (<0.2) were less frequently delivered by healthcare professionals (53.8%).

Secondary outcomes

Adverse incidents

Only six studies made explicit statements regarding adverse incidents; two studies, although not explicitly stated, documented adverse incidents. Allen et al. [43] reported four adverse incidents unrelated to the intervention; one study [51] reported no adverse incidents related to the exercise components. Relatively minor musculoskeletal complaints were reported in three studies [30, 52, 53]. Allergic reactions to pedometer clips [30] and minor cardiovascular events [53] were also reported. One author [52] noted that half of the participants in a walking group who developed increases in musculoskeletal complaints withdrew from the study. A fall resulting in a hip fracture sustained during a session was reported in one study [57] and three withdrawals due to increasing back pain were reported [42].

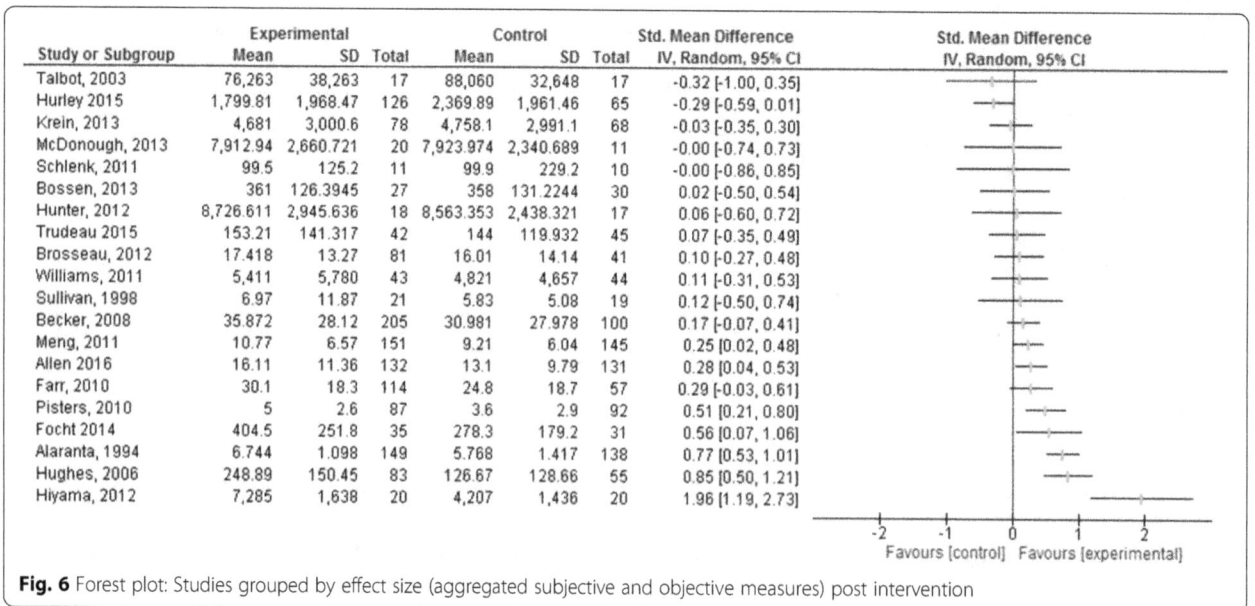

	Experimental			Control			Std. Mean Difference
Study or Subgroup	Mean	SD	Total	Mean	SD	Total	IV, Random, 95% CI
Talbot, 2003	76,263	38,263	17	88,060	32,648	17	-0.32 [-1.00, 0.35]
Hurley 2015	1,799.81	1,968.47	126	2,369.89	1,961.46	65	-0.29 [-0.59, 0.01]
Krein, 2013	4,681	3,000.6	78	4,758.1	2,991.1	68	-0.03 [-0.35, 0.30]
McDonough, 2013	7,912.94	2,660.721	20	7,923.974	2,340.689	11	-0.00 [-0.74, 0.73]
Schlenk, 2011	99.5	125.2	11	99.9	229.2	10	-0.00 [-0.86, 0.85]
Bossen, 2013	361	126.3945	27	358	131.2244	30	0.02 [-0.50, 0.54]
Hunter, 2012	8,726.611	2,945.636	18	8,563.353	2,438.321	17	0.06 [-0.60, 0.72]
Trudeau 2015	153.21	141.317	42	144	119.932	45	0.07 [-0.35, 0.49]
Brosseau, 2012	17.418	13.27	81	16.01	14.14	41	0.10 [-0.27, 0.48]
Williams, 2011	5,411	5,780	43	4,821	4,657	44	0.11 [-0.31, 0.53]
Sullivan, 1998	6.97	11.87	21	5.83	5.08	19	0.12 [-0.50, 0.74]
Becker, 2008	35.872	28.12	205	30.981	27.978	100	0.17 [-0.07, 0.41]
Meng, 2011	10.77	6.57	151	9.21	6.04	145	0.25 [0.02, 0.48]
Allen 2016	16.11	11.36	132	13.1	9.79	131	0.28 [0.04, 0.53]
Farr, 2010	30.1	18.3	114	24.8	18.7	57	0.29 [-0.03, 0.61]
Pisters, 2010	5	2.6	87	3.6	2.9	92	0.51 [0.21, 0.80]
Focht 2014	404.5	251.8	35	278.3	179.2	31	0.56 [0.07, 1.06]
Alaranta, 1994	6.744	1.098	149	5.768	1.417	138	0.77 [0.53, 1.01]
Hughes, 2006	248.89	150.45	83	126.67	128.66	55	0.85 [0.50, 1.21]
Hiyama, 2012	7,285	1,638	20	4,207	1,436	20	1.96 [1.19, 2.73]

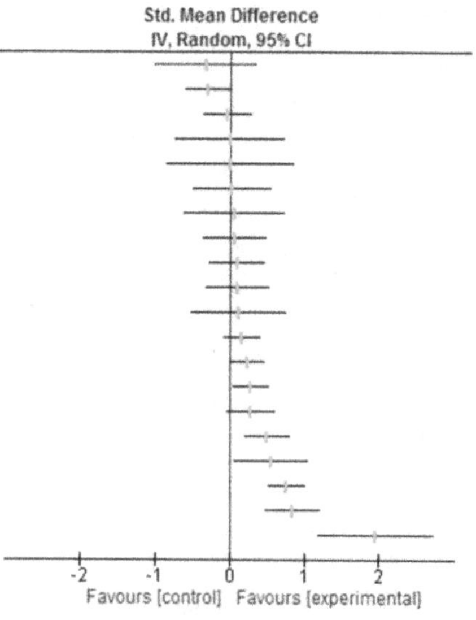

Fig. 6 Forest plot: Studies grouped by effect size (aggregated subjective and objective measures) post intervention

Discussion

Summary of findings

This is the first systematic review and meta-analysis examining the effectiveness of interventions in improving subjective and/or objective levels of PA in adults with PMP and possible associations between BCTs and other intervention characteristics on effect sizes.

In builds on the findings of two similar reviews; Williamson et al. [60] who assessed the effectiveness of behavioural PA interventions in participants with lower-limb osteoarthritis, and Oliveira et al. [33] who assessed the effectiveness of interventions in increasing objectively measured PA in chronic musculoskeletal pain. In contrast to the latter study this review makes a clear distinction between therapeutic exercise programmes and interventions specifically aimed at increasing PA levels or 'habitual PA behaviours'.

With respect to subjective PA, interventions were ineffective in the short term (up to 12 weeks, very low quality evidence); or had a small effect medium term (3–6 months: SMD 0.25, 95%CI 0.01 to 0.48, low quality evidence) and long term (SMD 0.21 95% CI 0.08 to 0.33, moderate evidence). Given the quality of the evidence further research is likely or very likely to have an important impact on our confidence in the estimate of effect and is likely to change the estimate. Analysis of the evidence for objective outcomes showed that interventions were not effective at any time point. These observations were based on very low to low quality evidence therefore the estimate of effect is very uncertain and further research is very likely to change the estimate.

Subgroup analyses indicated that interventions were more effective in improving PA levels in adults with osteoarthritis compared to those with persistent low back pain. Intervention effects were also consistently higher in interventions with a greater number of contact hours (> 8.3 h). These subgroup analyses should be interpreted with caution; as differences may not relate to their classifications. However, subgrouping participants by condition was clinically plausible and intervention intensity has previously been associated with effectiveness.

Comparison of subjective outcomes with published literature

Two reviews examining long term outcomes of PA interventions: a Cochrane review of face-to-face interventions to promote PA [61] and a systematic review of PA interventions for adults aged 55–70 years [62]: both reported significant, but very small effects (SMD 0.19) at 12 months. Similarly, this review found small effects for outcomes measured beyond six months (SMD 0.21 95% CI 0.08, 0.33). These findings may indicate that individuals with pain respond to PA interventions in a similar manner to non-pain populations.

In a subgroup analysis Williamson et al. [60] found intervention effects were greatest between 6 and 12 months (SMD 0.53, 95% CI 0.41 to 0.65) and that the effectiveness of interventions declined over time, reporting no significant benefit compared to controls in outcomes beyond 12 months. Similarly, in our osteoarthritis sub-group we found a moderate effect size for medium term outcomes (>3 months ≤6 months) (SMD 0.41, 95% CI 0.10, 0.72) that diminished over time (>6 months) (SMD 0.29, 95% CI 0.08, 0.49). These findings may suggest that individuals with osteoarthritis make changes to their PA levels gradually. However, without ongoing support or increased efforts directed towards maintenance of PA, individuals with osteoarthritis may struggle to sustain increased levels of PA.

Comparison of objective outcomes with published literature

In line with our own findings of no detectable effect on objectively measured PA, Oliveira et al. [33] also found no effect on short, intermediate or long term objective outcomes. Williamson et al. [60] were unable to conduct a meta-analysis using objective measures due to a lack of studies reporting objective measures. In contrast to our findings, the review of interventions aimed at increasing PA in adults aged 55 to 70 years, found larger effects for objective measures (steps per day) (SMD 1.08; 95%CI 0.16, 1.99) at 12 months [62]. A possible explanation for this difference could be that the participants included in this review by Hobbs et al. [62] were essentially 'healthy populations' in contrast, our review and that of Williamson et al. [60] and Oliveira et al. [33] all involved participants with PMP.

Intervention characteristics

We found interventions with a higher number of contact hours resulted in greater effect sizes. Similarly in a post hoc meta-regression, Williamson et al. [60] also found, that a higher number of contact hours had a significant influence on intervention effectiveness. In contrast Hobbs et al. [62] found less intensive interventions were more effective than higher intensity interventions. A plausible explanation for these contrasting findings, is that those with PMP may need additional interventional support, in order to successfully change their PA behaviours in comparison to healthy populations.

In this review the influence of BCTs on PA outcomes is unclear but the findings are consistent with those of previous reviews. Bishop et al. [63] published a review and meta-analysis exploring the effects of contextual and BCT content of control and target interventions in 42 trials included in a Cochrane review of interventions to improve adherence to exercise for chronic musculoskeletal pain [64]. In keeping with the findings from our review, among the most frequently coded BCT's were 'instruction on how to perform the behaviour' and 'behavioural practice and rehearsal'. A finding also reported by Keogh et al. [65] who reviewed BCTs utilised in chronic low back pain self-management programmes. We found 'self-monitoring of the behaviour' was amongst the most frequently coded techniques in interventions with greater effect sizes, a finding not replicated in the either the Bishop et al. [63] or the Keogh et al. [65] reviews, but consistent to findings of PA reviews in healthy populations [24], older adults [66], and in obese adults [28]. As our review was more narrowly focused on habitual PA as opposed to adherence to exercise or self-management, this finding (although tentative) lends some support to the evidence that this technique may be particularly useful in PA interventions.

Interventions included in this review were generally multifaceted often involving several modes of delivery with varying degrees of complexity. It was difficult to draw firm conclusions regarding which characteristics of interventions are associated with more effective interventions.

Few studies provided explicit statements regarding adverse incidents; where they were reported they were largely limited to minor musculoskeletal complaints. Although risk of adverse incidents in PA interventions is generally regarded as low; it is plausible that exacerbating pain may have a deleterious effect on participation, particularly in those with PMP.

Completeness and quality of the evidence

The quality of the evidence within this review ranged from moderate to very low across the different timepoints and outcomes. Effect sizes at best are small and limited to subjective measures. Key limiting factors leading to downgrading the quality of the evidence were, ROB, statistical heterogeneity in the observed effects and imprecision as evidenced by wide confidence intervals. With respect to ROB many studies were designed to identify changes in pain and function/disability as their primary outcomes and were thus underpowered to detect changes in physical activity levels; as such the results of this review should be interpreted with caution. Furthermore, a number of studies failed to provide adequate detail regarding blinding of outcome assessors and allocation concealment. In cluster randomised controlled trials it was often unclear if authors had considered the effect of trial design and the influence clustering may have had on results and whether this was considered when comparing effects with other trials.

Whilst the use of validated measures of PA, was in itself a strength, a more standardised approach to reporting PA data would have permitted a more robust statistical analysis, strengthening the evidence. Self-report measures are known to be prone to recall bias: it has been suggested that as both the intervention and control groups complete the measure any misclassification should be non-differential [67]. However, it could be argued, that using self-report measures in interventions where participants and providers are also unlikely to be blinded the potential of recall bias is increased. Only three studies included subjective and objective measures; this approach might be considered ideal given the relative strengths and limitations of each.

Descriptions of intervention content varied greatly impacting on the number of BCTs that could be reliably reported as occurring within an intervention. In this review we only coded BCTs clearly delivered to the participants and directed towards the target behaviour. As reported by others, [24, 63] this approach, although more rigorous, may result in less BCTs being coded than were actually delivered.

The variation noted across the control conditions could have influenced effect-estimates with smaller between group effects associated with comparisons against more active control treatments [68]. However, we did not detect this when reviewing individual effect size comparisons.

Six studies initially assessed as suitable for inclusion did not report means, standard deviations or sample sizes and requests to obtain this data from study authors were unsuccessful; this data could have added to the quality of the evidence in this review.

Study participants were largely recruited from primary or secondary care (General Practitioners, physiotherapy clinics): it is very possible that the effects seen in those recruited via these settings, differ to those accessing for example, specialist pain services.

Potential biases in the review process

Studies were primarily excluded from the review because a suitable measure of PA was not reported. This may reflect a selective reporting bias; however, it is suggested this is more likely to reflect the changing emphasis of healthcare interventions, particularly the drive towards self-management and a public health approach to managing long term conditions. Although databases were searched from inception only two studies included in the review were published prior to 2003 [42, 57].

Conclusions

Implications for practice

Based on the findings of this review it is not possible to conclude which characteristics of interventions are more effective. However, based on observational analysis and in line with findings of previous reviews, integration of behavioural techniques such as; 'self-monitoring of the behaviour', 'instruction on how to perform the behaviour' and 'goal setting (behaviour)' may be indicated. Higher intensity interventions - in terms of the estimated contact time with the intervention, may be more effective than less intensive interventions.

The emphasis of PA and exercise interventions in PMP has largely been directed at reducing pain and disability. However, these interventions may have little impact on the overall level of PA an individual engages. Targeted behaviour change interventions are likely to be required to address the risk of morbidity and mortality in this population.

Implications for research

Persistent pain, like many other non-communicable diseases is influenced by several determinants of health such as; socioeconomic status, education, employment and mental health [69]. There is a need for future studies to adopt methods to encourage and secure participation from individuals representing the broad spectrum of persistent pain patients. In particular, those accessing specialist pain services were under represented in this review. Individuals accessing specialist pain services are often deemed to be on the more severe end of the pain spectrum and typically report much higher levels of disability and poorer health related quality of life scores [2]. We agree with previous suggestions [70] that health inequalities may actually be increased because of differences in responses to recruitment. A clear finding from this review is the need to standardise the measurement of PA in PMP populations.

To improve the quality of evidence, future studies should be sufficiently powered, collect longer term follow up data and report on cost-effectiveness. Study authors should report methods for blinding outcome assessors clearly. Providing access to supplementary data such may improve the quality of coding and reporting of intervention content. Future reviews should consider incorporating meta-regression or moderator analysis to explore if specific components or characteristics of interventions are associated with more effective interventions.

Differences between published protocol and review

The review authors reappraised the decision to include unpublished studies and included only those that had been published.

Study authors were amended: SH was added to review team and coded intervention content. LA was added to the review team and provided expert input on aspects relating to coding of BCTs.

The review team agreed to limit the extraction of secondary outcomes to adverse incidents relating to the intervention. There were two main reasons; firstly, to maintain the focus and specificity of the review. Secondly a number of systematic reviews have recently been published describing many of the secondary measures; pain, disability and function, it was felt that extracting these outcomes would be of little additional value to readers of the review.

ROB: The validity of the PA outcome measure is not added as an additional domain within the ROB. This data was included in the data extraction forms and is discussed in relation to outcome measures. An additional domain of sample size calculation for the primary outcome (not specifically for PA) was added to the ROB table and a priori agreements were made during piloting of the ROB table with regards to agreed cut-offs for attrition bias.

The GRADE approach was adopted post-protocol to rate the quality of evidence generated within the review process.

Abbreviations

BCT: Behaviour change technique; GRADE: Grading of recommendations, assessment, development and evaluations; PA: Physical Activity; PABAK: Prevalence-adjusted bias-adjusted Kappa; PMP: Persistent musculoskeletal pain; RCT: Randomised controlled trials; ROB: Risk of bias; SMD: Standardised mean difference

Acknowledgements

The authors would like to express their gratitude to Miss Mary Rose Holman, subject librarian at Ulster University, for her help in developing the search strategies and Dr. Ian Bradbury, Frontier Science, Scotland for comments and advice on statistical analysis and assessing risk of bias in cluster randomized trials.

Funding

This research was funded by the Public Health Agency, HSC R&D Division through a Doctoral Fellowship awarded to JM.
SMcD and MAT are co-funded by the UKCRC Centre of Excellence for Public Health (Northern Ireland), a UKCRC Public Health Research Centre of Excellence. Funding from the British Heart Foundation, Cancer Research UK, Economic and Social Research Council, Medical Research Council, Research and Development Office for the Northern Ireland Health and Social Services, and the Wellcome Trust, under the auspices of the UK Clinical Research Collaboration, is gratefully acknowledged.

Authors' contributions

JM: conception and design of study, developed initial search strategy, collected background data, completed title and abstract screening, ROB assessments and statistical analysis, prepared first draft of manuscript. SMcD: conception and design of study, refinement of search strategy, reviewing drafts, inputting on methodology, title and abstract screening, ROB assessments, and intellectual content. MAT: refining search strategy, title and abstract screening, BCT coding advice, critical revisions, reviewing methodology and intellectual content. BB: provided input on methodology and statistical analysis. APA: refining search strategy and inputting on methodology. SH: completed dual coding of BCTs. LA: completed critical reviews and inputted on aspects of the review pertaining to BCTs. JO'H: inputted on the design of the study, provided content expertise from a clinical perspective. All authors critically reviewed the manuscript and approved the final version submitted for publication.

Competing interests

The authors declare no competing interests, two authors of this review are authors of studies included in the review (SMcD and MAT).

Author details
[1]Centre for Health and Rehabilitation Technologies, Institute of Nursing and Health, School of Health Sciences, Ulster University, Shore Road, Newtownabbey, Co Antrim BT37 0QB, UK. [2]Centre for Public Health, Queens University Belfast, Royal Victoria Hospital, Grosvenor Road, Belfast BT12 6BA, UK. [3]UKCRC Centre of Excellence for Public Health (Northern Ireland), Centre for Public Health, School of Medicine, Dentistry and Biomedical Sciences, Queens University Belfast Room 02020, Institute of Clinical Science B, Royal Victoria Hospital, Grosvenor Road, Belfast, BT 12 6BJ, UK. [4]Belfast Health and Social Care Trust, Chronic Pain Service, Belfast City Hospital, 51 Lisburn Road, Belfast BT9 7AB, UK. [5]Centre for Behaviour Change, University College London, 1-9 Torrington Place, London, UK. [6]Honorary Research Professor, School of Physiotherapy, University of Otago, Dunedin, New Zealand.

References

1. Breivik H, Collett B, Ventafridda V, Cohen R, Gallacher D. Survey of chronic pain in Europe: prevalence, impact on daily life, and treatment. Eur J Pain. 2006;10(4):287–333.
2. EFIC. Pain proposal improving the current and future management of chronic pain. A European Consensus Report, 2010.
3. IHME. The global burden of disease: generating evidence, guiding policy. European Union and European free trade association regional edition. Seattle: IHME, 2013: Institute For Health Metrics And Evaluation University of Washington; 2013.
4. IHME. The Global Burden Of Disease: Generating Evidence, Guiding Policy. European Union And European Free Trade Association Regional Edition. Seattle, WA: IHME, 2013: Institute For Health Metrics And Evaluation University of Washington.
5. Andersson HI. Increased mortality among individuals with chronic widespread pain relates to lifestyle factors: a prospective population-based study. Disabil Rehabil. 2009;31(24):1980–7.
6. Kadam UT, Jordan K, Croft PR. Clinical comorbidity in patients with osteoarthritis: a case-control study of general practice consulters in England and Wales. Ann Rheum Dis. 2004;63(4):408–14.
7. Nuesch E, Dieppe P, Reichenbach S, Williams S, Iff S, Juni P. All cause and disease specific mortality in patients with knee or hip osteoarthritis: population based cohort study. BMJ. 2011;342:d1165.
8. McBeth J, Symmons DP, Silman AJ, Allison T, Webb R, Brammah T, Macfarlane GJ. Musculoskeletal pain is associated with a long-term increased risk of cancer and cardiovascular-related mortality. Rheumatology. 2009;48(1):74–7.
9. Macfarlane GJ, McBeth J, Silman AJ. Widespread body pain and mortality: prospective population based study. BMJ. 2001;323(7314):662–5.
10. Airaksinen O, Brox JI, Cedraschi C, Hildebrandt J, Klaber-Moffett J, Kovacs F, Mannion AF, Reis S, Staal JB, Ursin H, Zanoli G, Pain CBWGoGfCLB. Chapter 4. European guidelines for the management of chronic nonspecific low back pain. Eur Spine J. 2006;15(Suppl 2):S192–300.
11. BPS. Core standards for pain management services in the UK. CSPMS. UK: British Pain Society; 2015.
12. Fernandes L, Hagen KB, Bijlsma JW, Andreassen O, Christensen P, Conaghan PG, Doherty M, Geenen R, Hammond A, Kjeken I, Lohmander LS, Lund H, Mallen CD, Nava T, Oliver S, Pavelka K, Pitsillidou I, da Silva JA, de la Torre J, Zanoli G, Vliet Vlieland TP. European league against R. EULAR recommendations for the non-pharmacological core management of hip and knee osteoarthritis. Ann Rheum Dis. 2013;72(7):1125–35.
13. NICE. Low back pain: early management of persistent non-specific low back pain. CG88. London: National Institute for Health and Care Excellence; 2009.
14. NICE. Osteoarthritis care and management in adults. CG177. London: National Institute for Health and Care Excellence; 2014.
15. NICE. Non-specific low back pain and sciatica: management. CG [in development]. London: National Institute for Health and Care Exellence; 2016.
16. SIGN. Management of Chronic Pain. Scottish Intercollegiate Guidelines Network: Scotland; 2013.
17. Zhang W, Nuki G, Moskowitz RW, Abramson S, Altman RD, Arden NK, Bierma-Zeinstra S, Brandt KD, Croft P, Doherty M, Dougados M, Hochberg M, Hunter DJ, Kwoh K, Lohmander LS, Tugwell P. OARSI recommendations for the management of hip and knee osteoarthritis: part III: changes in evidence following systematic cumulative update of research published through January 2009. Osteoarthr Cartil. 2010;18(4):476–99.
18. Warburton DE, Bredin SS. Reflections on physical activity and health: what should we recommend? Can J Cardiol. 2016;32(4):495–504.
19. Warburton DE, Nicol CW, Bredin SS. Health benefits of physical activity: the evidence. CMAJ. 2006;174(6):801–9.
20. Caspersen CJ, Powell KE, Christenson GM. Physical activity, exercise, and physical fitness: definitions and distinctions for health-related research. Public Health Rep. 1985;100(2):126–31.
21. WHO. Physical activity factsheet. Online: World Health Organisation, 2016.
22. Michie S, van Stralen MM, West R. The behaviour change wheel: a new method for characterising and designing behaviour change interventions. Implement Sci. 2011;6:42.
23. Abraham C, Michie S. A taxonomy of behavior change techniques used in interventions. Health Psychol. 2008;27(3):379–87.
24. Bird EL, Baker G, Mutrie N, Ogilvie D, Sahlqvist S, Powell J. Behavior change techniques used to promote walking and cycling: a systematic review. Health Psychol. 2013;32(8):829–38.
25. Fjeldsoe B, Neuhaus M, Winkler E, Eakin E. Systematic review of maintenance of behavior change following physical activity and dietary interventions. Health Psychol. 2011;30(1):99–109.
26. Greaves CJ, Sheppard KE, Abraham C, Hardeman W, Roden M, Evans PH, Schwarz P, Group IS. Systematic review of reviews of intervention components associated with increased effectiveness in dietary and physical activity interventions. BMC Public Health. 2011;11:119.
27. Michie S, Abraham C, Whittington C, McAteer J, Gupta S. Effective techniques in healthy eating and physical activity interventions: a meta-regression. Health Psychol. 2009;28(6):690–701.
28. Olander EK, Fletcher H, Williams S, Atkinson L, Turner A, French DP. What are the most effective techniques in changing obese individuals' physical activity self-efficacy and behaviour: a systematic review and meta-analysis. Int J Behav Nutr Phys Act. 2013;10:29.
29. NICE. Behaviour change: individual approaches. PH49. London: National Institute for Health and Care Excellence; 2014.
30. McDonough SM, Tully MA, Boyd A, O'Connor SR, Kerr DP, O'Neill SM, Delitto A, Bradbury I, Tudor-Locke C, Baxter GD, Hurley DA. Pedometer-driven walking for chronic low back pain: a feasibility randomized controlled trial. Clin J Pain. 2013;29(11):972–81.
31. Talbot LA, Gaines JM, Huynh TN, Metter EJ. A home-based pedometer-driven walking program to increase physical activity in older adults with osteoarthritis of the knee: a preliminary study. J Am Geriatr Soc. 2003;51(3):387–92.
32. Williams NH, Amoakwa E, Belcher J, Edwards RT, Hassani H, Hendry M, Burton K, Lewis R, Hood K, Jones J, Bennett P, Linck P, Neal RD, Wilkinson C. Activity increase despite arthritis (AIDA): phase II randomised controlled trial of an active management booklet for hip and knee osteoarthritis in primary care. Br J Gen Pract. 2011;61(589):e452–8.
33. Oliveira CB, Franco MR, Maher CG, Lin CC, Morelhao PK, Araujo AC, Negrao Filho RF, Pinto RZ. Physical activity interventions for increasing objectively measured physical activity levels in chronic musculoskeletal pain: systematic review. Arthritis Care Res. 2016;
34. Marley J, Tully MA, Porter-Armstrong A, Bunting B, O'Hanlon J, McDonough SM. A systematic review of interventions aimed at increasing physical activity in adults with chronic musculoskeletal pain–protocol. Syst Rev. 2014;3:106.
35. Michie S, Richardson M, Johnston M, Abraham C, Francis J, Hardeman W, Eccles MP, Cane J, Wood CE. The behavior change technique taxonomy (v1) of 93 hierarchically clustered techniques: building an international consensus for the reporting of behavior change interventions. Ann Behav Med. 2013;46(1):81–95.
36. Byrt T, Bishop J, Carlin JB. Bias, prevalence and kappa. J Clin Epidemiol. 1993;46(5):423–9.
37. Landis JR, Koch GG. The measurement of observer agreement for categorical data. Biometrics. 1977;33(1):159–74.
38. Higgins JPT, Green S. Cochrane handbook for systematic reviews of interventions version 5.1.0 [updated march 2011]: the Cochrane collaboration, 2011. .
39. Alonso-Coello P, Schünemann HJ, Moberg J, Brignardello-Petersen R, Akl EA, Davoli M, Treweek S, Mustafa RA, Rada G, Rosenbaum S, Morelli A, Guyatt GH, Oxman AD. GRADE evidence to decision (EtD) frameworks: a systematic and transparent approach to making well informed healthcare choices. 1: introduction. BMJ. 2016;353. doi:10.1136/bmj.i2016.

40. Oxman AD. Grading quality of evidence and strength of recommendations: GRADE working group. BMJ. 2004;328(7454):1490.
41. Cohen J. Statistical power analysis or the behavioural sciences: Lawrence Earlbaum associates, 1988.
42. Alaranta H, Rytokoski U, Rissanen A, Talo S, Ronnemaa T, Puukka P, Karppi S, Videman T, Kallio V, Slatis P. Intensive physical and psychosocial training program for patients with chronic low back pain: a controlled clinical trial. Spine. 1994;19(12):1339–49.
43. Allen KD, Yancy WS Jr, Bosworth HB, Coffman CJ, Jeffreys AS, Datta SK, McDuffie J, Strauss JL, Oddone EZ. A combined patient and provider intervention for Management of Osteoarthritis in veterans: a randomized clinical trial. Ann Intern Med. 2016;164(2):73–83.
44. Becker A, Leonhardt C, Kochen M, Keller S, Wegscheider S, Baum E, Donner-Banzhoff N, Pfingsten M, Hildebrandt J, Heinz-Dieter BW, Chenot J. Effects of two guideline implementation strategies on patient outcomes in primary care: a cluster randomized controlled trial. Spine. 2008;33(5):473–80.
45. Bossen D, Veenhof C, Van Beek KE, Spreeuwenberg PM, Dekker J, De Bakker DH. Effectiveness of a web-based physical activity intervention in patients with knee and/or hip osteoarthritis: randomized controlled trial. J Med Internet Res. 2013;15(11):e257.
46. Brosseau L, Wells GA, Kenny GP, Reid R, Maetzel A, Tugwell P, Huijbregts M, McCullough C, Angelis G, Chen L. The implementation of a community-based aerobic walking program for mild to moderate knee osteoarthritis: a knowledge translation randomized controlled trial: part II: clinical outcomes. BMC Public Health. 2012;12:1073.
47. Farr JN, Going SB, McKnight PE, Kasle S, Cussler EC, Cornett M. Progressive resistance training improves overall physical activity levels in patients with early osteoarthritis of the knee: a randomized controlled trial. Phys Ther. 2010;90(3):356–66.
48. Focht BC, Garver MJ, Devor ST, Dials J, Lucas AR, Emery CF, Hackshaw KV, Rejeski WJ. Group-mediated physical activity promotion and mobility in sedentary patients with knee osteoarthritis: results from the IMPACT-pilot trial. J Rheumatol. 2014;41(10):2068–77.
49. Hiyama Y, Yamada M, Kitagawa A, Tei N, Okada S. A four-week walking exercise programme in patients with knee osteoarthritis improves the ability of dual-task performance: a randomized controlled trial. Clin Rehabil. 2012;26(5):403–12.
50. Hughes SL, Seymour RB, Campbell RT, Huber G, Pollak N, Sharma L, Desai P. Long-term impact of fit and strong! On older adults with osteoarthritis. Gerontologist. 2006;46(6):801–14.
51. Hunter R, McDonough S, Bradbury I, Liddle S, Walsh D, Dhamija S, Glasgow P, Gormley G, McCann S, Park J. Exercise and auricular acupuncture for chronic low-back pain: a feasibility randomized-controlled trial. Clin J Pain. 2012;28(3):259–67.
52. Hurley DA, Tully MA, Lonsdale C, Boreham CA, van Mechelen W, Daly L, Tynan A, McDonough SM. Supervised walking in comparison with fitness training for chronic back pain in physiotherapy: results of the SWIFT single-blinded randomized controlled trial (ISRCTN17592092). Pain. 2015;156(1):131–47.
53. Krein SL, Kadri R, Hughes M, Kerr EA, Piette JD, Holleman R, Kim HM, Richardson CR. Pedometer-based internet-mediated intervention for adults with chronic low back pain: randomized controlled trial. J Med Internet Res. 2013;15(8):e181.
54. Meng K, Seekatz B, Roband H, Worringen U, Vogel H, Faller H. Intermediate and long-term effects of a standardized back school for inpatient orthopedic rehabilitation on illness knowledge and self-management behaviors: a randomized controlled trial. Clin J Pain. 2011;27(3):248–57.
55. Pisters M, Veenhof C, de BD SF, Dekker J. Behavioural graded activity results in better exercise adherence and more physical activity than usual care in people with osteoarthritis: a cluster-randomised trial. Aus J Physiother. 2010;56(1):41–7.
56. Schlenk E, Lias J, Sereika S, Dunbar-Jacob J, Kwoh C. Improving physical activity and function in overweight and obese older adults with osteoarthritis of the knee: a feasibility study. Rehabilitation Nursing. 2011;36(1):32–42.
57. Sullivan T, Allegrante JP, Peterson MG, Kovar PA, MacKenzie CR. One-year followup of patients with osteoarthritis of the knee who participated in a program of supervised fitness walking and supportive patient education. Arthritis Care Res. 1998;11(4):228–33.
58. Trudeau KJ, Pujol LA, DasMahapatra P, Wall R, Black RA, Zacharoff K. A randomized controlled trial of an online self-management program for adults with arthritis pain. J Behav Med. 2015;38(3):483–96.
59. Kovar PA, Allegrante JP, MacKenzie CR, Peterson MG, Gutin B, Charlson ME. Supervised fitness walking in patients with osteoarthritis of the knee. A randomized, controlled trial. Ann Intern Med. 1992;116(7):529–34.
60. Williamson W, Kluzek S, Roberts N, Richards J, Arden N, Leeson P, Newton J, Foster C. Behavioural physical activity interventions in participants with lower-limb osteoarthritis: a systematic review with meta-analysis. BMJ Open. 2015;5(8). doi:10.1136/bmjopen-2015-007642.
61. Richards J, Hillsdon M, Thorogood M, Foster C. Face-to-face interventions for promoting physical activity. Cochrane Database Syst Rev. 2013;9: CD010392.
62. Hobbs N, Godfrey A, Lara J, Errington L, Meyer TD, Rochester L, White M, Mathers JC, Sniehotta FF. Are behavioral interventions effective in increasing physical activity at 12 to 36 months in adults aged 55 to 70 years? A systematic review and meta-analysis. BMC Med. 2013;11:75.
63. Bishop FL, Fenge-Davies AL, Kirby S, Geraghty AW. Context effects and behaviour change techniques in randomised trials: a systematic review using the example of trials to increase adherence to physical activity in musculoskeletal pain. Psychol Health. 2015;30(1):104–21.
64. Jordan JL, Holden MA, Mason EE, Foster NE. Interventions to improve adherence to exercise for chronic musculoskeletal pain in adults. Cochrane Database Syst Rev. 2010;(1):Cd005956.
65. Keogh A, Tully MA, Matthews J, Hurley DA. A review of behaviour change theories and techniques used in group based self-management programmes for chronic low back pain and arthritis. Man Ther. 2015. doi:10.1016/j.math.2015.03.014.
66. French DP, Olander EK, Chisholm A, Mc SJ. Which behaviour change techniques are most effective at increasing older adults' self-efficacy and physical activity behaviour? A systematic review. Ann Behav Med. 2014;48(2):225–34.
67. Hillsdon M, Foster C, Thorogood M. Interventions for promoting physical activity. Cochrane Database Syst Rev. 2005;1:Cd003180.
68. Karlsson P, Bergmark A. Compared with what? An analysis of control-group types in Cochrane and Campbell reviews of psychosocial treatment efficacy with substance use disorders. Addiction. 2015;110(3):420–8.
69. Goldberg DS, McGee SJ. Pain as a global public health priority. BMC Public Health. 2011;11:770.
70. Foster CE, Brennan G, Matthews A, McAdam C, Fitzsimons C, Mutrie N. Recruiting participants to walking intervention studies: a systematic review. Int J Behav Nutr Phys Act. 2011;8:137.

14

Examination of concomitant glenohumeral pathologies in patients treated arthroscopically for calcific tendinitis of the shoulder and implications for routine diagnostic joint exploration

Gernot Lang[1*], Kaywan Izadpanah[1], Eva Johanna Kubosch[1], Dirk Maier[1], Norbert Südkamp[1] and Peter Ogon[1,2]

Abstract

Background: Glenohumeral exploration is routinely performed during arthroscopic removal of rotator cuff calcifications in patients with calcific tendinitis of the shoulder (CTS). However, evidence on the prevalence of intraarticular co-pathologies is lacking and the benefit of glenohumeral exploration remains elusive. The aim of the present study was to assess and quantify intraoperative pathologies during arthroscopic removal of rotator cuff calcifications in order to determine whether standardized diagnostic glenohumeral exploration appears justified in CTS patients.

Methods: One hundred forty five patients undergoing arthroscopic removal of calcific depots (CD) that failed conservative treatment were included in a retrospective cohort study. Radiographic parameters including number/localization of calcifications and acromial types, intraoperative arthroscopic findings such as configuration of glenohumeral ligaments, articular cartilage injuries, and characteristics of calcifications and sonographic parameters (characteristics/localization of calcification) were recorded.

Results: One hundred forty five patients were analyzed. All CDs were removed by elimination with a blunt hook probe via "squeeze-and-stir-technique" assessed postoperatively via conventional X-rays. Neither subacromial decompression nor refixation of the rotator cuff were performed in any patient. Prevalence of glenohumeral co-pathologies, such as partial tears of the proximal biceps tendon (2.1%), superior labral tears from anterior to posterior (SLAP) lesions (1.4%), and/or partial rotator cuff tears (0.7%) was low. Most frequently, glenohumeral articular cartilage was either entirely intact (ICRS grade 0 (humeral head/glenoid): 46%/48%) or showed very mild degenerative changes (ICRS grade 1: 30%/26%). Two patients (1.3%) required intraarticular surgical treatment due to a SLAP lesion type III ($n = 1$) and an intraarticular rupture of CD ($n = 1$).

Conclusions: Routine diagnostic glenohumeral exploration does not appear beneficial in arthroscopic treatment of CTS due to the low prevalence of intraarticular pathologies which most frequently do not require surgical treatment. Exploration of the glenohumeral joint in arthroscopic removal of CD should only be performed in case of founded suspicion of relevant concomitant intraarticular pathologies.

Keywords: Calcific tendinitis, Rotator cuff, Shoulder arthroscopy, Postoperative recovery, Outcome factors, Shoulder, Degeneration, Glenohumeral, Osteoarthritis, Diagnostic, Tendinopathy

* Correspondence: Gernot.michael.lang@uniklinik-freiburg.de
[1]Department of Orthopedics and Trauma Surgery, Medical Center - Albert-Ludwigs-University of Freiburg, Faculty of Medicine, Albert-Ludwigs-University of Freiburg, Hugstetter Strasse 55, 79106 Freiburg, Germany
Full list of author information is available at the end of the article

Background

Calcific tendinitis of the shoulder (CTS) is a common musculoskeletal disorder (2.7% to 20% of the population), usually affecting women more often than men [1, 2]. The pathogenesis of CTS is still poorly understood. To date, several theories on the development of CTS exist: while some authors propose that calcification of a tendon might occur due to vascular ischemia, repetitive micro trauma, or cellular necrosis of tissue, others believe that CTS might be an active cell mediated process (based on multiple factors, i.e. genetic disposition, environmental factors, metabolic disorders, etc.) resulting in alterations of cell and extracellular matrix differentiation [3]. Most frequently, CTS can be treated conservatively with satisfying outcome. Ultrasound-guided (US) needling and extracorporeal shock wave therapy (ESWT) have recently emerged as alternative therapies in CTS patients and demonstrated good to excellent clinical outcome [1, 4, 5]. When primary and secondary conservative treatments fail due to chronicity of symptoms, eventually more invasive treatment modalities are indicated in 10% to 15% of patients. To date, shoulder arthroscopy has been the preferred therapy as surgical treatment option, as it provides minimal invasive access to the glenohumeral joint, rotator cuff, and subacromial space, allowing for efficient removal of calcific deposits (CD) under direct visualization. In these cases, surgical procedures have proven to relief pain and improve function significantly [6–8]. Although arthroscopy includes a significant reduction of approach-related comorbidity compared to open procedures, aggressive arthroscopic CD removal often results in relevant rotator cuff defects including a variety of complications, such as arthrofibrosis and/or shoulder stiffness, conditions that potentially require additional surgical treatment and/or prolonged rehabilitation [7, 9–12]. Furthermore, shoulder arthroscopy is associated with certain inherent complications which can lead to devastating outcome [13–17]. In addition to that, the extent of CD removal as well as the clinical benefit of subacromial decompression and/or glenohumeral joint exploration remain elusive. Moreover, glenohumeral exploration accounts for additional operative time, which potentially translates into increased perioperative risk for complications as well as additional costs. As there is no evidence supporting that patients with CTS benefit from glenohumeral exploration during arthroscopic removal of calcifications, it is difficult to justify the supplemental approach to the joint.

Arthroscopic treatment of CTS usually starts with diagnostic glenohumeral joint exploration, followed by CD removal through a direct subacromial approach. Recently, Sirveaux et al. proposed that diagnostic glenohumeral arthroscopy should not be performed in routine manner when treating patients with CTS [18]. In this retrospective, comparative study, the cohort of 32 patients undergoing additional diagnostic glenohumeral arthroscopy showed significantly prolonged postoperative pain (11 weeks vs. 6 weeks) and a significant latency in return-to-work (12 weeks vs. 5 weeks). The authors concluded, that the additional intervention of diagnostic glenohumeral joint exploration would cause further harm rather than yielding improved clinical outcome [18]. The authors found concomitant pathologies in 5/32 (15.6%) cases. However, none of them required surgical intervention. In conclusion, the authors recommended excising as much of the CD as possible via a direct bursal approach without performing additional diagnostic glenohumeral arthroscopy. However, aggressive CD removal at expense of the affected rotator cuff's integrity might negatively influence postoperative recovery and outcome. In addition to the retrospective study design with a limited case number, this issue might have substantially biased the result of the study of Sirveaux et al.. Previously, it was demonstrated that blunt arthroscopic CD removal preserving the integrity of the rotator cuff resulted in good to excellent outcome in 90% of patients [6, 19]. The authors tolerated minor remnant calcifications in favor of rotator cuff integrity. None of the patients received an additional rotator cuff repair. The remaining calcifications did not impair functional outcome and had spontaneously resolved until follow-up.

To date, there is minimal knowledge on the prevalence of concomitant pathologies in CTS. The study of Sirveaux et al. described a prevalence of 15.6% but the case number is too low for a conclusive assessment. Given the controversial findings and argumentation throughout literature, it still remains questionable whether diagnostic glenohumeral arthroscopy is justified in arthroscopic treatment of CTS.

Therefore, the purpose of this study was to investigate the prevalence and clinical significance of concomitant glenohumeral pathologies assessed during arthroscopic treatment of rotator cuff calcifications in order to determine whether diagnostic glenohumeral exploration appears justified in routine manner. We hypothesized a low prevalence of concomitant pathologies in patients with CTS and assumed that diagnostic glenohumeral exploration might not be required in a standardized fashion.

Methods

Study population

We conducted a descriptive retrospective cohort study of patients presenting with symptomatic chronic CTS undergoing arthroscopic removal of CD between 2008 and 2011 that failed at least six months of conservative treatment. Patients had been referred by a general practitioner, rheumatologists, or orthopedic surgeon for treatment. Most common clinical findings were persistent shoulder pain, functional disability and the presence of symptomatic rotator cuff calcifications. Further inclusion criteria were the presence of radiographically and sonographically determined calcifications within the rotator cuff and the presence of clinically symptomatic CTS of the shoulder. Patients with previous ipsilateral shoulder surgeries or shoulder comorbidities were excluded. Calcifications were confirmed preoperatively by conventional radiographs (anterior-posterior) and bilateral ultrasound examination.

Preoperative localization of CD via quadrant technique

Preoperative ultrasound examination (1 to 2 days before surgery) of the rotator cuff was performed in a standardized manner by a board certified orthopedic surgeon who was experienced with musculoskeletal sonography. Calcific depositions were evaluated according to the quadrant technique within preoperative outpatient consultation [20]. The number of calcifications and dorsal attenuation were recorded accordingly. Additionally, ultrasound was used to assess the integrity of the rotator cuff and biceps tendon.

Radiographic evaluation

Radiographic parameters (based on standard anterior-posterior (a.-p.) and outlet radiographic views) were measured at two time points: preoperatively (1 to 2 days before surgery) and postoperatively (within 2 to 3 days after surgery). The number of calcific lesions and localization of calcifications (medial/lateral) were assessed using standardized a.-p. films. Acromion morphology was classified according to Bigliani et al. on outlet radiographs [21]. Postoperative radiographs were performed to determine the amount of CD removal.

Surgical procedure

All surgeries were performed by the same board-certified orthopedic surgeon experienced in shoulder arthroscopies (PO). Our surgical procedure of shoulder arthroscopy in patients with CTS has previously been described in detail [6]. Briefly, under general anesthesia patients were positioned laterally in a decubitus position with slight extension to the arm. Preoperatively, the exact localization of CD was determined by utilization of ultrasonographical mapping according to the quadrant technique [20]. As the patient's arm was resting in the neutral position, the intraoperative anatomy was configured in the same exact fashion as performed for preoperative localization of the rotator cuff calcifications, which facilitated in situ localization of CD significantly. The calcifications were identified and marked with respect to the affected quadrants.

A stab skin incision was made followed by careful advancement of the scope into the glenohumeral joint through a posterior portal. The diagnostic arthroscopy was carried out in a conventional manner to rule out relevant intraarticular concomitant pathologies. Then, the subacromial space was identified and exposed using the same approach. Additionally, a lateral approach was used to insert a blunt trocar and subsequently gain access to the bursa. As the bursa was frequently hypertrophic and/or hypervascularized due to the chronic proinflammatory stimulus of the irritating intraarticular calcifications (Fig. 1), we performed a partial bursectomy by utilization of the arthroscopic shaver. The respective CD was then identified via needling and the center of the calcification was localized and incised with a needle (Fig. 1b). Calcific remnants in the needle's tip indicated correct localization. Hereafter, a blunt hook probe was carefully advanced in order to gently release and eliminate (squeeze-and-stir-technique) the calcifications (Fig. 1c, d). Additionally, the superficial membrane was elevated in order to flush the joint followed by intermittent squeezing of the CD with the probe. This procedure was repeated until the calcific deposit was removed in a blunt fashion (Fig. 1e). Finally, a thorough irrigation of the "calcific cave" was performed by utilization of a syringe to ensure proper elimination of small calcific particles. Finally, the continuity of the affected rotator cuff tendon was confirmed precisely (risk for underestimation of rotator cuff tears following CD removal) before the wound was closed. No tendon repair was performed after CD removal.

Assessment of concomitant glenohumeral pathologies

Intraarticular concomitant pathologies were assessed within glenohumeral arthroscopy. The configuration of glenohumeral ligaments were evaluated according to Morgan et al. [22]. Glenohumeral cartilage injuries were assessed according to the International Cartilage Repair Society (ICRS, Table 1) cartilage injury classification (Fig. 2) [23]. Consistency and characteristics of calcifications were evaluated by macroscopic assessment and/or manipulation via blunt probe. Superior labral tears from anterior to posterior (SLAP lesions) were classified according to Snyder et al. (Fig. 3) [24]. Tears of the proximal biceps tendon were graded according to the thickness of injury (superficial, 25%, 50%, 75%, and full thickness rupture (100%). Rotator cuff lesions were classified according to Ellman et al. for partial tears and Bateman et al. for full thickness tears including indication of the affected tendon [25, 26].

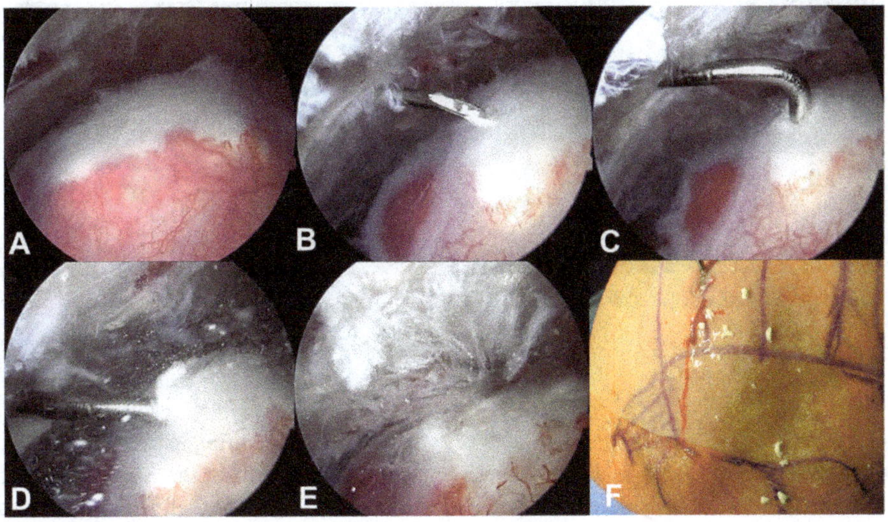

Fig. 1 Surgical steps for minimally invasive arthroscopic removal of rotator cuff calcifications. **a**. Identification of the calcific deposit. **b**. Localization of the calcific deposit's center via needling. **c**. and **d**. A blunt hook probe is carefully advanced in order to gently release and eliminate the calcifications. **d**. "Snowstorm-phenomenon" - initial release of calcific particles. **e**. "Calcific cave" after removal of calcifications **f**. Macroscopic demonstration of removed calcific deposits on the patient's skin

Statistical analysis

Continuous variables are shown as mean ± standard error of the mean. For categorical variables percentages were calculated. All analyses were performed using SPSS version 20 (IBM, Armonk, NY, USA).

Ethical considerations

The study was approved by our local institutional review board and informed consent was obtained from all patients before surgery (protocol number: 598/16).

Table 1 International Cartilage Repair Society (ICRS) Hyaline Cartilage Lesion Classification System [23]

Grade	Subgrade	Definition	Characteristics
0		Normal	Normal
1	A	Nearly Normal	Superficial lesions. Soft indentation
	B		A + and/or superficial fissures and cracks
2		Abnormal	Lesions extending down to <50% of cartilage depth
3	A	Severely Abnormal	Cartilage defects extending down to >50% of cartilage depth
	B		A + Cartilage defects extending down to calcified layer
	C		A + B + not extending through the subchondral bone
	D		A + B + C+ blisters are included
4		Severely Abnormal	

Results

Baseline characteristics

145 patients were enrolled in the study (66.2% female, Table 2). Mean age at surgery was 50.9 ± 8.9 years (range: 32–76). The major indication for arthroscopic removal of CD was symptomatic chronic CTS. The mean symptomatic time until patients decided to undergo surgical removal of CD was 3.5 years. 2.6% of patients had a previous shoulder surgery on the contralateral shoulder in the past. The most commonly treated side due to symptomatic CTS was the right shoulder in 54.5% of patients (Table 2). The dominant shoulder was affected in 33.1% (48/151).

Preoperative radiographic assessment of calcifying tendinitis

Preoperative radiographic assessment of CTS was performed 1 to 2 days before surgery. As demonstrated in Tables 3, 72% of calcifications were localized laterally while 19.4% of calcific depots were found within the medial part of the rotator cuff. Few patients (8.3%) presented a bilateral configuration of the calcification (i.e. lateral +50% medial). Furthermore, the majority of patients (94.5%) featured a single calcific depot within the preoperative radiographic evaluation. Distribution of acromion morphology according to Bigliani et al., resulted in 31.7%, 59.3%, and 9% for a flat (type I), curved (type II) and hooked (type III) acromial shape (Table 3).

Concomitant glenohumeral pathologies

The articular cartilage of the humeral head was intact in 45.5% of patients (Table 2). While mild cartilage injury

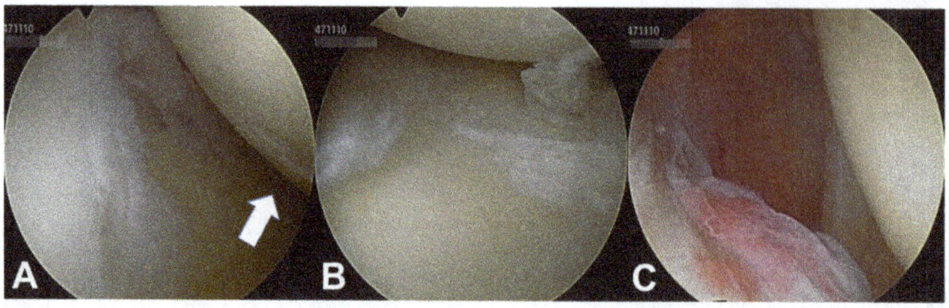

Fig. 2 Cartilage lesions in a patient with calcifying tendinitis. **a**. Mild cartilage defect on the humeral head. **b**. Mild cartilage defect at the glenoid. **c**. Intact biceps and supraspinatus tendon

at the humeral head (grade 1 and 2) was found in 29.7% and 23.4%, respectively, severe cartilage lesions were only detected in 1.4% (grade 4) of patients (Fig. 2). Moreover, 48.3% of glenoids did not reveal any cartilage injury at all. Mild cartilage lesions on glenoid articular surfaces were diagnosed in 26.2% (grade 1) and 24.1% (grade 2) of patients (Table 2). Severe glenoid lesions (grade 3) were recorded in 2 (1.4%) patients. Typical copathologies that were identified during arthroscopy were partial tears of the proximal biceps tendon (2.1%), SLAP lesions (1.4%), and rotator cuff defects (0.7%; Fig. 4). SLAP lesions and partial tears of the proximal biceps tendon were incidental findings. Furthermore, the glenohumeral capsular type was evaluated according to Morgan et al. (Table 2) [22]. The vast majority of our patients were classified as capsular type I (93.1%). Capsular type II and III were recorded in 1.4% and 4.8% of patients, respectively. Sublabral foramen were observed in 6.9% of cases, whereas over 90% of patients did not present any sublabral lesions. Two of our patients (1.4%) required specific glenohumeral surgical treatment due to a SLAP lesion type III and an intraarticular rupture of calcific deposits (Figs. 4, 5, and 3). As the other SLAP lesion in our study population was mild (type I) a debridement was not indicated. Neither did the patients with SLAP lesions complain about specific symptoms preoperatively nor have the SLAP lesions been detected via ultrasound (i.e. joint effusion) before surgery. One patient (0.7%) showed a tear of the rotator cuff interval without involvement of the subscapularis or supraspinatus tendon. CD removal was confirmed postoperatively by conventional X-rays.

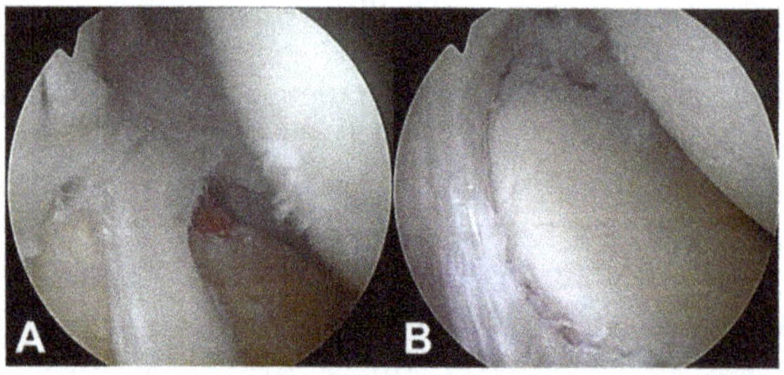

Fig. 3 SLAP lesion type III according to Snyder et al. [18]. **a**. Intraoperative detection of a SLAP lesion type III which required surgical treatment. **b**. SLAP lesion type III after debridement and resection

Intraoperative assessment of calcifying tendinitis

During arthroscopic removal of CD, rotator cuff calcifications typically presented with a tough and "toothpaste"-like consistency (63.4%; mixed-forms were described); Table 4 and Figs. 1 and 5). We observed two cases (1.4%) of CD perforations into adjacent anatomical structures. One patient showed an extensive calcific bursitis as a result of CD rupture and perforation into the subacromial bursa. We observed CD perforation into the glenohumeral joint with both adhesive and free floating calcific components inside the joint in another patient.

Discussion

The purpose of the present study was to investigate whether glenohumeral arthroscopic exploration is justified in patients with CTS based on the prevalence of intraarticular pathologies that require surgical treatment. This study adds evidence that glenohumeral pathologies have a low prevalence in patients undergoing arthroscopic removal of rotator cuff calcifications. Outcome of this study suggests that a standardized diagnostic glenohumeral exploration may not be mandatory as a routine procedure during arthroscopic treatment of CTS. As far as we are aware, there is no previous investigation specifically analyzing the prevalence of intraarticular glenohumeral pathologies during arthroscopic removal of rotator cuff calcifications.

Minimally invasive removal of rotator cuff calcifications

Most commonly, treatment of symptomatic CTS can be managed non-operatively (90% of patients) by

Table 2 Patient demographics

Parameter		*N* = 145	%
Gender	Male	49	33.8
	Female	96	66.2
Mean age at surgery in years[1]	Max: 76 - Min: 32	50.9 ± 8.9	
ICRS cartilage injury – humeral head [23]	0	66	45.5
	1	43	29.7
	2	34	23.4
	3	0	0
	4	2	1.4
ICRS cartilage injury – glenoid [23]	0	70	48.3
	1	38	26.2
	2	35	24.1
	3	2	1.4
	4	0	0
Previous shoulder surgery	At the contralateral side	4	2.6
Intraarticular lesions		2	1.4
Intraarticular Co-pathology	Partial tear of the proximal biceps tendon (30% - 50% in relative width)	3	2.1
	SLAP lesion	2	1.4
	Interval rotator cuff lesion	1	0.7
Capsular type (n = 1 missing) [22]	1	135	93.1
	2	2	1.4
	3	7	4.8
	4	0	0
Intraoperative sublabral foramen	Yes	10	6.9
	No	131	90.3
	Buford complex	4	2.8
Side of injury	Left shoulder	66	45.5
	Right shoulder	79	54.5
	Dominant shoulder	48	33.1

Demographic characteristics of the study population
ICRS International Cartilage Repair Society, *SLAP* Superior labral tear from anterior to posterior, [1] Mean ± SD

Table 3 Preoperative radiographic assessment of calcifying tendinitis

Parameter		N = 145	%
Localization (missing: n = 1)	Medial	28	19.4
	Lateral	104	72.2
	Lateral +50% medial	11	7.6
	Medial +50% lateral	1	0.7
Number of calcifications	1	137	94.5
	2	6	4.1
	3	0	0
	4	2	1.4
Acromion morphology [21]	1 – Flat	46	31.7
	2 – Curved	86	59.3
	3 – Hooked	13	9
Ultrasound – affected quadrants	1	115	79.3
	2	41	28.3
	3	10	6.9
	4	11	7.6
Ultrasound	Total number of lesions	139	
	Dorsal attenuation	118	81.4

physiotherapy, analgesics, and injections [27]. Surgical treatment is reserved for patients in which conservative therapy has failed, such as prolonged periods of functional disability, severe pain, and when calcific deposits do not resolve spontaneously. To date, most surgeons perform an arthroscopic removal of CD with/without subacromial decompression and glenohumeral exploration [7]. Recently, our group demonstrated that good to excellent results can be achieved in 90% of patients with blunt arthroscopic removal of calcific lesions, without performing a subacromial decompression. Therefore, we pursue a minimal-invasive strategy which rather tolerates minor remnant calcifications in favor of rotator cuff integrity [6]. In the present study, the vast majority of our patients did not present any intraarticular pathologies requiring surgical treatment. If intraarticular pathologies were detected, most likely these lesions did not cause any symptoms. Our results confirm the conclusion of Sirveaux et al., who compared clinical and radiographic outcome in patients with CTS treated either by CD removal alone via an arthroscopic bursal approach or CD removal combined with a standardized glenohumeral exploration [18]. The authors did not identify a single glenohumeral injury that required surgical treatment. Moreover, duration of postoperative pain and latency of return-to-work were significantly shorter in patients who received CD removal solely compared to patients that underwent CD removal including an additional glenohumeral exploration. After 6-month follow-up, functional outcome and radiographic CD disappearance did not reveal significant differences. Therefore, we agree on the authors' statement, that a glenohumeral exploration can be avoided as the additional approach might include an increased risk for complications as well as it presumably leads rather to prolonged rehabilitation than clinical benefit. Furthermore, prolonged duration of surgery, increased postoperative pain and subsequently prolonged length of stay potentially cause higher costs [28, 29]. A glenohumeral exploration may be justified in specific scenarios: I.e. if a relatively large and consistent CD removal has been performed and an intra-articular assessment of the rotator cuff's integrity is pursued. A thorough evaluation of the rotator cuff (especially

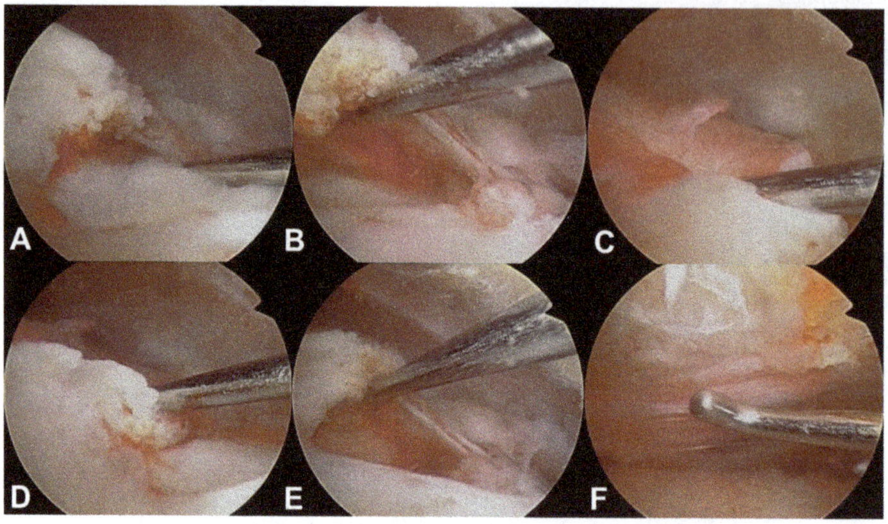

Fig. 4 Acute bursal rupture of calcifications. **a**. – **f**. Intraoperative images display an acute intraarticular rupture of calcifications. The supraspinatus tendon demonstrates tears and fatty degeneration. A "cave" of the former calcifications remains as a partial bursal-sided tear

of deep layers) may be facilitated by means of arthroscopic visualization. Nevertheless, for the majority of patients with CTS, an additional glenohumeral exploration seems to be an unnecessary and an expandable risk for complications as it contains an additional approach to the joint.

The amount of CD removal is another matter of debate: several authors favor a complete removal of CD while other authors presented good outcome with incomplete excision of CD [6, 7, 10, 30–32]. A total removal of CD may potentially result in a full thickness rotator cuff tear. Evidence is lacking whether an immediate reconstruction or no repair at all leads to superior outcome [6, 9, 31, 33, 34]. Last but not least, the size and consistency of CD lesions are highly important for the removal of rotator cuff calcifications. In the present study, the vast majority of CD lesions was either tough and tooth paste-like or presented as snowy powder, indicating that an

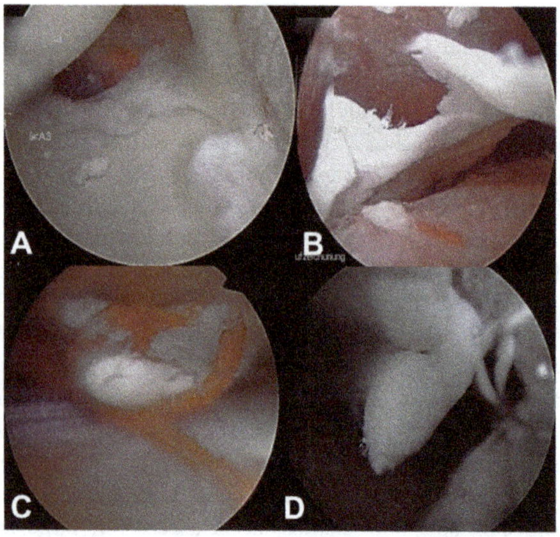

Fig. 5 Intraoperative findings during removal of rotator cuff calcifications. **a**. Intraarticular calcific deposits in the glenohumeral joint space. **b**. - **d**. Large pieces of calcific deposits

Table 4 Intraoperative macroscopic characteristics of calcifying tendinitis

Parameter			N = 145	Percent
Consistency of calcification	Tooth paste		10	6.9
	Tough + Tooth paste		92	63.4
	Tough + Tooth paste + streaks		1	0.7
	Tough + Tooth paste + clods		1	0.7
	Snow		20	13.8
	Snow + flaky		12	8.3
	Snow + streaks		2	1.4
	Snow + toothpaste		3	2.1
	Red/brown "sauce"		1	0.7
	Calcification of bursa + snow		1	0.7
	Flakes on RC		1	0.7
	Cloudy		1	0.7
Structure of calcification	From very fine (1) to rough (5)	1	39	26.9
		2	1	0.7
		3	98	67.6
		4	2	1.4
		5	5	3.4

easy removal is feasible without the application of intense forces.

In summary, instead of a standardized glenohumeral exploration within arthroscopic removal of CD lesions, we suggest a patient-specific treatment algorithm, that is individualized on the patient's presenting complains in order to optimize the risk-benefit-ratio.

Increased risk for complications due to glenohumeral exploration

CTS is predominantly an extraarticular phenomenon rather than a glenohumeral joint disease [1, 34]. Consequently, we expect an equivalent prevalence of glenohumeral pathologies in patients with CTS compared to healthy subjects. Certainly, an arthroscopic glenohumeral exploration provides the opportunity to detect intraarticular co-pathologies. However, our and previous data demonstrate that intraarticular co-pathologies in patients with CTS were hardly detected and moreover, if an intraarticular pathology was present, this almost never caused any procedural alteration [18]. Therefore, it is reasonable to question whether an additional glenohumeral arthroscopy can be justified in patients with CTS considering the increased risk for complications such as infection or shoulder stiffness against the lack of a true benefit through arthroscopy [18]?

The overall risk for complications in shoulder arthroscopy ranges between 4.8% and 10.6% [35–37]. Typical complications in patients having CTS are prolonged pain, secondary adhesive capsulitis, rotator cuff tears, ossifying tendinitis, and osteolysis of the greater tuberosity [38]. The incidence of a frozen shoulder after shoulder arthroscopy is 2% to 5% in the general population [39, 40]. Postoperative shoulder stiffness after rotator cuff repair ranges between 4.9% and 32.7% [41–43]. Shoulder stiffness is not well tolerated by patients with CTS; it does not resolve easily and may require long-term rehabilitation [44]. Reasons for shoulder stiffness are supposed to be the manipulation of capsule and/or residual calcium debris [6, 34]. Moreover, postoperative shoulder stiffness may be related to rotator cuff tear morphology, postoperative immobilization, glenohumeral adhesion, capsular contracture, or underlying predisposing patient comorbidities [42, 44, 45]. Reduction of approach-related comorbidity may potentially reduce complication rates and offers the opportunity to perform this procedure as an outpatient surgery that allows for immediate rehabilitation, which subsequently reduces the risk for postoperative stiffness [18]. Our current rate of postoperative arthrofibrosis is relatively low compared to previous studies – however, if the risk for postoperative arthrofibrosis can be further reduced without performing a glenohumeral approach while at the same time achieving equivalent outcome, one may assume that it might be reasonable to abstain from a glenohumeral exploration in routine fashion when treating patients with CTS arthroscopically [46]. However, this needs to be further confirmed in prospective comparative investigations.

Furthermore, infection following shoulder arthroscopy is another relevant risk factor. Pauzenberger et al. observed infections following arthroscopic rotator cuff repair in 0.009% [47]. The authors identified sex (male), age (≥60 years), and length of surgery (≥90 min) to be significantly associated with postoperative infection. Other groups reported overall infection rates after shoulder arthroscopy between 0.03% and 3.4% [37, 48–50]. Especially, joint infections due to Propionibacterium acne (P. acne) are currently controversially discussed in association with shoulder arthroscopy as conventional perioperative antibiotic- or preoperative prophylaxis do not seem to sufficiently decrease the risk for postoperative infections [47, 51]. Moreover, presurgical skin preparations do not entirely eliminate P. acne [52–54]. Current evidence suggests P. acne being the most frequent identified organism in shoulder infections [51, 55, 56]. Both, open and arthroscopic surgery provide approach related-opportunities for P. acne to be transferred from skin to deep layers and thus potentially causing glenohumeral joint infections [57]. Seth et al. observed differences in positive skin cultures contaminated by P. acne that were assessed before skin incision (15.8%) and directly before wound closure (40.4%), which underlines the association between length of surgery and potential risk for surgical side infections [58]. In order to minimize the risk for infections by P. acne, it is suggested to reduce the size and contamination of surgical approaches [59]. Due to the fact that glenohumeral joint infections are associated with disability and significant direct and indirect socioeconomic costs, we suggest to perform a glenohumeral joint exploration only if an intraarticular injury that requires surgical treatment is highly expected.

In general, the impact of glenohumeral exploration within arthroscopic removal of calcifications in CTS remains an under-investigated issue. To date, postoperative pain and latency of return-to-work were found to be significantly shorter in patients who received CD removal solely compared to patients that received an additional glenohumeral exploration [18]. It is reasonable that any additional manipulation/invasive maneuver during shoulder surgery might affect the clinical and/or functional outcome and potentially increases the likelihood of complications since this has already been demonstrated in various other surgical procedures [13, 37, 60, 61]. Investigations comparing complications of different arthroscopic approaches have not been performed yet. Sufficient data exist on 30-day readmission rates as well as risk factors for postoperative complications following shoulder arthroscopy as described by

Shields et al. [45]. The authors found shoulder arthroscopy to have a 1% thirty-day complication rate. Age ≥ 60 years, operating room (OR) time ≥ 90 min, chronic obstructive pulmonary disease, inpatient status, disseminated cancer, and nicotine abuse are risk factors for postoperative complications [60]. These results have been confirmed by other authors such as Moody et al. who demonstrated, that prolonged operative time, more invasive and/or additional surgical approaches increase the risk for complications as well as health care expenditures [29, 60].

In the present study, intraarticular pathologies that needed surgical treatment have only been observed in few patients. For the majority of patients with CTS, an additional glenohumeral exploration might be an unnecessary risk and would most likely not translate into a clinical benefit. As patients undergoing surgery in CTS already reflect a "negative selection" due to failed conservative treatment, a reasonable risk-benefit-ratio by means of minimal approach-related comorbidity and perioperative risk for complications should be pursued. As there is currently no evidence supporting that patients with CTS benefit from glenohumeral explorations during arthroscopic removal of calcifications, the additional glenohumeral approach should only be performed in case of founded suspicion of relevant concomitant intraarticular pathologies.

Limitations and strength

The retrospective study design is associated with certain limitations, such as loss of information (missing reports), heterogeneous preoperative conservative treatment, and unequal group power (i.e. gender, affected shoulder, etc.). Additionally, functional and clinical outcome data was not implemented into this study. Moreover, this study was of descriptive nature and did not include a control group. Nevertheless, as far as we are aware, there is no previous study specifically investigating intraarticular glenohumeral pathologies during CD removal in patients with calcifying tendinitis. Furthermore, a huge advantage of the present study is that all patients were treated by the same orthopedic surgeon resulting in high consistency and homogeneous evaluation of intraarticular conditions.

Conclusion

Glenohumeral co-pathologies in CTS are rare and most commonly do not require surgical treatment. Routine diagnostic glenohumeral exploration does not appear mandatory in arthroscopic treatment of CTS. Exploration of the glenohumeral joint in arthroscopic removal of CD should only be performed when relevant intraarticular injuries with therapeutic relevance are highly expected.

Abbreviations

CD: Calcific depots; CTS: Calcific tendinitis; OR: Operating room; SLAP: Superior labral tears from anterior to posterior lesions

Acknowledgements

Not applicable.

Funding

No funding was obtained for this study.

Authors' contributions

GL: research hypothesis, data acquisition, analysis and interpretation of data, draft of manuscript. KI: study design, analysis and interpretation of data, revision of manuscript. EJK: research hypothesis, data acquisition, analysis and interpretation of data, draft of manuscript. DM: study design, analysis and interpretation of data, revision of manuscript. NS: study design, analysis and interpretation of data, revision of manuscript. PO: research hypothesis and design of study, data acquisition, analysis and interpretation of data, draft of manuscript. All authors critically reviewed and approved the final manuscript.

Competing interests

Gernot Lang, M.D. has the following financial disclosures:
Educational grants: DePuy-Synthes.
Travel grants: GSK Foundation, DePuy-Synthes.
The authors declare that they have no competing interests.

Author details

[1]Department of Orthopedics and Trauma Surgery, Medical Center - Albert-Ludwigs-University of Freiburg, Faculty of Medicine, Albert-Ludwigs-University of Freiburg, Hugstetter Strasse 55, 79106 Freiburg, Germany. [2]Center of Orthopedic Sports Medicine Freiburg, Breisacher Strasse 84, 79110 Freiburg, Germany.

References

1. Bosworth B. Calcium deposits in the shoulder and subacromial bursitis: a survey of 12,122 shoulders. J Am Med Assoc. 1941;116:2477–82.
2. Rupp S, Seil R, Kohn D. Tendinosis calcarea der Rotatorenmanschette. Orthopade. 2000;29:852–67.
3. Oliva F, Via AG, Maffulli N. Physiopathology of intratendinous calcific deposition. BMC Med. 2012;10:95.
4. Del Castillo-Gonzalez F, Ramos-Alvarez JJ, Rodriguez-Fabian G, Gonzalez-Perez J, Calderon-Montero J. Treatment of the calcific tendinopathy of the rotator cuff by ultrasound-guided percutaneous needle lavage. Two years prospective study. Muscles Ligaments Tendons J. 2014;4:407–12.
5. Gatt DL, Charalambous CP. Ultrasound-guided barbotage for calcific tendonitis of the shoulder: a systematic review including 908 patients. Arthroscopy. 2014;30:1166–72.
6. Maier D, Jaeger M, Izadpanah K, Bornebusch L, Suedkamp NP, Ogon P. Rotator cuff preservation in arthroscopic treatment of calcific tendinitis. Arthroscopy. 2013;29:824–31.
7. Ark JW, Flock TJ, Flatow EL, Bigliani LU. Arthroscopic treatment of calcific tendinitis of the shoulder. Arthroscopy. 1992;8:183–8.
8. Gschwend N, Patte D, Zippel J. Therapy of calcific tendinitis of the shoulder. Arch Orthop Unfallchir. 1972;73:120–35.
9. Yoo JC, Park WH, Koh KH, Kim SM. Arthroscopic treatment of chronic calcific tendinitis with complete removal and rotator cuff tendon repair. Knee Surg Sports Traumatol Arthrosc. 2010;18:1694–9.
10. Porcellini G, Paladini P, Campi F, Paganelli M. Arthroscopic treatment of calcifying tendinitis of the shoulder: clinical and ultrasonographic follow-up findings at two to five years. J Shoulder Elb Surg. 2004;13:503–8.
11. Peng X, Feng Y, Chen G, Yang L. Arthroscopic treatment of chronically painful calcific tendinitis of the rectus femoris. Eur J Med Res. 2013;18:49.

12. Louwerens JK, Veltman ES, van Noort A, van den Bekerom MP. The effectiveness of high-energy extracorporeal shockwave therapy versus ultrasound-guided needling versus arthroscopic surgery in the Management of Chronic Calcific Rotator Cuff Tendinopathy: a systematic review. Arthroscopy. 2016;32:165–75.
13. Moen TC, Rudolph GH, Caswell K, Espinoza C, Burkhead WZ, Jr., Krishnan SG: Complications of shoulder arthroscopy. J Am Acad Orthop Surg 2014, 22:410–419.
14. Cogan A, Boyer P, Soubeyrand M, Hamida FB, Vannier JL, Massin P. Cranial nerves neuropraxia after shoulder arthroscopy in beach chair position. Orthop Traumatol Surg Res. 2011;97:345–8.
15. Park TS, Kim YS. Neuropraxia of the cutaneous nerve of the cervical plexus after shoulder arthroscopy. Arthroscopy. 2005;21:631.
16. Bhatti MT, Enneking FK. Visual loss and ophthalmoplegia after shoulder surgery. Anesth Analg. 2003;96:899–902. table of contents
17. Zmistowski B, Austin L, Ciccotti M, Ricchetti E, Williams G Jr. Fatal venous air embolism during shoulder arthroscopy: a case report. J Bone Joint Surg Am. 2010;92:2125–7.
18. Sirveaux F, Gosselin O, Roche O, Turell P, Mole D. postoperative results after arthroscopic treatment of rotator cuff calcifying tendonitis, with or without associated glenohumeral exploration. Rev Chir Orthop Reparatrice Appar Mot. 2005;91:295–9.
19. Maier D, Jaeger M, Izadpanah K, Kostler W, Bischofberger AK, Sudkamp NP, Ogon P. Arthroscopic removal of chronic symptomatic calcifications of the supraspinatus tendon without Acromioplasty: analysis of postoperative recovery and outcome factors. Orthop J Sports Med. 2014;2: 2325967114533646.
20. Ogon P, Ogon M, Jager A. Technical note: the quadrant technique for arthroscopic treatment of rotator cuff calcifications. Arthroscopy. 2001;17:E13.
21. Bigliani LUMD, April EW. He morphology of the acromion and its relationship to rotator cuff tears. Orthop Trans. 1986;(1986):10–228.
22. Morgan CDRR, Snyder SJ. Arthroscopic assessment of the glenohumeral ligaments associated with recurrent anterior shoulder instability. Washington, DC: Paper presented at the Fifty-NInth Annual Meeting of the American Academy of Orthopaedic Surgeons; 1992.
23. Brittberg M, Winalski CS. Evaluation of cartilage injuries and repair. J Bone Joint Surg Am. 2003;85-A(Suppl 2):58–69.
24. Snyder SJ, Karzel RP, Pizzo WD, Ferkel RD, Friedman MJ. SLAP lesions of the shoulder. Arthroscopy. 1990;6:274–9.
25. Ellman H. Diagnosis and treatment of incomplete rotator cuff tears. Clin Orthop Relat Res. 1990:64–74.
26. Bayne OBJ. Long-term results of surgical repair of full-thickness rotator cuff tears. Philadelphia. 1984;
27. Oliva F, Via AG, Maffulli N. Calcific tendinopathy of the rotator cuff tendons. Sports Med Arthrosc. 2011;19:237–43.
28. Dhupar R, Evankovich J, Klune JR, Vargas LG, Hughes SJ. Delayed operating room availability significantly impacts the total hospital costs of an urgent surgical procedure. Surgery. 2011;150:299–305.
29. Moody AE, Moody CE, Althausen PL. Cost savings opportunities in perioperative Management of the Patients with Orthopaedic Trauma. J Orthop Trauma. 2016;30(Suppl 5):S7–s14.
30. Hofstee DJ, Gosens T, Bonnet M, De Waal Malefijt J. Calcifications in the cuff: take it or leave it? Br J Sports Med. 2007;41:832–5.
31. Rizzello G, Franceschi F, Longo UG, Ruzzini L, Meloni MC, Spiezia F, Papalia R, Denaro V. Arthroscopic management of calcific tendinopathy of the shoulder–do we need to remove all the deposit? Bull NYU Hosp Jt Dis. 2009;67:330–3.
32. Hurt G, Baker CL, Jr.: Calcific tendinitis of the shoulder. Orthop Clin North Am 2003, 34:567–575.
33. Seyahi A, Demirhan M. Arthroscopic removal of intraosseous and intratendinous deposits in calcifying tendinitis of the rotator cuff. Arthroscopy. 2009;25:590–6.
34. Jacobs R, Debeer P. Calcifying tendinitis of the rotator cuff: functional outcome after arthroscopic treatment. Acta Orthop Belg. 2006;72:276–81.
35. Randelli P, Castagna A, Cabitza F, Cabitza P, Arrigoni P, Denti M. Infectious and thromboembolic complications of arthroscopic shoulder surgery. J Shoulder Elb Surg. 2010;19:97–101.
36. Borgeat A, Bird P, Ekatodramis G, Dumont C. Tracheal compression caused by periarticular fluid accumulation: a rare complication of shoulder surgery. J Shoulder Elb Surg. 2000;9:443–5.
37. Weber SC, Abrams JS, Nottage WM. Complications associated with arthroscopic shoulder surgery. Arthroscopy. 2002;18:88–95.
38. Merolla G, Bhat MG, Paladini P, Porcellini G. Complications of calcific tendinitis of the shoulder: a concise review. J Orthop Traumatol. 2015; 16:175–83.
39. Hsu JE, Anakwenze OA, Warrender WJ, Abboud JA. Current review of adhesive capsulitis. J Shoulder Elb Surg. 2011;20:502–14.
40. White D, Choi H, Peloquin C, Zhu Y, Zhang Y. Secular trend of adhesive capsulitis. Arthritis Care Res (Hoboken). 2011;63:1571–5.
41. Brislin KJ, Field LD, Savoie FH 3rd. Complications after arthroscopic rotator cuff repair. Arthroscopy. 2007;23:124–8.
42. Huberty DP, Schoolfield JD, Brady PC, Vadala AP, Arrigoni P, Burkhart SS. Incidence and treatment of postoperative stiffness following arthroscopic rotator cuff repair. Arthroscopy. 2009;25:880–90.
43. Constant CR, Murley AH. A clinical method of functional assessment of the shoulder. Clin Orthop Relat Res. 1987:160–4.
44. Itoi E, Arce G, Bain GI, Diercks RL, Guttmann D, Imhoff AB, Mazzocca AD, Sugaya H, Yoo YS. Shoulder stiffness: current concepts and concerns. Arthroscopy. 2016;32:1402–14.
45. Shields E, Thirukumaran C, Thorsness R, Noyes K, Voloshin I. An analysis of adult patient risk factors and complications within 30 days after arthroscopic shoulder surgery. Arthroscopy. 2015;31:807–15.
46. Seil R, Litzenburger H, Kohn D, Rupp S. Arthroscopic treatment of chronically painful calcifying tendinitis of the supraspinatus tendon. Arthroscopy. 2006;22:521–7.
47. Pauzenberger L, Grieb A, Hexel M, Laky B, Anderl W, Heuberer P. Infections following arthroscopic rotator cuff repair: incidence, risk factors, and prophylaxis. Knee Surg Sports Traumatol Arthrosc. 2017;25:595–601.
48. Brislin KJ, Field LD, Savoie FH. Complications after arthroscopic rotator cuff repair. Arthroscopy. 2007;23:124–8.
49. Johnson LL, Shneider DA, Austin MD, Goodman FG, Bullock JM, DeBruin JA. Two per cent glutaraldehyde: a disinfectant in arthroscopy and arthroscopic surgery. J Bone Joint Surg Am. 1982;64:237–9.
50. McFarland EG, O'Neill OR, Hsu CY. Complications of shoulder arthroscopy. J South Orthop Assoc. 1997;6:190–6.
51. Namdari S, Nicholson T, Parvizi J, Ramsey M. Preoperative doxycycline does not decolonize Propionibacterium acnes from the skin of the shoulder: a randomized controlled trial. J Shoulder Elb Surg. 2017;26:1495–9.
52. Murray MR, Saltzman MD, Gryzlo SM, Terry MA, Woodward CC, Nuber GW. Efficacy of preoperative home use of 2% chlorhexidine gluconate cloth before shoulder surgery. J Shoulder Elb Surg. 2011;20:928–33.
53. Savage JW, Weatherford BM, Sugrue PA, Nolden MT, Liu JC, Song JK, Haak MH. Efficacy of surgical preparation solutions in lumbar spine surgery. J Bone Joint Surg Am. 2012;94:490–4.
54. Saltzman MD, Nuber GW, Gryzlo SM, Marecek GS, Koh JL. Efficacy of surgical preparation solutions in shoulder surgery. J Bone Joint Surg Am. 2009;91:1949–53.
55. Dodson CC, Craig EV, Cordasco FA, Dines DM, Dines JS, DiCarlo E, Brause BD, Warren RF. Propionibacterium acnes infection after shoulder arthroplasty: a diagnostic challenge. J Shoulder Elb Surg. 2010;19:303–7.
56. Horneff JG, Hsu JE, Huffman GR. Propionibacterium acnes infections in shoulder surgery. Orthop Clin N Am. 2014;45:515–21.
57. Mook WR, Klement MR, Green CL, Hazen KC, Garrigues GE. The incidence of Propionibacterium acnes in open shoulder surgery: a controlled diagnostic study. J Bone Joint Surg Am. 2015;97:957–63.
58. Sethi PM, Sabetta JR, Stuek SJ, Horine SV, Vadasdi KB, Greene RT, Cunningham JG, Miller SR. Presence of Propionibacterium acnes in primary shoulder arthroscopy: results of aspiration and tissue cultures. J Shoulder Elb Surg. 2015;24:796–803.
59. Matsen FA, Butler-Wu S, Carofino BC, Jette JL, Bertelsen A, Bumgarner R. Origin of Propionibacterium in surgical wounds and evidence-based approach for culturing Propionibacterium from surgical sites. J Bone Joint Surg Am. 2013;95:e181.
60. Olsen MA, Nepple JJ, Riew KD, Lenke LG, Bridwell KH, Mayfield J, Fraser VJ. Risk factors for surgical site infection following orthopaedic spinal operations. J Bone Joint Surg Am. 2008;90:62–9.
61. Peersman G, Laskin R, Davis J, Peterson MG, Richart T. Prolonged operative time correlates with increased infection rate after total knee arthroplasty. HSS J. 2006;2:70–2.

15

Contact stresses, pressure and area in a fixed-bearing total ankle replacement: a finite element analysis

Nicolo Martinelli[1*], Silvia Baretta[1,2], Jenny Pagano[1,2], Alberto Bianchi[1], Tomaso Villa[1,2], Gloria Casaroli[1] and Fabio Galbusera

Abstract

Background: Mobile-bearing ankle implants with good clinical results continued to increase the popularity of total ankle arthroplasty to address endstage ankle osteoarthritis preserving joint movement. Alternative solutions used fixed-bearing designs, which increase stability and reduce the risk of bearing dislocation, but with a theoretical increase of contact stresses leading to a higher polyethylene wear. The purpose of this study was to investigate the contact stresses, pressure and area in the polyethylene component of a new total ankle replacement with a fixed-bearing design, using 3D finite element analysis.

Methods: A three-dimensional finite element model of the Zimmer Trabecular Metal Total Ankle was developed and assembled based on computed tomography images. Three different sizes of the polyethylene insert were modeled, and a finite element analysis was conducted to investigate the contact pressure, the von Mises stresses and the contact area of the polyethylene component during the stance phase of the gait cycle.

Results: The peak value of pressure was found in the anterior region of the articulating surface, where it reached 19. 8 MPa at 40% of the gait cycle. The average contact pressure during the stance phase was 6.9 MPa. The maximum von Mises stress of 14.1 MPa was reached at 40% of the gait cycle in the anterior section. In the central section, the maximum von Mises stress of 10.8 MPa was reached at 37% of the gait cycle, whereas in the posterior section the maximum stress of 5.4 MPa was reached at the end of the stance phase.

Discussion: The new fixed-bearing total ankle replacement showed a safe mechanical behavior and many clinical advantages. However, advanced models to quantitatively estimate the wear are need.

Conclusion: To the light of the clinical advantages, we conclude that the presented prosthesis is a good alternative to the other products present in the market.

Keywords: Contact stress, Ankle arthroplasty ankle osteoarthritis

Background

Total Ankle Arthroplasty (TAA) has become a valuable procedure to relieve pain and restore functions in patients with osteoarthritis or rheumatoid arthritis. Newer implant designs with improved clinical results and longer term outcomes studies with satisfactory survival rates, increased the popularity of TAA to address end-stage ankle osteoarthritis preserving joint movement [15, 16]. In the past, high failure rates were associated to the first generation of implants due to loosening and subsidence at the bone-implant interface as a consequence of abnormal shear, compression and rotations [2–4, 8, 9, 11]. Loosening rates of the first generation two-component implants were found to be 60% and 90% after 5 and 10 years, respectively [11]. Further knowledge of the biomechanics associated with TAA, resulted in the second generation of implants that involved less bony resection and avoided cemented components with stem or peg fixation for primary stability. Second generation of TAAs was fixed-bearing, semi-constrained and two-component systems. These

* Correspondence: N.Martinelli@unicampus.it
[1]IRCCS Istituto Ortopedico Galeazzi, Milan, Italy
Full list of author information is available at the end of the article

implants had the advantages to increase stability and reduce the risk of bearing dislocation. However, this second generation of implants led to increased polyethylene wear, symptomatic impingement and subluxation or dislocation of the components [11, 12]. The third generation of implants was less constrained, two- or three-component design. Although these implants offer majors advantages over the past designs which commonly failed due to loosening and osteolysis, the clinical outcomes are still less satisfactory than total hip and total knee arthroplasty [14]. A randomized prospective study conducted on 200 ankle replacements of the three-component Buechel-Pappas (BP) and the Scandinavian Total Ankle Replacement (STAR), found a six year survivor-ship of 86.5% [25].

The Zimmer Trabecular Metal Total Ankle (ZTMTA) replacement, available in the United States and in Europe, is the newest total ankle arthroplasty system. This implant belongs to the third generation of TAAs. The theoretical advantages, which are clinically unproven yet, are indeed attractive: the lateral transfibular surgical approach would enable surgeons to better visualize the anatomic center of rotation of the ankle, and due to the use of an assisted external fixator alignment system, bony resections are guided during the entire procedure, thus maintaining the integrity of the blood supply to the skin and potentially reducing the risk of wound complications [23]. Moreover, the lateral approach permits an extensive exposure to the ankle and to the subtalar joint in the surgical plane between angiosomes, thus maintaining the integrity of the blood supply to the skin and potentially reducing the risk of wound complications. However, due to the fixed-bearing design, there are some concerns related to polyethylene wear as possible consequences of high contact pressure [17].

Finite Element (FE) analysis is a consolidated method to investigate the mechanical behavior of prostheses and biological tissues because it has many advantages. First, it reveals all the mechanical parameters (e.g. stresses and strains) that are not always experimentally measurable; second, it allows performing parametric studies and doing structural analysis, in order to highlight areas of design weakness and suggest improvement possibilities; third, it allows performing quicker and cheaper analyses with respect to experimental testing. Although in vivo and in vitro conditions are not completely reproducible in finite element models, this method can give a clear view of the mechanical effect of a specific loading condition, and it can be used as a supporting tool by the industries and surgeons. In the last decades, some numerical studies have been performed to investigate the effect of the design features of each component, of the polyethylene thickness and of the ankle flexion angle [15]. It has been showed that, in a mobile-bearing implant, increasing the polyethylene thickness causes a more uniform distribution of the contact pressure, but increases the von Mises stresses at the edges [15]. In a semiconstrained prosthesis, Miller et al. [19] found the peak von Mises stress beneath the contact surface in two different configurations of the talar component. Jay et al. [13] compared the contact pressure, von Mises stresses and contact area in seven different implants, concluding that increasing the liner thickness and the articulating-surface area, the contact stresses may significantly decrease. A main problem in TAA studies is that a direct comparison is not always possible to do, due to the different investigated implants and the different boundaries and loading conditions. Indeed, many studies applied simple loading conditions and did not consider the action of the ligamentus apparatus. Reggiani et al. [21] investigated the effect of the gait cycle in a three component TAA including the ligaments, finding an uneven distribution of the contact pressure with small peaks in the demanding loading experience of gait. Thus, finite element analysis is a useful tool to compare the biomechanical behavior of a new prosthesis and to compare it with the other implants available on the market.

The objective of this study was therefore to investigate the contact pressure, the von Mises stresses and the contact area in the polyethylene component of the new ZTMTA with three different thicknesses, using a 3D finite element analysis.

Methods

A size two left ZTMTA and "zero" size of the polyethylene component (Fig. 1) provided by the manufacturer were digitally scanned (Scanprobe ST Nivol Scansystems, Pisa, Italy) and the initial Computer Aided Drafting (CAD) models were created (SolidWorks, Dassault Systemes S.A., Vlizy, France). The talar, the tibial and the polyethylene components were then smoothed and the imperfections due to the scanning process were removed.

Computed Tomography (CT) images, one in the sagittal and one in the frontal view, were acquired from a selected patient to assess the consolidation of the fibular

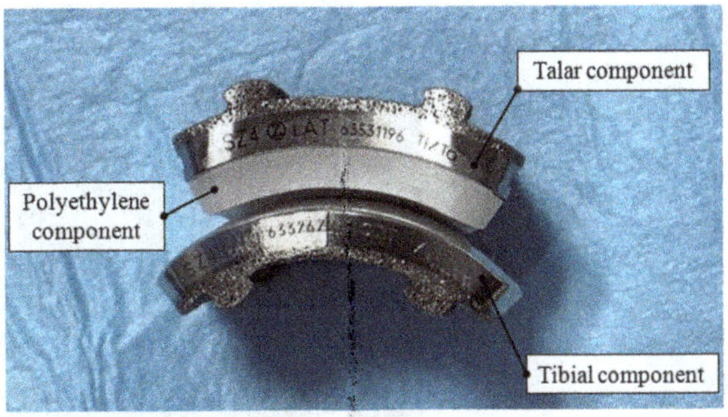

Fig. 1 Zimmer Trabecular Metal Total Ankle Arthroplasty (TMTA). The implant is composed by the talar and the tibial component with a fixed-polyethylene bearing

osteotomy at the IRCCS Istituto Ortopedico Galeazzi (Milan, Italy). Written informed consent for the use of the data for research purposes was obtained and the patient's data were anonymized. Because the patient was not involved in the study and the data were anonymized, ethics approval was not requested (CPMP/ICH/135/95, Good Clinical Practice GCP: Consolidated Guidance, European Directive 75/318/EEC). CT images were used to locate the ZTMTA model in neutral position using the software Mimics (Materialise, Leuven, Belgium) (Fig. 2). Then, 3D models were imported into ABAQUS (Version 6.12–1, Dassault Systemes) and meshed. The final assembled model was composed by 23,631 linear hexahedral elements.

All the materials in the finite element model were homogenous, isotropic and linear elastic, except for the Ultra High Molecular Weight Polyethylene (UHMWPE) component that was modeled as an ideal elastic-plastic material [19] (Table 1). The stress-strain curve of the UHMWPE was taken from the literature and the yield stress was fixed to 10.86 MPa[19] (Fig. 3). A surface to surface contact behavior was defined between the talar and the polyethylene components, with a friction coefficient of 0.04 [10]. Normal hard contact-overclosure behavior was assigned with the talar surface as master. To enforce the contact, a penalty method was applied. The tibial and the UHMWPE components were totally constrained and belong to the same mesh.

The five major ligaments which surround the ankle joint complex were included into the model: the Anterior Talofibular (ATaFi), the Tibiocalcaneal (TiCa), the Calcaneofibular (CaFi), the Tibionavicular (TiNa) and the Superior Tibiotalar (sTiTa) (Fig. 4). The ligaments were modeled using non-linear, one dimensional spring elements, and their mechanical behavior was described by the constitutive law suggested by Funk and colleagues [7]. The ligaments were assumed having an elastic response described by the formulation

$$F(\varepsilon) = A\left(e^{B\varepsilon}-1\right)$$

Table 1 Material properties assigned to the Zimmer Trabecular Metal Total Ankle components and to the bearing

Component	Material	Young Modulus (GPa)	Poisson ratio
Tibial	Ti-6Al-4 V	115	0.36
Talar	CoCrMo	241	0.3
Polyethylene	UHMWPE	Stress-strain curve taken from Miller et al. (2004) [17]	

where ε was the strain and A and B were taken from the literature (Table 2) [7].

The locations of the ligaments insertions in the ankle neutral position were taken from previous studies [5, 21]. Since this model did not include any bones, a kinematic constraint was established between each insertion of ligament and one of the two components of the prosthesis. The origin of each ligament was linked to groups of nodes on the tibial component through a continuum-distributing coupling, whereas each insertion was constrained to a node set on the talus component (Fig. 4). According to Wei et al., in order to simulate the pretension of the ankle ligaments ε was set to zero for a spring element 2% shorter than the distance between the insertion points [24].

In order to apply rotations to the components of the prosthesis, a tibial and a talar control points were defined and kinematically constrained to the relative parts. The tibial component was constrained in the anteroposterior and mediolateral direction, whereas the talar component was constrained in the axial and in the mediolateral directions. The loading scenario proposed by Bell and colleagues [2] was applied: it included the axial compression and the internalexternal rotation of the tibial component, and the plantar dorsiflexion rotation and anteroposterior displacement of the talus (Fig. 5). The mechanical actions of muscles and tendons were included in the applied loads [1]. Each load was described by an independent time history (Fig. 6) [2]. Only the stance phase of the gait was investigated, which represented the 60% of the entire gait cycle. To ensure that the results of the simulations were independent on

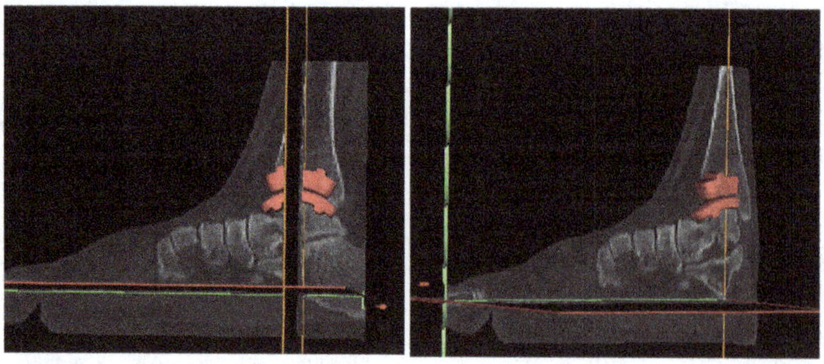

Fig. 2 Schematic representation of the implant positioning using the CT images

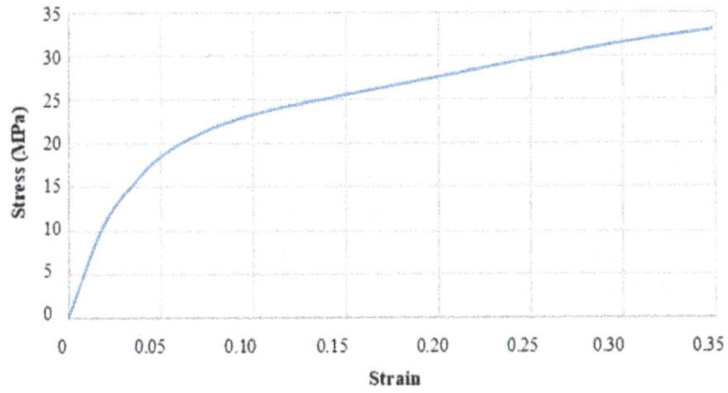

Fig. 3 Stress-strain curve of the polyethylene material [16]

the element size, a mesh sensitivity study has been carried out. The maximum contact area between the talar and the polyethylene components, the maximum von Mises stress of the bearing and the peak contact pressure were evaluated for five element sizes equal in the entire assembly (1.35 mm; 1.3 mm; 1.0 mm; 0.7 mm; 0.6 mm). Because the value of the peak contact area converged to less than 0.3%, the von Mises stress converged to less than 0.2% and the maximum contact pressure converged to 1% difference upon the further mesh, the mesh with 1 mm element size was used.

The influence of polyethylene height was evaluated by analyzing two additional configurations, one 2 mm and one 4 mm thicker than the standard size. Thus, two additional models were created extruding the surface of the polyethylene component. The new assembled models were composed by 26,621 and 29,676 linear hexahedral elements, respectively. All the other parameters, as well the ligaments initial strain, were left unchanged.

For a more precise prediction of the stress distribution, the anterior, central and posterior cross sectional areas of the polyethylene component were investigated.

Table 2 Elastic response function data of the ligaments (Funk et al.)

Ligaments	A(N)	B
ATaFi	7.18	12.50
CaFi	0.20	49.63
TiCa	0.51	45.99
TiNa	0.51	45.99
sTiTa	2.06	20.11

Results

The average and the maximum von Mises stress and contact pressure value were found between the 30–50% of the entire gait cycle in the anterior and in the central section (Table 3). The contact pressure distribution was higher in the anterior part during the most of the stance phase (Fig. 7). The peak values were found in the anterior region of the articulating surface, where reached 19.8 MPa at 40% of the gait cycle (Fig. 8). The average contact pressure during the stance phase of gait was 6.9 MPa.

In the anterior section, the maximum von Mises stress of 14.1 MPa was reached at 40% of the gait cycle. In the central section, the maximum von Mises stress of 10.8 MPa was reached at 37% of the gait cycle, whereas in the posterior section the maximum of 5.4 MPa was reached at the end of the stance phase (60% of the gait cycle) (Figs. 9 and 10).

The contact area increased up to 296 mm^2 (about 40% of the contact surface) until 35% of the gait cycle. This result was consistent with the maximum value of the set of loads and boundaries on the polyethylene bearing, in particular with the axial force. At the beginning of the stance phase, when heel strike occurred and the minimum solicitations acted on the polyethylene bearing, the minimum value of 28 mm^2 (about the 4% of the contact surface) was reached.

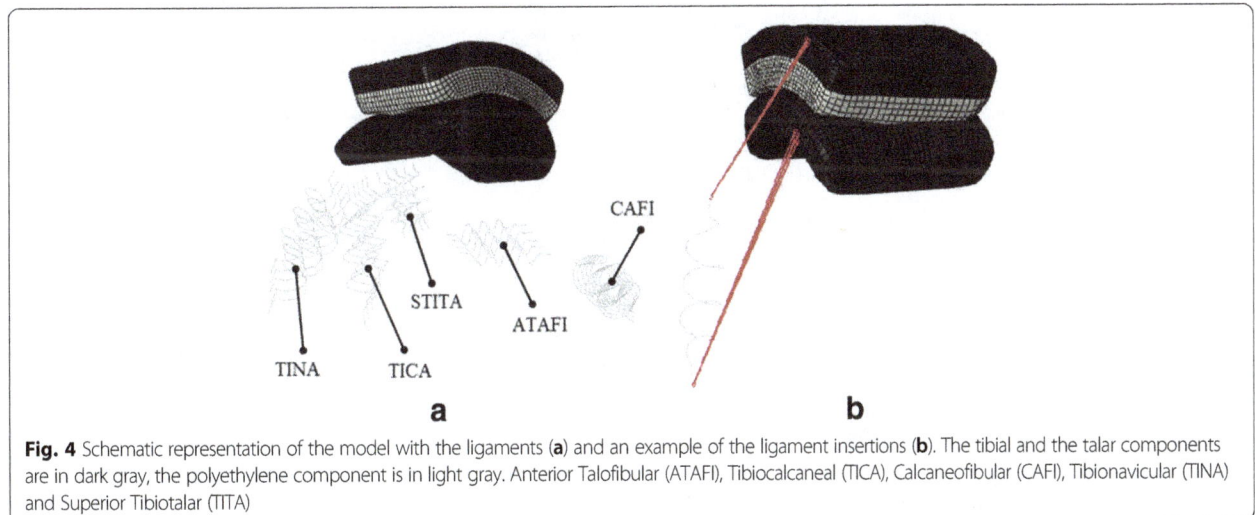

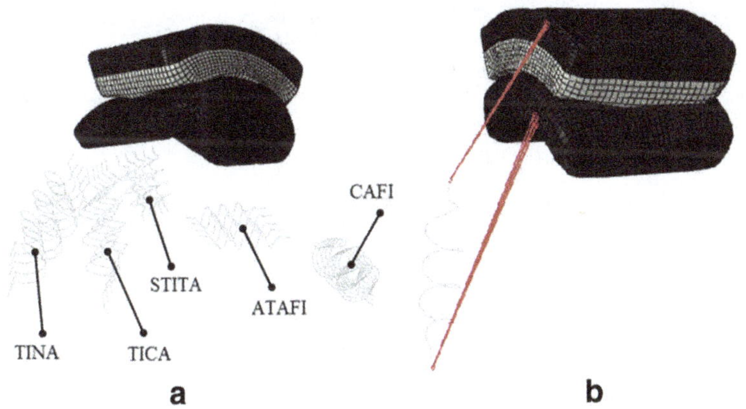

Fig. 4 Schematic representation of the model with the ligaments (**a**) and an example of the ligament insertions (**b**). The tibial and the talar components are in dark gray, the polyethylene component is in light gray. Anterior Talofibular (ATAFI), Tibiocalcaneal (TICA), Calcaneofibular (CAFI), Tibionavicular (TINA) and Superior Tibiotalar (TITA)

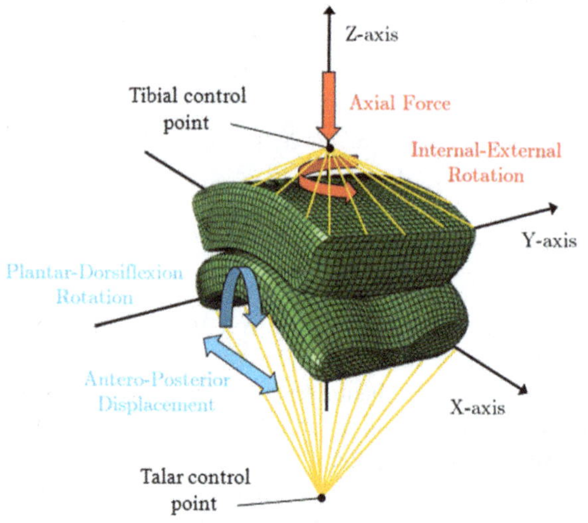

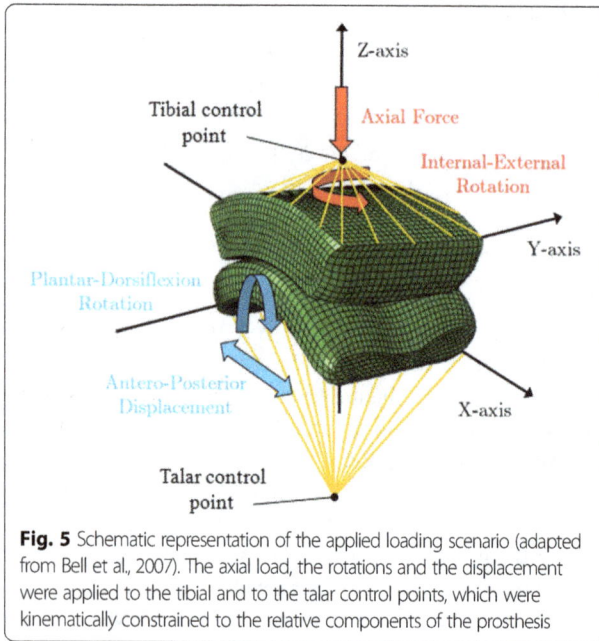

Fig. 5 Schematic representation of the applied loading scenario (adapted from Bell et al., 2007). The axial load, the rotations and the displacement were applied to the tibial and to the talar control points, which were kinematically constrained to the relative components of the prosthesis

The maximum lateral displacement and the maximum rotation of the polyethylene bearing were 1.67 mm and 1.4°, and were reached at about 40% and 62% of the gait cycle, respectively.

The talar component had a maximum internal rotation of 4.9° at about 18% of the gait cycle and a maximum external rotation of 3.8° at about 62% of the gait cycle.

Increasing the thickness of the polyethylene bearing did not significantly influence the von Mises stress and the pressure in the polyethylene bearing. The average and peak pressure values were 6.93, 6.32 and 6.78 MPa and 12.19, 11.50 and 12.33 MPa for the standard, 2 mm and 4 mm thicker polyethylene bearing, respectively. Von Mises stress was higher in the anterior section with respect to the lateral and the posterior ones in all cases, and was higher in the medial and in the lateral regions than in the central one. Increasing the thickness of the polyethylene component caused a reduction of the 2% and of the 9% the maximum von Mises stress in the anterior section in the 2 mm and 4 mm thicker bearing, respectively.

Discussion

This study presents a numerical model of a novel TAR with three different sizes of fixed polyethylene bearing. Contact pressure, von Mises stresses and contact area were predicted during the stance phase of the gait cycle. The knowledge of these mechanical parameters is important because they are related to wear problems as well as to the risk of loosening and osteolysis.

In general, the model predictions were in a good agreement with previous studies [19, 22, 23] conducted on other total ankle replacements. However, the comparison of the present results with the literature was difficult due to the different designs analyzed, to the different loading protocols and boundary conditions and to the presence (or lack) of ligamentous apparatus.

For each studied configuration, it was showed that the average pressure value at the interfaces of ZTMTA was less than 10 MPa, which is generally considered a critical

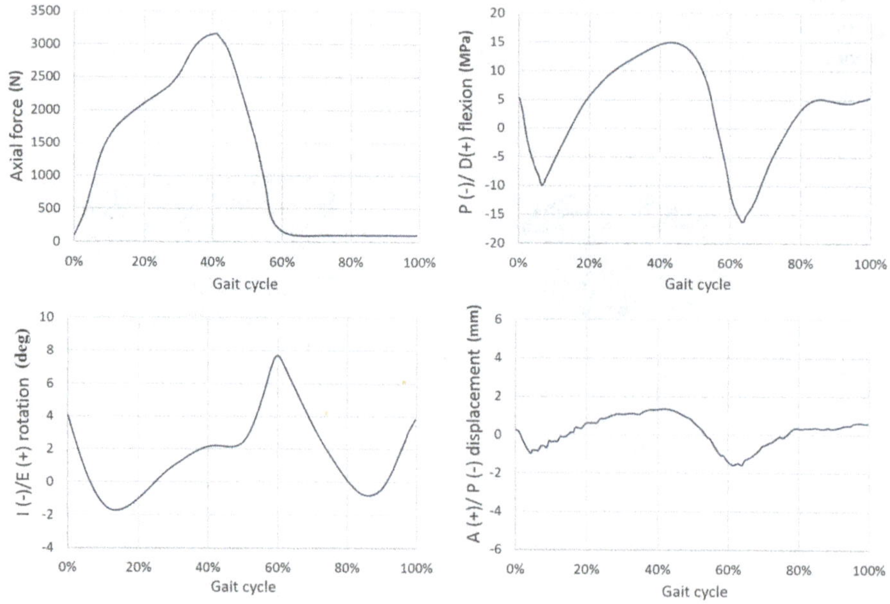

Fig. 6 Time-histories of the applied boundary conditions during the gait cycle. A/P means Anterior/Posterior, I/E means internal/external, P/D means plantar/dorsiflexion. Adapted from Bell et al. (2007)

Table 3 Average and maximum von Mises stress and contact pressure in the anterior, central and posterior section of the polyethylene component between 10 and 70% of the gait cycle

	Anterior				Central				Posterior			
	von Mises (MPa)		Contact pressure (MPa)		von Mises (MPa)		Contact pressure (MPa)		von Mises (MPa)		Contact pressure (MPa)	
	Average	Max	Average	Max	Average	Max	Average	Max	Average	Max	Average	Max
10%	1.3	4.9	1.2	7.6	4.2	9.4	5.7	12.4	0.8	2.3	0.0	0.0
20%	4.1	10.3	5.6	12.6	3.7	8.6	5.0	11.7	0.5	1.6	0.0	1.0
30%	6.1	11.9	8.4	16.2	2.7	7.5	3.3	11.0	0.3	1.0	0.0	2.0
40%	7.5	14.1	10.0	19.8	2.7	7.6	2.9	11.0	0.3	1.0	0.0	3.0
50%	2.8	6.9	3.4	8.6	4.3	9.7	6.1	13.2	0.6	2.2	0.4	4.9
60%	0.3	2.1	0.0	0.0	0.4	2.1	0.1	0.9	0.6	5.4	0.0	0.0
70%	0.4	2.5	0.1	2.5	0.2	0.9	0.1	0.9	0.1	0.2	0.0	0.0

value for polyethylene integrity [9, 19]. However, peaks pressure higher than 10 MPa were recorded in small areas. High peaks pressure indicated local high stress concentrations of the polyethylene, which could cause wear, accelerated component loosening and clinical failure. Many contrast results were found in the literature. Some studies reported a yield stress values for medical grade polyethylene in the range from 15 to 23 MPa [19, 20]. Espinosa et al. [6] performed a finite element comparison between two validated models of the Agility two-component prosthesis (size 4 - DePuy) and the Mobility three-component prosthesis (size 3, 3 × 7 mm mobile-bearing - DePuy). They measured the contact pressure under standard position and under misalignments deviated from this relative position. The three-component Mobility TAA showed a contact pressure more evenly distributed and threefold lower than the two-component Agility, which exceeded the yield stress of 18 MPa for all tested configurations. Reggiani et al. showed that in the three-component Bologna-Oxford prosthesis [21] (BOX) the average contact pressure experienced by a lower surface of the polyethylene bearing was 10.3 MPa, with a peak value of 16.1 MPa at 79% of the stance phase (about 40% of the entire gait cycle). However, the applied loads and boundary conditions differed from this study: in particular, a lower axial load of 1600 N in combination with an anteriorposterior force on the talar component and an internal/external torque were applied. Saad et al. developed a FE model of the BOX implant and predicted a peak contact pressure of 18.4 MPa at 79% of the stance phase [21]. Differently from our study, they applied an internal/external rotation instead of a torque moment.

Von Mises stress is a mechanical condition used to indicate the state of stress in ductile materials and it is used to investigate the failure processes. In biomechanics, von Mises stress is a valuable indicator of the immediate post-operative period and for the implant failure. The von Mises stress values predicted in the current study were similar to the outcomes of previous FE models. Indeed, Miller et al., in an Agility FE model, found von Mises stress values in the range from 19.5 to 16.3 MPa in the edge and from 11.4 to 9.3 MPa in the center of the polyethylene bearing [19]. Jay et al. [13] analyzed the average von Mises cross-sectional stresses on

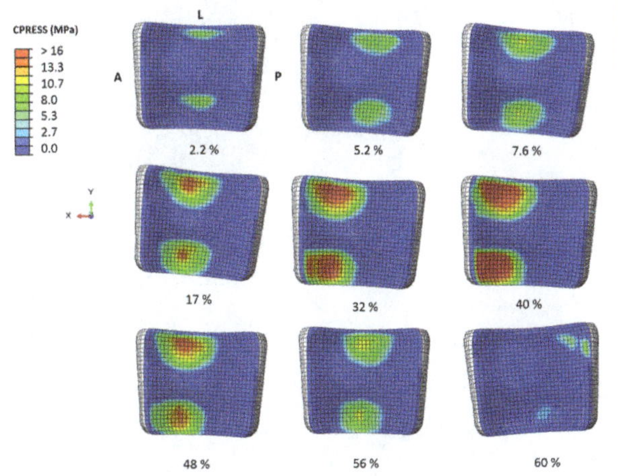

Fig. 7 Contact stresses on the polyethylene bearing at different percentage of gait cycle. A = anterior, P = posterior, L = lateral

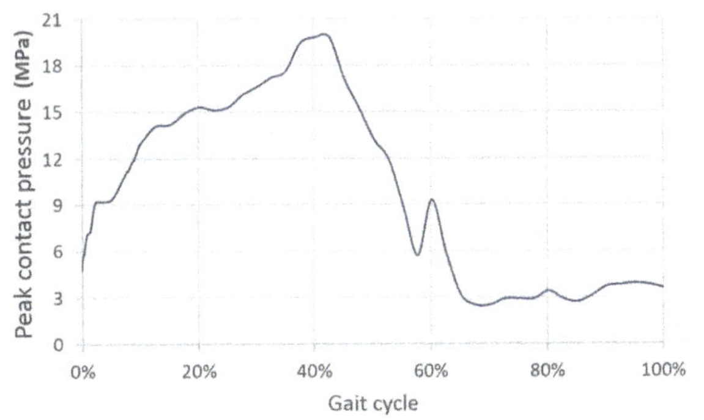

Fig. 8 Peak contact pressure on the articulating surface during the entire gait cycle

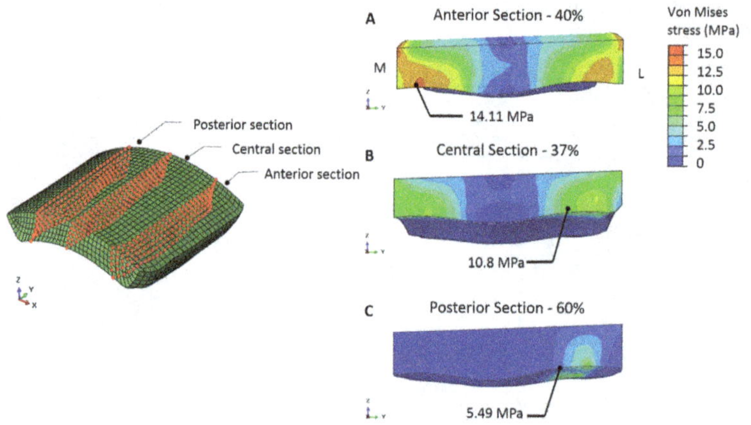

Fig. 9 Sections for the investigation of stresses distribution on polyethylene component and maximum von Mises cross-sectional values for the anterior (A), central (B) and posterior (C) section, from the medial (M) to the lateral (L) side

the ankle joint subjected to an uniform pressure corresponding to the normal component of the ankle gait with a maximum value of 4400 N. The values reported ranged from 4 to 14 MPa; in our model, the average von Mises stresses on the polyethylene bearing ranged from 7 to 12 MPa.

Increasing the thickness of the polyethylene bearing showed a slight decrease of the von Mises stresses. This outcome was in agreement with the study of Bartel and collegues [1], which showed that in total knee replacement a polyethylene insert with a thickness of more than eight to ten millimeters should be maintained. This result suggested that the choice of the bearing size can be made on the basis of clinical reasons. On contrast, McIff and colleagues [18] found a noticeable effect of the polyethylene insert on pressure distribution: in particular they concluded that with a thicker polyethylene insert the pressure was more evenly distributed in the anteroposterior direction, while a thinner polyethylene resulted in higher stresses at the midline of the insert. The contact area between the talar and the polyethylene component has two conflicting mechanical aspects related: indeed, an extended contact area enhances the stability of the prosthesis, preventing possible dislocation of the implant. On the other hand, when the surface increases also the area subjected to wear could increase. It was showed that the contact surface increased with the load and it was always about the 25% of the natural ankle joint. This outcome ensured the stability of the prosthesis [1], but further studies should be done to

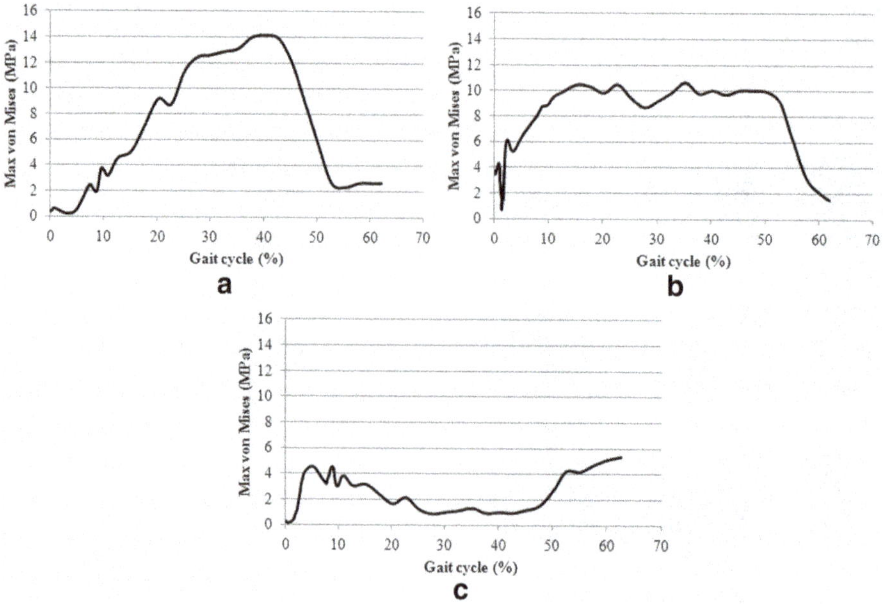

Fig. 10 Maximum von Mises stress in the stance phase in anterior (**a**), central (**b**) and posterior section (**c**)

investigate the wear generation. Jay et al. [13] conducted a FE investigation on seven Wright State University patented TAA models belonging to two different generations of implants. They found that neither coefficient of friction nor material properties differences of the talar and tibial component contributed to significantly change the stress state in the UHMWPE liner. They hypothesized, it was due to the fact that geometry had a major role in determining the stress state, concluding that increasing the liners thickness and the contact area could significantly decrease the cross-sectional von Mises stresses.

Some limitations related to the modeling approach should be highlighted. First, bones were not taken into account in the present model [9, 19]. However, this simplification was not expected to have a major impact on the prediction of the stresses on the contact surfaces because of the high Young modulus of the ZTMTA components (Table 1). Therefore, for mechanical reasons the load is supported by the implant, making the absence of bone a reasonable assumption. Moreover, a total osteointegration between the implant and the bone has been supposed, since any relative motions were neglected. Thus, we believe that this is a reasonable simplification, since the main purpose of the study was the evaluation of contact outputs on the polyethylene bearing components and not to investigate the state of stress in the bone. Caution may be taken to interpret the results because the model was not validated and an in vitro study may be performed to validate the current numerical findings. However, the ligaments properties were taken from the literature and the implants geometrical and mechanical parameters were given by the manufacturer; therefore we assumed the presented model reliable.

A major limitation of the present study regards the lack of a general consensus about the boundary and loading conditions to be used to simulate the gait cycle. Indeed, there are wide differences in the ankle loads used by various authors (e.g. among Bell and Reggiani), which may have a significant impact on the stress predictions [2, 21]. An additional limitation is that we analyzed only one size implant. In fact, the dimensions of the prosthesis may influence the pressure in the polyethylene component; however, it can be argued that larger implants are generally used for heavier patients, therefore a higher compressive force should be applied and the pressure distribution should result similar.

Conclusions

In conclusion, taking into account these limitations of the modeling approach, the present results showed that the von Mises stresses and pressure values of the ZTMTA are generally similar to those calculated in previous studies for other implants, and a similar wear behavior in the long term might be expected. It should be noted that other factors not related to the biomechanical ones (e.g. invasivity, safety of the surgical access, etc.) should be taken into account when selecting a TAA and might provide advantages for the ZTMTA with respect to alternative implants. However, to the light of the clinical advantages, the minimum bone resection requirement and the similar mechanical outcomes between this study and others present in the literature, we conclude that the ZTMTA is a good alternative to the other prostheses present in the market.

Potential benefits need however to be proven by means of long term clinical studies.

Abbreviations

ATaFi: Anterior Talofibular; BOX: Bologna-Oxford prosthesis; BP: Buechel-Pappas; CAD: Computer Aided Drafting; CaFi: Calcaneofibular; CGP: Good Clinical Practice; CT: Computed Tomography; FE: Finite Element; STAR: Scandinavian Total Ankle Replacement; sTiTa: Superior Tibiotalar; TAA: Total Ankle Arthroplasty; TiCa: Tibiocalcaneal; TiNa: Tibionavicular; UHMWPE: Ultra High Molecular Weight Polyethylene; ZTMTA: Zimmer Trabecular Metal Total Ankle

Acknowledgements

Not Applicable.

Funding

Expenses related to the publication of the present article were supported by the Italian Ministry of Health.

Authors' contributions

NM made substantial contributions to conception and design, acquisition and interpretation of data and was involved in revising the manuscript critically for important intellectual content; SB and JP made substantial contributions to conception and design, analysis and interpretation of data and in manuscript drafting; AB made substantial contributions to acquisition and interpretation of data; TV made substantial contributions to conception, analysis of the data and general supervision; GC made substantial contributions to analysis and interpretation of data and was involved in drafting and revising the manuscript critically; FG made substantial contributions to conception and design, interpretation and analysis of the data, and gave a general supervision. All the authors have given final approval of the version to be published.

Competing interests

Zimmer provided the ZTMTA device for the study. However, Zimmer did not take part in any steps of the current study and no funds were received. All the authors declared no conflict of interest related with this paper. No financial relationship exists between Zimmer and the authors.

Author details

[1]IRCCS Istituto Ortopedico Galeazzi, Milan, Italy. [2]Laboratory of Biological Structure Mechanics (LaBS), Department of Chemistry, Materials and Chemical Engineering "Giulio Natta , Politecnico di Milano, 20133 Milan, Italy.

References

1. Bartel DL, Bicknell VL, Wright TM. The effect of conformity, thickness and material on stresses in ultra-high molecular weight components for total joints replacements. J Bone Joint Surg Am. 1986;68(7):1041–51.
2. Bell CJ, Fisher J. Simulation of polyethylene wear in ankle joint prostheses. J Biomed Mater Res B Appl Biomater. 2007;81(1):162–7.

3. Bolton-Maggs BG, Sudlow RA, Freeman MA. Total ankle arthroplasty. A long-term review of the London hospital experience. J Bone Joint Surg Br. 1985;67(5):785–90.
4. Buechel FF, Pappas MJ. Survivorship and clinical evaluation of cementless, meniscal-bearing total ankle replacements. Semin Arthroplast. 1992;3(1):43–50.
5. Corazza F, O'Connor J, Leardini A, Parenti CV. Ligaments fibre recruitment and forces for the anterior drawer test at the human ankle joint. J Biomech. 2003;36(3):363–72.
6. Espinosa N, Walti M, Favre P, Snedeker JG. Misalignment of total ankle components can induce high joint contact pressures. J Bone Joint Surg Am. 2010;92(5):1179–87.
7. Funk JR, Hall GW, Crandall JR, Pilkey WD. Linear and quasi-linear viscoelastic characterization of ankle ligaments. J Biomech Eng. 2000;122(1):15–22.
8. Giannini S, Leardini A, O'Connor JJ. Total ankle replacement: review of the designs and of the current status. Foot Ankle Surg. 2000;6(2):77–88.
9. Gill LH. Challenges in total ankle arthroplasty. Foot Ankle Int. 2004;25(4):195–207.
10. Godest AC, Beaugonin M, Haug E, Taylor M, Gregson PJ. Simulation of a knee joint replacement during a gait cycle using explicit finite element analysis. J Biomech. 2002;35(2):267–75.
11. Gougoulias NE, Khanna A, Maffulli N. History and evolution in total ankle arthroplasty. Br Med Bull. 2009;89(1):111–51.
12. Guyer AJ, Richardson G. Current concepts review: total ankle arthroplasty. Foot Ankle Int. 2008;29(2):256–64.
13. Jay Elliot B, Gundapaneni D, Goswami T. Finite element analysis of stress and wear characterization in total ankle replacements. J Mech Behav Biomed Mater. 2014;34:134–45.
14. Jastifer JR, Coughlin MJ. Long-term follow-up of mobile bearing total ankle arthroplasty in the United States. Foot Ankle Int. 2015;36(2):143–50.
15. Kakkar R, Siddique MS. Stresses in the ankle joint and total ankle replacement design. Foot and Ankle Surgery. 2011;17(2):58–63.
16. Kerkhoff YRA, Kosse NM, Metsaars WP, Louwerens JWK. Long-term functional and radiographic outcome of a mobile bearing ankle prosthesis. Foot Ankle Int. 2016;37(12):1292–302.
17. Martinelli N, Baretta S, Bianchi A, Malerba F, Bonifacini CC, Galbusera F. Contact Stresses in a Fixed-Bearing Total Ankle Replacement: A Finite Element Analysis. Foot & Ankle Orthopaedics. 2017; 2(3).
18. McIff T, Saltzman C, and Brown T. Contact pressure and internal stresses in a mobile bearing total ankle replacement. In Proceedings of the 47th Annual Meeting, Orthopaedic Research Society, San Francisco, CA, page 191, 2001.
19. Miller MC, Smolinski P, Conti S, Galik K. Stresses in polyethylene liners in a semiconstrained ankle prosthesis. J Biomech Eng. 2004;126(5):636–40.
20. Plank GR, Estok DM 2nd, Muratoglu OK, O'Connor DO, Burroughs BR, Harris WH. Contact stress assessment of conventional and highly crosslinked ultra high molecular weight polyethylene acetabular liners with finite element analysis and pressure sensitive film. J Biomed Mater Res B Appl Biomater 2007;80(1):1–10.
21. Reggiani B, Leardini A, Corazza F, Taylor M. Finite element analysis of a total ankle replacement during the stance phase of gait. J Biomech. 2006;39(8):1435–43.
22. Saad APBM, Syahrom A, Harun MN, Kadir MRA. Contact pressure of Total ankle replacement (TAR): Springer International Publishing; 2016.
23. Tan EW, Maccario C, Talusan PG, Schon LC. Early complications and secondary procedures in Transfibular Total ankle replacement. Foot Ankle Int. 2016;37(8):835–41.
24. Wei F, Braman JE, Weaver BT, Haut RC. Determination of dynamic ankle ligament strains from a computational model driven by motion analysis based kinematic data. J Biomech. 2011;44(15):2636–41.
25. Wood PLR, Sutton C, Mishara V, Suneja R. A randomized, controlled trial of two-mobile bearing total ankle replacements. J Bone Joint Surg (Br). 2009;91-B:69–74.

16

The impact of rheumatologist-performed ultrasound on diagnosis and management of inflammatory arthritis in routine clinical practice

Stephen Kelly[1*], Brian Davidson[2], Sarah Keidel[3], Stephan Gadola[2], Claire Gorman[4], Gary Meenagh[5] and Piero Reynolds[4]

Abstract

Background: Rheumatologists increasingly perform ultrasound (US) imaging to aid diagnosis and management decisions. There is a need to determine the role of US in facilitating early diagnosis of inflammatory arthritis. This study describes the impact of US use by rheumatologists on diagnosis and management of inflammatory arthritis in routine UK clinical practice.

Methods: We conducted a prospective study in four secondary care rheumatology clinics, each with one consultant who routinely used US and one who did not. Consenting patients aged > 18, newly referred with suspected inflammatory arthritis were included. Data were collected both retrospectively from medical records and via a prospectively-completed physician questionnaire on US use. Analyses were stratified by US/non-US groups and by sub-population of rheumatoid arthritis (RA)-diagnosed patients.

Results: 258 patients were included; 134 US and 124 non-US. 42% (56/134) of US and 47% (58/124) of non-US were diagnosed with RA. Results described for US and non-US cohorts, respectively as follows. The proportion of patients diagnosed at their first clinic visit was 37% vs 19% overall ($p = 0.004$) and 41% vs 19% in RA-diagnosed patients ($p = 0.01$). The median time to diagnosis (months) was 0.85 vs 2.00 (overall, $p = 0.0046$) and 0.23 vs 1.38 (RA-diagnosed, $p = 0.0016$). Median time (months) to initiation on a DMARD (where initiated) was 0.62 vs 1.41 (overall, $p = 0.0048$) and 0.46 vs 1.81 (RA-diagnosed, $p = 0.0007$).

Conclusion: In patients with suspected inflammatory arthritis, routine US use in newly referred patients seems to be associated with significantly earlier diagnosis and DMARD initiation.

Keywords: Arthritis, Ultrasound, DMARD

Background

It is widely accepted that early detection of persistent synovitis and initiation of disease-modifying anti-rheumatic drugs (DMARDS) in patients with Rheumatoid Arthritis (RA) is of critical importance [1, 2]. Assessment and initiation of DMARD therapy in RA at an early juncture has beneficial effects on both long-term clinical outcomes for patients and socioeconomic benefits [3, 4]. However there is still need to clarify the role of US imaging in the assessment of patients within early arthritis clinics as suggested by the 2016 update of the EULAR recommendations for the management of early arthritis [5].

Ultrasonography and MRI have consistently been shown to be more sensitive than clinical examination in detecting synovitis and predicting progression to persistent arthritis or RA [6, 7]. Previous studies have demonstrated that the use of ultrasound (US) improves diagnostic certainty in new patients presenting with seronegative early arthritis [8]. Additionally, US imaging has been consistently proven to be superior to plain

* Correspondence: Stephen.kelly@bartshealth.nhs.uk
[1]Barts Health NHS Trust, London, UK
Full list of author information is available at the end of the article

radiographs in detecting erosions in the setting of early inflammatory arthritis [9, 10].

The aim of this study was to describe the impact of rheumatologist-performed US on the diagnosis and management of patients with early inflammatory arthritis in routine clinical practice. Our objectives were to compare 1) the time from first visit to treatment initiation (DMARDS) and 2) the time from first visit to formal diagnosis between patients with and without rheumatologist-performed US assessment; both overall and in a sub-population of patients with a final diagnosis of RA.

Methods

This multi-centre prospective observational study was undertaken in four UK secondary/tertiary care rheumatology clinics (London [2 sites], Antrim and Southampton). All centres included a consultant who routinely used US at initial presentation to early arthritis clinics and at least one who did not, allowing comparison of decision making with respect to diagnosis and management.

Participants

Patient aged ≥ 18 years at the time of presentation to the clinic and presenting with suspected new onset of inflammatory arthritis based upon the referral letter were recruited. At each participating centre, consultants received referrals form a similar pool of patients. All patients were unselected and were a true representation of the clinical workload undertaken in the study period.

All patients being referred to the early arthritis clinic were approached for recruitment. Patients were reviewed in consultant clinics where; 1) diagnosis and management decisions were routinely made with the use of rheumatologist-performed US (*US group*) **or** 2) diagnosis and management decisions were routinely made without the use of US (*non-US group*). Patients were randomly allocated into these groups without selection bias. Some patients had received investigations by their primary care physician prior to attending the Rheumatology service and these have been documented in Table 1.

Ethical approval

Research ethics committee approval was obtained from the East London REC 2 (reference 10/H0704/25) prior to commencing the study. The study was carried out according to the principles of Good Clinical Practice. All participants provided written informed consent.

Data collection

Data were collected from the initial clinic visit and three further subsequent visits, or until 1 year after the initial clinic visit. An independent *data collector* collected data from the medical notes of patients in both groups and the final locked database was provided to the statistician independent of any of the participating clinicians. The observation period varied depending on the timing of a patient's clinic visits. For all patients diagnosed with RA, outcome data at one year after their initial clinic visit

Table 1 Patient demographics and sample characteristics at baseline, including tests carried out prior to initial clinic visit by referring primary physician

	US	Non-US	RA US	RA Non-US
Total no. Patients	134	124	56	58
Mean (standard deviation) age (years) at initial clinic visit	51.28 (15.75)	53.12 (17.34)	54.42 (17.21)	54.19 (17.75)
N (%)Male	42 (31%)	43 (35%)	17 (30%)	14 (24%)
N (%) Female	92 (69%)	81 (65%)	39 (70%)	44 (76%)
Median (IQR) time (months) from onset of symptoms to first clinic visit	5.98 (3.66 to 14.26)	5.26 (2.89 to 7.62)	5.36 (3.61 to 12.87)	4.78 (3 to 10.56)
Tests carried out prior to initial clinic visit by referring GP[a]				
N (%) Rheumatoid Factor	82 (61%)	81 (65%)	42 (75%)	45 (78%)
N (%) Anti-CCP	8 (6%)	9 (7%)	4 (7%)	6 (10%)
N (%) CRP	90 (67%)	78 (63%)	42 (75%)	36 (62%)
N (%) ESR	92 (69%)	84 (68%)	40 (71%)	41 (71%)
N (%) FBC	98 (73%)	74 (60%)	41 (73%)	40 (69%)
N (%) Joint x-ray (any joint)	39 (29%)	37 (30%)	17 (30%)	18 (31%)
ANA	51 (38%)	54 (44%)	26 (46%)	28 (48%)
Other[b]	67 (50%)	60 (48%)	27 (48%)	28 (48%)

[a]Abbreviations: anti-CCP = anti-cyclic citrullinated peptides; CRP = C-Reactive Protein; ESR = Erythrocyte sedimentation rate; FBC = full blood count; ANA = antinuclear antibodies

[b]Most commonly liver function, renal function and bone profile

were also collected (sub-population). For patients in the US group, a physician questionnaire was used to evaluate the extent to which diagnosis and management decisions were affected by the results of their US scan (Additional file 1). All centres were blinded to the recruitment and diagnosis of patients within the Early Arthritis Clinics at other participating centres during the study period. Additional data on US technique, joints scanned and US findings were also collected. Investigations requested by primary care physicians, prior to attendance at an early arthritis clinic, was recorded.

Statistical analysis

The sample size for the study was based on the historical frequency of patients with specific diagnosis and this informed the power of the study and sites selected. Analyses were stratified for the US and non-US groups. It was expected that there would be variation in the speed of diagnosis over time with an estimated initial 20% difference in diagnosis and treatment rates between each cohort. A sample size was submitted to the ethics committee with at least 100 patients in each arm providing sufficient power to demonstrate a difference in both the primary end point (time to treatment) and secondary end point (time to diagnosis).

Data for RA-diagnosed patients were analysed separately (sub-population). The non-parametric Mann-Whitney U test was used to test for significant differences between the US and non-US groups (both overall and for the RA-diagnosed subgroup) for time to diagnosis and time to treatment initiation (DMARDS). Only patients who received DMARDS during the follow up period were analysed for the time to treatment analysis. Fisher exact testing was used to compare percentages of patients diagnosed at their initial appointment and within one month.

Results

A total of 258 patients were included in the study (134 US managed [range 7–55 per centre] and 124 non-US managed [range 6–65 per centre]).

The proportion of patients receiving a diagnosis of an inflammatory arthritis during the study period was 62% (83/134) in the US group and 65% (81/124) in the non-US group. 42% (56/134) of patients in the US group compared to 47% (58/124) in the non-US group were diagnosed with RA. Baseline patient characteristics are presented in Table 1 and a comprehensive list of diagnosis can be found in Table 2.

Median time between symptom onset and initial clinic visit in the US and non-US groups was 5.98 months and 5.26 months, respectively and 5.36 months and 4.78 months in the RA sub-population (Table 1).

Eleven patients were excluded from the US group and seven from the Non-US group subsequent analysis because of either a lack of data recorded or the referral to the early arthritis clinic was deemed inappropriate as symptoms and diagnosis had previously been established (Table 2). Analysis based on 123 patient in US and 117 in Non-US arm.

Table 2 Final diagnosis after 12 months of follow up by clinicians

Diagnosis	US	Non-US
Rheumatoid arthritis	56	58
Primary inflammatory arthritis (other than RA)	27	23
Mechanical or degenerative disorder	24	21
Connective tissue disease	4	3
Other systemic inflammatory disorder	2	4
Crystal arthritis	3	3
Metabolic disorder	2	3
Pain syndrome	4	2
Drug reaction	1	0
Not specified / unknown	11	7
Total	134	124

All patients – US managed vs non-US managed groups

Both the median time to formal diagnosis and the time to treatment initiation (starting DMARDs) in the US group were less than in the non-US group: time to formal diagnosis 0.85 months versus 2.00 months ($p = 0.0046$); time to treatment initiation 0.62 months versus 1.41 months ($p = 0.0048$) (Table 3).

In the US group 37% (45/123) of patients received a formal diagnosis at their initial clinic visit compared to 19% (22/117) in the non-US group (Fisher's exact test $p = 0.004$); 54% (67/123) versus 32% (38/117) (US and non-US, respectively) received a formal diagnosis within one month of their initial clinic visit ($p = 0.003$). 60% (44/73) of US patients commenced treatment within 1 month of their initial clinic visit compared to 35% (27/77) of non-US (Fisher's exact test, $p = 0.006$) as described in Table 3.

RA diagnosed patient subgroup– US vs non-US managed groups

In the RA subpopulation the median time to formal diagnosis was 0.23 months and 1.38 months for the US and non-US groups, respectively ($p = 0.016$). The time to treatment initiation was also significantly lower in the US than in the non-US group (0.46 months versus 1.81 months, respectively, $p = 0.0007$) (Table 2).

For RA-diagnosed patients, a significantly greater proportion of patients in the US group than in the non-US group, 41% (23/56) versus 19% (11/58), received a formal diagnosis at their initial clinic visit (Fisher's exact test $p = 0.01$) (Fig. 1). 66% (37/56) and 36% (21/58) of patients (respectively) received a formal diagnosis within one month of their initial clinic visit ($p < 0.001$) (Fig. 1). 61% (34/56) in the US group initiated treatment within one

Table 3 Time (months) from initial clinic visit to diagnosis and treatment initiation (i.e. starting DMARDS)

	Time (months) to formal diagnosis				Time (months) to treatment initiation with DMARDS			
	US	Non-US	RA US	RA Non-US	US	Non-US	RA US	RA Non-US
Total	123	117	56	58	73	77	56	58
Mean	2.18	2.76	1.18	1.94	1.49	2.29	1.10	2.38
Median	0.85	2.00	0.23	1.38	0.62	1.41	0.46	1.81
SD	3.02	2.74	2.09	1.90	2.31	2.44	1.65	2.34
IQR	0.0 to 3.22	0.49 to 4.14	0.0 to 1.25	0.46 to 3.15	0.0 to 1.74	0.46 to 3.25	0.0 to 1.38	0.51 to 3.42
P value (Mann-Whitney U)	0.0046		0.0016		0.0048		0.0007	

month of their initial clinic visit compared to 31% (18/58) in the non-US group ($p = 0.002$) (Fig. 2).

Physician US questionnaires

Physicians completed 162 ultrasound scan questionnaires in respect of 162 patient visits: 1st US scans ($n = 120$); 2nd US scans ($n = 28$); 3rd US scans ($n = 12$); and 4th US scans ($n = 2$). The majority of scans were used to aid diagnosis (93% of 1st scans and 75% of subsequent scans).

The joints most commonly scanned with US were the MCP and wrist joints (> 70% of US scans); the PIP joints (50–60% of US scans) and the IP joints (40–50% of US scans), with one centre routinely scanning all hand and wrist joints (Table 4). Joints scanned less frequently (< 10% of US scans) included the elbow, shoulder, knee, ankle and MTP joints. Mean (SD) number of joints scanned: all scans 13.5 (8.8), RA scans 12.1 (9.2) and first scans 16.1 (7.8). More than 20 joints were scanned at 55% of 1st scans.

For 69 US scans (43% of the 159 with data recorded) it was recorded by the physician that the US scan result had made a difference to the patient's diagnosis when performed. The joints scanned and abnormalities detected in these cases (in terms of synovial thickening (ST) and positive power doppler (PD) signal) are shown in Table 5.

Discussion

Main findings

This study provides real life data from four different UK Rheumatology centres on the impact of rheumatologist-performed US on the diagnosis and management of patients with inflammatory arthritis.

Data were collected for 258 patients; 134 had been referred to rheumatologists who routinely use US to aid diagnosis and management and 124 to rheumatologists who do not. Patients in both groups were similar in age (mean (SD) 51.3 (15.8) vs 53.1 (17.3) years in the US and non-US groups respectively) and gender distribution (69% and 65% females). In addition there was no significant difference in disease duration prior to presentation, inflammatory markers and clinical assessments as outlined in Table 1. The proportion of patients finally

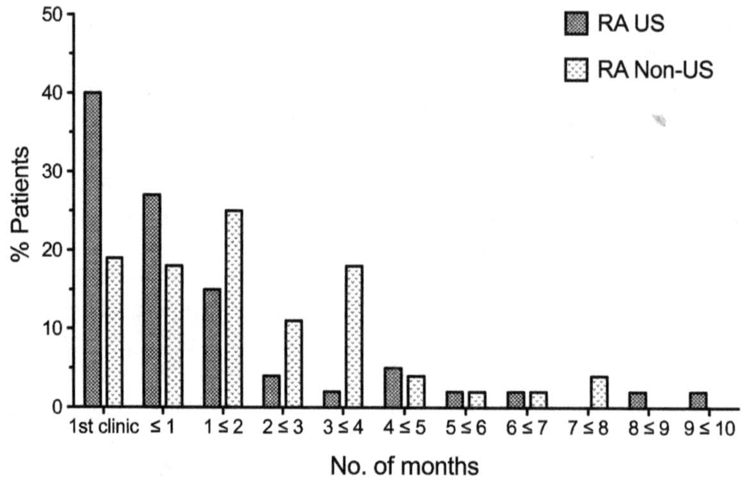

Fig. 1 Distribution of time (months) from initial clinic visit to formal diagnosis – RA diagnosed patients only. Median time to formal diagnosis was 0.23 months and 1.38 months for the US and non-US groups, respectively ($p = 0.014$). 66% of US patients were diagnosed with in month (41% at their 1st clinic visit) compared to 36% of non-US patients (19% at their 1st clinic visit)

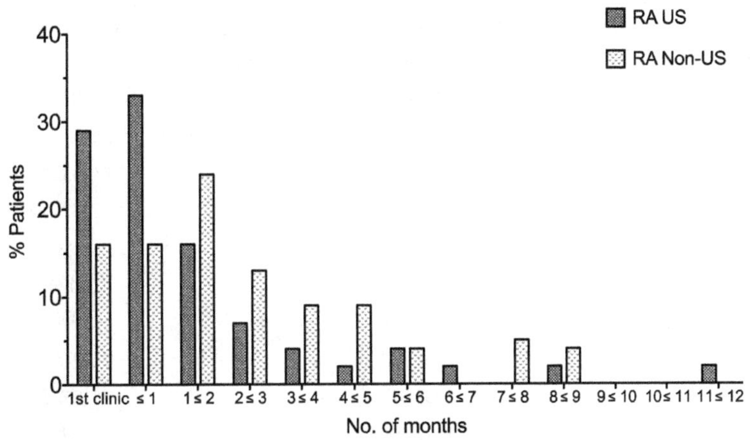

Fig. 2 Distribution of time (months) from initial clinic visit to treatment initiation (DMARDS) – RA diagnosed patients only. Median time to treatment initiation was also significantly lower in the US than in the non-US group (0.46 months versus 1.81 months, respectively, $p = 0.003$). 61% of US cohort was treated within a month versus 31% of non-US cohort

Table 4 Ultrasound data of all imaged joints. Data for 162 US scans were collected and frequency of scanning was calculated for each joint. One centre routinely scanned all wrist and hand joints. A high percentage of small joints of the hands with the right MCP 2 and both wrist joints being most frequently assessed

Joint[a]	LEFT SIDE ($n = 162$)	RIGHT SIDE ($n = 162$)
MCP 1	99 (61%)	102 (63%)
MCP 2	112 (69%)	122 (75%)
MCP 3	108 (67%)	117 (72%)
MCP 4	104 (64%)	110 (68%)
MCP 5	104 (64%)	114 (70%)
IP	70 (43%)	68 (42%)
PIP 2	88 (54%)	90 (56%)
PIP 3	87 (54%)	89 (55%)
PIP 4	74 (46%)	76 (47%)
PIP 5	74 (46%)	75 (46%)
Wrist	118 (73%)	121 (75%)
Elbow	5 (3%)	7 (4%)
Shoulder	2 (1%)	1 (1%)
Knee	10 (6%)	8 (5%)
Ankle	6 (4%)	6 (4%)
Mid-foot	1 (1%)	1 (1%)
MTPs	9 (6%)	12 (7%)
Other[b]	12 (7%)	

[a]Abbreviations: MCP = metacarpophalangeal; IP = interphalangeal; PIP = proximal interphalangeal; MTP = metatarsophalangeal
[b]Other joints recorded as: flexor tendon, post. Tibial, hip, epicondyle, carpometacarpal, distal interphalangeal, toe

receiving a diagnosis of RA was not significantly different between populations at 12 months. The predominance of female patients and age of symptom onset are in line with previous literature reports [11, 12].

The importance of early detection of persistent synovitis and initiation of DMARDS in patients with RA is well documented [9, 13, 14]. Early diagnosis enables prompt initiation of disease modifying therapy, which can slow or halt disease progression and is associated with improved long-term functional and radiological outcomes. 92% of patients subsequently diagnosed clinically with RA fulfilled the ACR / EULAR 2010 criteria at 12 months. In this study, patients managed by rheumatologists who routinely used US to aid diagnosis and management received a formal diagnosis and were initiated on DMARDs significantly earlier than those managed by rheumatologists who did not use US routinely. These differences were significant both in the overall group (median time to diagnosis 0.85 months US vs 2.00 non-US; median time to treatment initiation 0.62 months US vs 1.41 non-US) and in the subpopulation of RA-diagnosed patients (median time to diagnosis 0.23 months US vs 1.38 non-US; median time to treatment initiation 0.46 months US vs 1.81 non-US). While the time to diagnosis encompasses both inflammatory and non-inflammatory conditions, the difference to time of formal diagnosis seems to translate to earlier initiation of DMARD therapy. The proportion of patients who initiated treatment within one month of first outpatient appointment was significantly higher in the US when compared to the US group (57% vs 35% overall; 62% vs 33% RA).

However, although there were statistically significant differences in time to diagnosis and treatment initiation in the US vs the non-US group, the clinical significance of a 6 week reduction in time to DMARD initiation (as observed in the RA subgroup in this study) in terms of

Table 5 Abnormalities detected at US scans reported as making a difference to diagnosis at that clinic visit. US abnormalities were commonly found at both sets of MCPs, PIPs and wrists. Lower limb joints are under represented in the ultrasound data set

Joint[a]	No. (%) joint scanned ($n = 68$)[b]	No. (%)[c] with US abnormality	No. (%) ST only	No. (%) ST + PD
MCP1 L	47 (69.1%)	6 (12.8%)	5 (10.6%)	1 (2.1%)
MCP2 L	53 (77.9%)	19 (35.8%)	6 (11.3%)	13 (24.5%)
MCP3 L	51 (75.0%)	29 (56.9%)	17 (33.3%)	12 (23.5%)
MCP4 L	49 (72.1%)	21 (42.9%)	16 (32.7%)	5 (10.2%)
MCP5 L	50 (73.5%)	8 (16.0%)	1 (2.0%)	7 (14.0%)
MCP1 R	47 (69.1%)	3 (6.4%)	3 (6.4%)	0 (0.0%)
MCP2 R	52 (76.5%)	16 (30.8%)	2 (3.8%)	14 (26.9%)
MCP3 R	53 (77.9%)	20 (37.7%)	9 (17.0%)	11 (20.8%)
MCP4 R	48 (70.6%)	16 (33.3%)	9 (18.8%)	7 (14.6%)
MCP5 R	48 (70.6%)	11 (22.9%)	1 (2.1%)	10 (20.8%)
IP L	31 (45.6%)	1 (3.2%)	0 (0.0%)	1 (3.2%)
PIP2 L	40 (58.8%)	9 (22.5%)	2 (5.0%)	7 (17.5%)
PIP3 L	39 (57.4%)	10 (25.6%)	4 (10.3%)	6 (15.4%)
PIP4 L	37 (54.4%)	9 (24.3%)	3 (8.1%)	6 (16.2%)
PIP5 L	36 (52.9%)	9 (25.0%)	3 (8.3%)	6 (16.7%)
IP R	33 (48.5%)	1 (3.0%)	0 (0.0%)	1 (3.0%)
PIP2 R	39 (57.4%)	10 (25.6%)	4 (10.3%)	6 (15.4%)
PIP3 R	39 (57.4%)	15 (38.5%)	9 (23.1%)	6 (15.4%)
PIP4 R	35 (51.5%)	8 (22.9%)	3 (8.6%)	5 (14.3%)
PIP5 R	36 (52.9%)	8 (22.2%)	3 (8.3%)	5 (13.9%)
Wrist L	52 (76.5%)	18 (34.6%)	3 (5.8%)	15 (28.8%)
Wrist R	49 (72.1%)	19 (38.8%)	7 (14.3%)	12 (24.5%)
MTPs L	5 (7.4%)	5 (100.0%)	3 (60.0%)	2 (40.0%)
MTPs R	7 (10.3%)	7 (100.0%)	5 (71.4%)	2 (28.6%)

[a]Results presented for joints scanned at ≥ 5 US scans
[b]n = 68 (one questionnaire not included due to incomplete US findings)
[c]% of US scans at which each joint was imaged (e.g. for MCP1 (left) abnormalities were detected at 6 (12.8%) of 47 US scans)

impact on radiographic erosions, functional outcomes and economic burden, is unclear and requires further investigation. Moreover, the potential delays in referrals from primary care physicians is likely to presents a significant challenge to clinicians in achieving further reductions in time to treatment initiation.

In this study 162 prospective physician questionnaires were completed, providing valuable information about the current use of US in routine UK clinical practice. In most cases US scans were used to aid diagnosis (93% of 1st scans, 75% of all scans). The stated reason for US was to assess or monitor for sub-clinical disease (35%) in more cases than to inform treatment changes (7%). Physicians reported that in 43% of cases, US scans had made a difference to the diagnosis, indicating that US is linked to clinical decision making processes. The difference appears to be in the time to diagnosis rather than the diagnosis itself, since the proportion of patients diagnosed with RA was similar in the US and non-US groups (42% vs 47%, respectively).

In terms of the number and types of joints scanned; there was a tendency to scan more joints at 1st scans (more than 20 joints were scanned at 55% of 1st scans, for all scans this was 43%) with overall, a mean of 13.5 joints scanned at each US assessment. The MCPs (particularly 2nd and 3rd), wrist and PIP joints were heavily represented, both in terms of joints scanned and detection of abnormalities (for the US scans which were reported as having made a difference to diagnosis), with the 2nd and 3rd MCPs and wrists scanned at over 70% of all US scans. There is currently a lack of consensus about the joint regions and optimal or minimum number of joints, which should be targeted for routine US data set collection, and work is currently underway to develop a single standardised US scoring system that can be used in routine practice to reflect overall disease activity [15, 16]. Whilst a weakness of this study may be the lack of standardised data set scanning across sites, the primary focus of this work was to gather real world information regarding the practicalities of US imaging in early arthritis clinics and the feasibility of performing a wide data set collection. In the context of a prospective randomised trial a limited core data set would improve the study design. The relatively under imaged MTP joints may have provided additional information to clinicians improving the time to diagnosis and treatment in the US cohort. Recently published work has demonstrated that US evaluation of a specific core joint group could potentially be used to assess overall inflammatory activity [17]. Proposed scores include a 12 joint assessment score using the wrists, second and third MCP, second and third PIP of the hands and knee joints (Naredo et al.) [7] and the US7, a 7 joint score (Backhaus et al.) which uses the following joints of the clinically dominant hand and foot: wrist, second and third MCP and PIP and second and fifth MTP joints [18, 19]. Our study supports the inclusion of these joints in a core dataset with a high incidence of significant of ultrasonographic abnormalities detected and the incorporation of these findings into management decisions. The findings indicate that this approach is both feasible in real world clinical practice and yields good dividends where there is a reasonable index of suspicion.

Limitations

This study was undertaken in only four secondary/tertiary care centres. Nevertheless, some significant differences between groups were observed, with important implications for clinical practice. Patients were recruited to this study in a prospective fashion in an unselected manner, however, data were collected retrospectively from patient notes and it was not possible to obtain any missing data items.

Different rheumatologists managed patients in each group. Therefore the results may have been affected by confounding factors related to other differences between the practices of the rheumatologists. However the effect of a single rheumatologist, or single site, was minimised by a multi-centre collaboration in 4 centres and a prospective unselected patient recruitment to the study.

Conclusion

In this study of newly referred patients with inflammatory arthritis, use of US was associated with more rapid diagnosis of synovitis and earlier initiation of DMARDS; this is known to have beneficial effects on patient outcomes and its importance has been recognised by NICE, the National Audit office and the Department of Health in recent changes to commissioning guidance. Overall, the findings of the study support the use of US by rheumatologists at the bedside and reflect the growing interest in the use of US to assess joint inflammation.

Abbreviations

DMARDS: Disease-modifying anti-rheumatic drugs; RA: Rheumatoid Arthritis

Acknowledgments

The authors wish to thank pH associates, a company specialising in real world evaluation, who supported Abbvie and the authors in development of the protocol, conduct of the study and analysis of the results.

Funding

This study was sponsored by AbbVie and financial support for the study was provided by Abbvie. Abbvie participated in the analysis and interpretation of data.

Authors' contributions

Substantial contributions to study design conception and design: SK1, BD, SK2, SG. Substantial contributions to acquisition of data: SK1, BD, SK2, SG, CG, GM, PR. Substantial contributions to analysis and interpretation of data: SK1, BD, SK2, SG, CG, GM, PR. Drafting the article or revising it critically for important intellectual content: SK1, BD, SK2, SG, CG, GM, PR. Final approval of the version of the article to be published: SK1, BD, SK2, SG, CG, GM, PR.

Competing interests

SK1: Consulting/Honoraria/Research grants from UCB, Janssen, Pfizer and, AbbVie.
SG: Consulting/Honoraria/Research grants from Abbott Laboratories, Cellestis and Qiagen, Cellestis, and Pfizer.
The authors declare that there are no non-financial competing interests or financial competing interests from the publication of this manuscript.

Author details

[1]Barts Health NHS Trust, London, UK. [2]University Hospital Southampton NHS Foundation Trust, Southampton, UK. [3]Abbvie Limited, Maidenhead, UK. [4]Homerton University Hospital NHS Foundation Trust, London, UK. [5]Antrim Area Hospital, Antrim, Northern Ireland, UK.

References

1. NICE: Rheumatoid arthritis: the management of rheumatoid arthritis in adults. CG79. **Available at:** http://www.nice.org.uk/Guidance/CG79/NiceGuidance/pdf/English **(accessed 20.3.16)**. 2009.
2. NationalAuditOffice: Services for people with rheumatoid arthritis – report by the comptroller and auditor general (accessed 25.10.16). 2009.
3. Symmons DP, Jones MA, Scott DL, Prior P. Longterm mortality outcome in patients with rheumatoid arthritis: early presenters continue to do well. J Rheumatol. 1998;25(6):1072–7.
4. van der Linden MP, le Cessie S, Raza K, van der Woude D, Knevel R, Huizinga TW, van der Helm-van Mil AH. Long-term impact of delay in assessment of patients with early arthritis. Arthritis Rheum. 2010; 62(12):3537–46.
5. Combe B, Landewe R, Daien CI, Hua C, Aletaha D, Alvaro-Gracia JM, Bakkers M, Brodin N, Burmester GR, Codreanu C, et al. 2016 update of the EULAR recommendations for the management of early arthritis. Ann Rheum Dis. 2017;76(6):948-59. doi: 10.1136/annrheumdis-2016-210602. Epub 2016 Dec 15.
6. Ten Cate DF, Luime JJ, Swen N, Gerards AH, De Jager MH, Basoski NM, Hazes JM, Haagsma CJ, Jacobs JW. Role of ultrasonography in diagnosing early rheumatoid arthritis and remission of rheumatoid arthritis–a systematic review of the literature. Arthritis research & therapy. 2013;15(1):R4.
7. Naredo E, Gamero F, Bonilla G, Uson J, Carmona L, Laffon A. Ultrasonographic assessment of inflammatory activity in rheumatoid arthritis: comparison of extended versus reduced joint evaluation. Clin Exp Rheumatol. 2005;23(6):881–4.

8. Freeston JE, Wakefield RJ, Conaghan PG, Hensor EM, Stewart SP, Emery P. A diagnostic algorithm for persistence of very early inflammatory arthritis: the utility of power Doppler ultrasound when added to conventional assessment tools. Annals of the rheumatic diseases. 2010;69(2):417-9.
9. Weidekamm C, Koller M, Weber M, Kainberger F. Diagnostic value of high-resolution B-mode and doppler sonography for imaging of hand and finger joints in rheumatoid arthritis. Arthritis Rheum. 2003;48(2):325–33.
10. Funck-Brentano T, Etchepare F, Joulin SJ, Gandjbakch F, Pensec VD, Cyteval C, Miquel A, Benhamou M, Banal F, Le Loet X, et al. Benefits of ultrasonography in the management of early arthritis: a cross-sectional study of baseline data from the ESPOIR cohort. Rheumatology (Oxford, England). 2009;48(12):1515–9.
11. Goemaere S, Ackerman C, Goethals K, De Keyser F, Van der Straeten C, Verbruggen G, Mielants H, Veys EM. Onset of symptoms of rheumatoid arthritis in relation to age, sex and menopausal transition. J Rheumatol. 1990;17(12):1620–2.
12. Symmons D, Turner G, Webb R, Asten P, Barrett E, Lunt M, Scott D, Silman A. The prevalence of rheumatoid arthritis in the United Kingdom: new estimates for a new century. Rheumatology (Oxford, England). 2002;41(7):793–800.
13. Finckh A, Liang MH, van Herckenrode CM, de Pablo P. Long-term impact of early treatment on radiographic progression in rheumatoid arthritis: a meta-analysis. Arthritis Rheum. 2006;55(6):864–72.
14. Gremese E, Salaffi F, Bosello SL, Ciapetti A, Bobbio-Pallavicini F, Caporali R, Ferraccioli G. Very early rheumatoid arthritis as a predictor of remission: a multicentre real life prospective study. Ann Rheum Dis. 2013;72(6):858–62.
15. Mandl P, Naredo E, Wakefield RJ, Conaghan PG, D'Agostino MA. A systematic literature review analysis of ultrasound joint count and scoring systems to assess synovitis in rheumatoid arthritis according to the OMERACT filter. J Rheumatol. 2011;38(9):2055–62.
16. Ohrndorf S, Backhaus M. Advances in sonographic scoring of rheumatoid arthritis. Ann Rheum Dis. 72 Suppl 2:ii69-75. doi: 10.1136/annrheumdis-2012-202197. Epub 2012
17. Hammer HB, Kvien TK. Comparisons of 7- to 78-joint ultrasonography scores: all different joint combinations show equal response to adalimumab treatment in patients with rheumatoid arthritis. Arthritis research & therapy. 2011;13(3):R78.
18. Backhaus M, Ohrndorf S, Kellner H, Strunk J, Backhaus TM, Hartung W, Sattler H, Albrecht K, Kaufmann J, Becker K, et al. Evaluation of a novel 7-joint ultrasound score in daily rheumatologic practice: a pilot project. Arthritis Rheum. 2009;61(9):1194–201.
19. Backhaus TM, Ohrndorf S, Kellner H, Strunk J, Hartung W, Sattler H, Iking-Konert C, Burmester GR, Schmidt WA, Backhaus M. The US7 score is sensitive to change in a large cohort of patients with rheumatoid arthritis over 12 months of therapy. Ann Rheum Dis. 2013;72(7):1163–9.

Co-expression of 1α-hydroxylase and vitamin D receptor in human articular chondrocytes

Ann Kristin Hansen[1,2*], Yngve Figenschau[3,4,5] and Inigo Zubiaurre-Martinez[2]

Abstract

Background: The aim was to investigate whether resident chondrocytes in human articular cartilage and in subculture express vitamin D receptor (VDR) and the enzyme that hydroxylates the prohormone $25(OH)D_3$ to the active hormone $1\alpha,25(OH)_2D_3$, namely 1α-hydroxylase (CYP27B1). Any putative effects of vitamin D on chondrocytes were also explored.

Methods: Cartilage from human osteoarthritic knee joints, cultured chondrocytes and cells grown in 3D spheroids were examined for the expression of VDR and 1α-hydroxylase by PCR, Western blots and immunolabelling. Receptor engagement was judged by visualizing nuclear translocation. The effects of $25(OH)D_3$ and $1\alpha,25(OH)_2D_3$ on chondrocyte functions were assessed in proliferation-, chondrogenesis- and cartilage signature-gene expression assays. The capability of chondrocytes to hydroxylate $25(OH)D_3$ was determined by measuring the concentration of metabolites. Finally, a putative regulation of receptor and enzyme expression by $1\alpha,25(OH)_2D_3$ or interleukin (IL)-1β, was investigated by Western blot.

Results: Gene expression was positive for VDR in freshly isolated cells from native cartilage, cells subcultured in monolayers and in spheroids, whereas protein expression, otherwise judged low, was apparent in monolayers. Nuclear translocation of VDR occurred upon $1\alpha,25(OH)_2D_3$ treatment. Transcripts for 1α-hydroxylase were detected in freshly isolated cells, cultured cells and spheroids. Western blots and immunolabelling detected 1α-hydroxylase protein in all materials, while staining of tissue appeared confined to cells at the superficial layer. A dose-dependent $1\alpha,25(OH)_2D_3$ production was measured when the enzyme substrate was supplied to cell cultures. Western blots revealed that the VDR, but not 1α-hydroxylase, was induced by IL-1β treatment in adherent cells. Proliferation in monolayers was enhanced by both $25(OH)D_3$ and $1\alpha,25(OH)_2D_3$, and both compounds had negative effects on chondrogenesis and cartilage-matrix genes.

Conclusions: VDR expression in resident cartilage chondrocytes, generally considered differentiated cells, is elusive. A similar pattern applies for redifferentiated chondrocytes in spheroid cultures, whereas dedifferentiated cells, established in monolayers, stably express VDR. Both $25(OH)D_3$ and $1\alpha,25(OH)_2D_3$ are able to potentiate cell proliferation but have a negative impact in proteoglycan synthesis. Chondrocytes express 1α-hydroxylase and may contribute to the production of $1\alpha,25(OH)_2D_3$ into the joint environment. Effects of vitamin D could be unfavourable in the context of cartilage matrix synthesis.

Keywords: Vitamin D, $1\alpha,25(OH)_2D_3$, $25(OH)D_3$, VDR, CYP27B1, Chondrocyte, Cartilage, Osteoarthritis, Pellet culture, Static suspension culture

* Correspondence: ann.k.hansen@uit.no
[1]Department of Orthopaedic Surgery, University Hospital of North Norway, Tromsø, Norway
[2]Bone and joint research group, Institute of Clinical Medicine, Faculty of Health Sciences, University of Tromsø, Tromsø, Norway
Full list of author information is available at the end of the article

Background

Osteoarthritis (OA) is a debilitating degenerative disease of the joint affecting middle-aged and older people and the pathogenesis is considered multifactorial [1]. Over the last decades, mounting evidence suggests that OA develops as a cause of inflammation in addition to the mechanical aspects [2]. Vitamin D is a predecessor of the secosteroid hormone 1α,25(OH)$_2$D, which plays a pivotal role for appropriately regulated calcium required for a normal bone turnover. Of importance, 1α,25(OH)$_2$D has been suggested to dampen inflammation-driven diseases such as rheumatoid- and osteoarthritis [3]. Exogenous sources of vitamin D_3 are mainly fatty fish and fortified food items, whereas the predominant source is the endogenous production from cholesterol in sun-exposed skin. After hydroxylation in the liver, the vitamin circulates as the prohormone 25(OH)D_3 bound to D-binding protein (90%) and albumin (10%). Likewise, the active hormone 1α,25(OH)$_2D_3$ is transported by these proteins, but circulates in a concentration < 0.1% of that of the prohormone. Less than 1% of both metabolites are unbound by carrier proteins. The hydroxylation of 25(OH)D_3 to 1α,25(OH)$_2D_3$ is facilitated by the enzyme 1α-hydroxylase, which is primarily located in the kidneys. However, there is compelling evidence of an extra-renal distribution of the enzyme, including local induction by the immune system [4]. The effect of vitamin D in the extra-renal compartments are considered auto- or paracrine, and represent an entirely new paradigm of vitamin D actions compared to the endocrine action of renal vitamin D [5]. The active hormone binds the vitamin D receptor (VDR), which is abundantly expressed in the intestine, kidneys, parathyroid and bone; while it is expressed in costal cartilage, its presence in articular cartilage is less settled [6].

Several studies have suggested a link between vitamin D status and OA; some have found that individuals deficient in vitamin D have an increased risk of progressive knee-osteoarthritis, and there are reports of a pain reducing effect of oral supplementation [7, 8]. Both 25(OH)D_3 and 1α,25(OH)$_2D_3$ have been detected in synovial fluid [4, 9]. The presence of the receptor in human articular cartilage and chondrocytes has been previously investigated with divergent outcomes [10, 11], and the biological effect of vitamin D on cartilage pathophysiology remains uncertain. In rat chondrosarcoma cells, 1α,25(OH)$_2D_3$ dose-dependently induced MMP13, a matrix metalloprotease which degrades the extracelluar matrix [12]. 1α,25(OH)$_2D_3$ has also been associated with hypertrophy and mineralization of OA chondrocytes [13].

The aim of this study was to investigate whether the previously described expression patterns of VDR in human articular cartilage and subcultured cells could be confirmed by PCR, Western blots and immunolabelling. It was also questioned whether receptor activation occurred upon ligand binding, and whether this could be recorded by biological readouts such as promoted chondrogenesis, cell proliferation or cartilage signature gene expression. Furthermore, in view of the previously reported presence of 1α,25(OH)$_2D_3$ in synovial fluid, it was addressed whether the sole source was the circulation or if the hormone could also be attributed to a local production by chondrocytes expressing 1α-hydroxylase. Previous experiments are described using cartilage tissues and chondrocytes expanded in adherent monolayer cultures. Since chondrocytes are known to dedifferentiate upon monolayer expansion, thus undermining the extrapolation of findings to cartilage conditions, we included assays utilizing freshly isolated chondrocytes in a differentiated stage, and 3D culture assays where the chondrocyte redifferentiate to a chondrocyte-like phenotype [14].

Methods

Human material

Cartilage tissues were collected from macroscopically healthy looking areas of cartilage on the lateral femoral condyle of patients with osteoarthritis undergoing total knee replacement procedures (N = 13, age: 40–78). Patient records were searched to exclude any patients with rheumatic disease, while both secondary posttraumatic and primary osteoarthritis patients were included. The material was collected with the patient's written consent and all samples were anonymized at time of collection. All methods were performed in accordance with the relevant guidelines and regulations, and the study was approved by the regional ethics committee (2015/1730/REK Nord).

Chondrocytes isolation and culturing

Suspension cultures

Cartilage biopsies, in which bone was meticulously excluded, were minced into ~1mm^3 pieces and enzymatically digested in Collagen type XI (Cat. no. C9407, Sigma Aldrich) for 4–6 h until 95% degraded. Cells were counted using a haemocytometer, and suspension cultures were established in 24-well ultra-low binding plates (Cat. no. 3473, Corning, VWR) at 4 × 10^5 cells/well in DMEM (Cat. no. D5796, SigmaAldrich) supplemented with 62 mg/L ascorbic acid (Cat. no. 103033E, BDH Laboratories), 1% penicillin/streptomycin (P/S, Cat. no. P0781, Sigma-Aldrich) and 1% Fetal Bovine Serum (FBS, Cat. no. S0615, Biochrom). Suspension cultures were allowed to equilibrate for 24 h in at 37 °C and 5% O_2 before being treated with IL-1β (Cat. no. 200-01B, Peprotech) at 10 ng/mL, 1α,25(OH)$_2D_2$ (Cat. no. 11174, Cayman Chemical) or 1α,25(OH)$_2D_3$ (Cat. no. 71820, Cayman Chemical) at 10 $^{-8}$ M for 24 h.

Monolayer cultures

Immediately after tissue digestion, chondrocytes were seeded in polystyrene T25 flasks and serially expanded in monolayer cultures in DMEM supplemented with ascorbic acid, P/S and 10–20% FBS until confluence in T175 cultures flasks. Monolayer cells were used for experimentation at passages 2–5. Pieces of bone removed from cartilage biopsies were minced and explant cultured in DMEM supplemented with 20% FBS for 2 weeks to obtain the osteoblasts used as controls in Western blots.

3D cultures

Scaffold-free multicellular spheroid cultures of chondrocytes were established from chondrocytes expanded in the presence of vehicle, $25(OH)D_3$ or $1\alpha,25(OH)_2D_3$ at 10^{-7} M until confluency. The cells were detached from the culture flasks using an enzyme-free dissociation solution (Cat. no. S-014-B, Merck Millipore) and transient trypsinization (Trypsin-EDTA, T4049, Sigma-Aldrich) before plating in round bottom ultra-low attachment 96-well plates (Cat. no. 7007, Costar) at a density of 5×10^4 in 150 μL DMEM supplemented with 10 ng/mL TGF-β3 (Cat. no. 100-21C, Peprotech), 10 ng/mL BMP-2, 1:1000 Insulin-Transferrin-Selenium (ITS, Cat. no. 354351, BD Biosciences). The augmentation with vehicle, $25(OH)D_3$ or $1\alpha,25(OH)_2D_3$ at 10^{-7} M was continued through 3D culturing for 2 weeks for spheroids used to evaluate chondrogenesis. Spheroids used for immunolabelling of VDR and 1α-hydroxylase were propagated for 2 days or 3 weeks in chondrogenic medium alone.

Histology and immunohictochemistry

Cartilage biopsies, two-day spheroids and three-week spheroids were fixed in 4% formalin overnight. Spheroids were embedded in 1% agarose before, along with the cartilage biopsies, they were cast and cut into 4 μm sections. Slides were rehydrated and antigen retrieval was achieved by placing the slides in a 60 °C citrate buffer for 60 min. The SuperPicture kit (Cat. no. 879673, Novex, LifeTechnologies) was used, along with specific antibodies targeting 1α-hydroxylase (Cat. no. ABIN2118284, Antibodies-online.com) and VDR (Cat. no. Sc-13,133, Santa Cruz) [15]. As previously described [16], slides from two-day and three-week controls and vitamin D-treated spheroids were prepared and stained with Alcian blue to detect glycosaminoglycan production. Pictures were developed using the Zeiss Axiophot photomicroscope (Carl Zeiss, Oberkochen, Germany), and the images were evaluated by three investigators using the Bern score to assess chondrogenicity [17].

Immunofluorescence

Chondrocytes were cultured until confluency seeded on 2-well chamber slides (Cat. no. 177429; NUNC Lab Tek), and incubated for 24 h before being treated with vehicle or $1\alpha,25(OH)_2D_3$ at 10^{-8} M for 2 h, and subsequently subjected to fixation. Concomitant fixation-permeabilization of cells was done using 100% ice-cold methanol for 8 min, followed by serial washings with PBS for the rehydration of cells. For protein detection, fixed cells were incubated with primary antibodies against 1α-hydroxylase and VDR. Alexa 546-conjugated secondary antibodies targeting rabbit (Cat. no. A11010, Life Technologies) or mouse IgG (Cat. no. A11003, Life Technologies), respectively, were used to visualize 1α-hydroxylase and VDR in an appropriate microscope.

Western blot

Protein was extracted from freshly isolated chondrocytes, suspension cultures and monolayer- expanded cultures using the NP-40 buffer (150 nM NaCl, 50 mM Tris-HCl, 1% Igepal), supplemented with protease inhibitor (Complete, EDTA-free, Cat. no. 11873580001, Roche). Protein concentration was measured using a colorimetric assay (Cat. no. 500-0116, BioRad), and separated along with BLUeye Prestained Protein Ladder (Cat. no. PM007-0500, Sigma-Aldrich) and MagicMark™ XP Western Protein Standard Ladder (Cat. no. LC5602, Novex, Life Technologies) using TruPage gels (Cat. no. PCG2003, Sigma-Aldrich). The protein input was 40 μg/lane for cartilage samples, 45 μg/lane for suspension cultures and 20 μg/lane for cultured cell samples. Proteins were transferred to PVDF membranes, incubated for 1 h in a dry milk buffer and incubated overnight at 4 °C with 1α-hydroxylase (1:200 in BSA buffer) or VDR antibody (1:100 in dry milk buffer). Next, the membranes were incubated with secondary α-rabbit antibody (Cat. no. sc-2004, Santa-Cruz) and α-mouse antibody (Cat. no. sc-2005, Santa-Cruz) for 1 h at room temperature, and lastly, a chemiluminescence detection solution (Cat. no. 170-5040, BioRad) was applied before images were procured using an ImageQuant LAS 4000 CCD camera. Beta-actin antibody (Cat. no. SAB5500001, Sigma-Aldrich) was used as a loading control, relative density was assessed using Image Studio Lite 5.2 and a Dunnett's test used to compare the treated groups to the control group.

PCR

Suspension cultured cells and three-weeks spheroid cultures were harvested, and RNA was extracted using the RNeasy Micro Kit (Cat. no. 74004, Qiagen). Lysates were dissolved in TissueLyser (Qiagen), homogenized using QiaShredder columns (Cat. no. 79654, Qiagen), and cleaned and eluted according to the manufacturer's instructions. RNA from monolayer expanded chondrocytes was extracted using the PerfectPure Cultured Cell Kit (Cat. no. 2900319, 5prime) according to the manufacturer's protocol. RNA concentration was measured by Nano-Drop

2000 and 35 ng of each sample was reverse-transcribed to cDNA using qScript (Cat. no. 95047, Quanta Biosciences, VWR). The PCR reaction included JumpStart REDTaq ReadyMix, cDNA and specific primers targeting 1α-hydroxylase (CYP27B1) and VDR (Table 1), and was amplified for 35 cycles using an MJ Research thermal cycler. Products were separated in FlashGels (Cat. no. 57023, Lonza, Fisher Scientific), and images were obtained using an ImageQuant LAS4000 camera system.

qPCR

RNA was extracted from monolayer cultures propagated in 6-well plates and treated with vehicle, $25(OH)D_3$ or $1\alpha,25(OH)_2D_3$ at 10^{-6} M and 10^{-7} M for 72 h. Extracts were used in a qPCR assay where each reaction contained 5 μL Precision Fast ROX MasterMix (Primer Design), 0.5 μL hydrolysis probe (Invitrogen), 2.5 μL H_2O and 2 μL cDNA. Hydrolysis probes (Life Technologies by Fisher Scientific) include: collagen type I alpha 1 chain (*COL1A1*, Assay ID: Hs00164004_m1), collagen type II alpha 1 chain (*COL2A1*, Hs00264051_m1), aggrecan (*ACAN*, Hs00153936_m1), versican (*VCAN*, Hs00171642_m1), SRY-box 9 (*SOX9*, Hs00165814_m1), cytochrome P450 family 24 subfamily A member 1 (CYP24A1, Hs00167999_m1), vitamin D receptor (VDR, Hs01045843_m1) and ribosomal protein L13a (*RPL13A*, Hs04194366_g1, reference gene). Reactions were run in BrightWhite 96-well plates (PrimerDesign) using a StepOnePlus™ Real-Time PCR System. The dCq was calculated by subtracting the reference gene from the gene of interest so that a higher dCq value represents an upregulation and vice versa. A Dunnett's test was used to compare treated samples to the control samples.

$25(OH)D_3$ hydroxylation assay

To detect the hydroxylation of $25(OH)D_3$ to $1\alpha,25(OH)_2D_3$, parallel 6-well plates with and without confluent chondrocytes were challenged with $25(OH)D_3$ at 0, 50, 250 and 500 nM for 24 h. Supernatants were collected, and $1\alpha,25(OH)_2D_3$ was measured using an automated immunometric assay (Diasorin) at the Hormone Laboratory, Oslo University Hospital, Norway. Conversion attributed to 1α-hydroxylase activity was calculated as the difference between $1\alpha,25(OH)_2D_3$ in wells with and without cells in order to cancel out any spontaneous conversion. A linear model was used to evaluate the correlation between $25(OH)D_3$ and $1\alpha,25(OH)_2D_3$.

Table 1 PCR Primers

VDR F	5'-ACC AAG CTC ACA GTT CCT CG-3'
VDR R	5'-CGG CAG GGA GAT CAT GAC TC-3'
CYP27B1 F	5'-ACC ATG GTC TCT CTG CTT GC-3'
CYP27B1 R	5'-GCC CAA AGA TGT CTC TGC CT-3'
APRT F	5'-CCCGAGGCTTCCTCTTTG GC-3'
APRT R	5'-CTCCCTGCCCTTAAGCGAGG-3'

Proliferation assay

Chondrocytes from two donors were plated in E-plate VIEW 16 (Cat. no. 06324746001, ACEA Biosciences) at 3000 cells per well in 100 μL DMEM, supplemented with 10% FBS and vehicle, $25(OH)D_3$ or$1\alpha,25(OH)_2D_3$ at 10^{-6} M for 80 h and real-time proliferation was monitored using the xCELLigence RTCA system (Roche Diagnostics). The cell-index was normalized to 25 h (1 h after treatment) and log 2 converted to more accurately display growth rate [18].

Immunoelectron microscopy

Chondrocytes cultures from two different donors established in 10 cm Ø dishes were fixed in 8% formaldehyde in a 200 mM HEPES buffer, pH 7.5, for 24 h, collected by gently scraping of cells and centrifuged in an Eppendorf microfuge. After infusion for 30 min with 2.3 mol/L sucrose containing 20% polyvinylpyrrolidone, pellets were mounted on a specimen holder and frozen in liquid nitrogen. Cryosections were prepared, and immunolabeling was performed as described elsewhere [19]. Antibodies against VDR and 1α-hydroxylase (diluted 1:25) were detected by protein A-gold complexes, and the dried sections were then examined in a JEOL JEM 1010 transmission electron microscope (JEOL, Tokyo, Japan) operating at 80 kV. Moreover, negative controls were routinely included in parallel by the omission of primary antibodies.

Statistics

Data analysis and figures were acquired using RStudio [20], with tidy, plyr, dplyr, broom, data.table, purrr, ggplot2 and ggthemes packages [21–28]. Differences were considered significant at $p < 0.05$.

Results

Chondrocyte dedifferentiation and redifferentiation

In this study, we have investigated the expression of vitamin D receptor and 1a-hydroxylase on human articular chondrocytes established in different experimental conditions comprising native tissue, suspension cultures, adherent cells/monolayer cultures and 3D spheroids cultures. This approach is relevant if we take into consideration that chondrocytes change their phenotype during cell expansion in vitro (dedifferentiation) and that they are able to gain (at least in part) their phenotypic traits in 3D cultures (redifferentiation) [14]. A qPCR assay was performed, comparing gene expression of cartilage signature genes between suspension cultures and monolayer cultures, and the results indicate that the suspension cultures were indeed in a differentiated stage compared to the dedifferentiated monolayers (Additional file 1: Figure S1).

Expression of 1α-hydroxylase in cartilage tissue and cells

By using conventional PCR, 1α-hydroxylase mRNA was detected in freshly isolated cells from native cartilage, chondrocytes in monolayers and in 3D spheroids cultivated for 3 weeks in chondrogenic conditions (Fig. 1f). By immunolabelling of native cartilage, 1α-hydroxylase appears confined to chondrocytes residing in the superficial layer (in Fig. 1a and b). Chondrocytes in monolayers and in spheroids were also positively stained (Fig. 1c and d). In Western blots, an expected 58 kD band in protein extracts from native cartilage, suspension and monolayer cells as well as in a positive control, i.e. osteoblast culture, was confirmed (Fig. 1e). In subcellular distribution experiments, utilizing immunoelectron microscopy, 1α-hydroxylase was found in the cytoplasm and in electron-dense mitochondria-like structures (Fig. 3b).

Expression of VDR in cartilage tissue and cells

Results show that mRNA transcripts encoding VDR was detected in all samples, i.e. in freshly isolated chondrocytes, monolayer cultured cells and three-weeks spheroids (Fig. 2f). As judged by immunolabelling, no staining of the VDR protein was identified in cartilage (Fig. 2a) in contrast to the staining observed in intestinal mucosa used as a positive control (Fig. 2b). In monolayer expanded cells, staining was apparent in the cytoplasm and the nucleus (Fig. 2c). In 3D spheroid cultures, immunostaining was negative already 2 days after 3D culture initiation (Fig. 2d). Western blotting confirmed these findings by the occurrence of an expected 53 kD band in extracts from monolayer cells and the positive control, primary osteoblasts culture (Fig. 2e). Of note, the nearly invisible band corresponding to the loading control beta-actin in cartilage samples underscores the low levels of cell-associated proteins compared to extracellular matrix (ECM) proteins in such samples. At the subcellular level, VDR was found primarily in cytoplasmic regions and sporadically in the nucleus (Fig. 3a).

Receptor and enzyme are functional

VDR engagement was investigated by immunolabelling of nuclear translocation of the receptor upon ligand binding. In Fig. 4c and d, the predominant-nuclear staining of VDR after 2 h of treatment with 1α,25(OH)$_2$D$_3$ can be observed, compared to the mixed cytoplasmic-nuclear staining of VDR from untreated cells (Fig. 4a and b).

Evidence for 1α-hydroxylase activity was arranged by supplementing cultured cells with its substrate 25(OH)D$_3$ followed by the assessment of 1α,25(OH)$_2$D$_3$ concentration after 24 h. It was revealed that 1α,25(OH)$_2$D$_3$ was dose-dependently produced in cell supernatants (Fig. 4e).

Induced expression of VDR, but not 1α-hydroxylase by IL-1β

Aiming at exploring potential receptor and/or enzyme regulation during inflammatory conditions, VDR and 1α-hydroxylase expression was judged by Western blotting in freshly isolated cells and in monolayers after treatment with the pro-inflammatory cytokine IL-1β or the active hormone 1α,25(OH)$_2$D$_3$. Bands occurring after blotting from three randomly chosen donors were subjected to densitometric assessment. In suspension culture preparations, an increased expression of 1α-hydroxylase (CYP27B1) was detected in two out of three samples, but the lack of regulation in one donor made the total effect not significant. In contrast, the expression of VDR was uniform across treated and untreated samples (Fig. 5a). In monolayer samples, the VDR expression was amplified almost three-fold after IL-1β stimulation, an alteration that was judged as statistically significant (Fig. 5b), while the expression of 1α-hydroxylase was unaltered by IL-1β or 1α,25(OH)$_2$D$_3$.

Both 25(OH)D$_3$ and 1α,25(OH)$_2$D$_3$ influence chondrogenesis and expression of cartilage signature genes

Last, the potential effects of 25(OH)D$_3$ and 1α,25(OH)$_2$D$_3$ on major chondrocyte functions was investigated. Since the expression of the VDR receptor was more evident in monolayer cells, and scarcely detectable in freshly isolated or 3D conditions, we resorted to chondrocytes in monolayers to study vitamin D effects. For chondrogenesis, cells established in monolayers were incubated in the presence or absence of 25(OH)D$_3$ or 1α,25(OH)$_2$D$_3$ for 1 week prior to 3D spheroids formation and incubation for 2 weeks in a chondrogenic environment supplemented with 25(OH)D$_3$, 1α,25(OH)$_2$D$_3$ or vehicle. The resulting 3D structures were stained with the glycosaminoglycan marker Alcian blue (Fig. 6a-c). A semi-quantitative visual scoring of Alcian blue-stained spheroids from three different donors (Bern score) indicated a detrimental effect of both 25(OH)D$_3$ and 1α,25(OH)$_2$D$_3$ on proteoglycan synthesis and chondrogenesis (Fig. 6d).

Effects of 25(OH)D$_3$ or 1α,25(OH)$_2$D$_3$ on cartilage-signature gene expression were studied by qPCR (Fig. 6f). Regulation of CYP24A1 expression was used as an internal positive control for 1α,25(OH)$_2$D$_3$ action. Cultures treated with 25(OH)D$_3$ or 1α,25(OH)$_2$D$_3$ both exhibit a significant increase in expression of CYP24A1 compared to the untreated cultures, while the VDR transcript remained unaffected. Both 25(OH)D$_3$ and 1α,25(OH)$_2$D$_3$ significantly increased the expression of VCAN, whereas the expression of ACAN (the cartilage proteoglycan) was significantly reduced compared to the

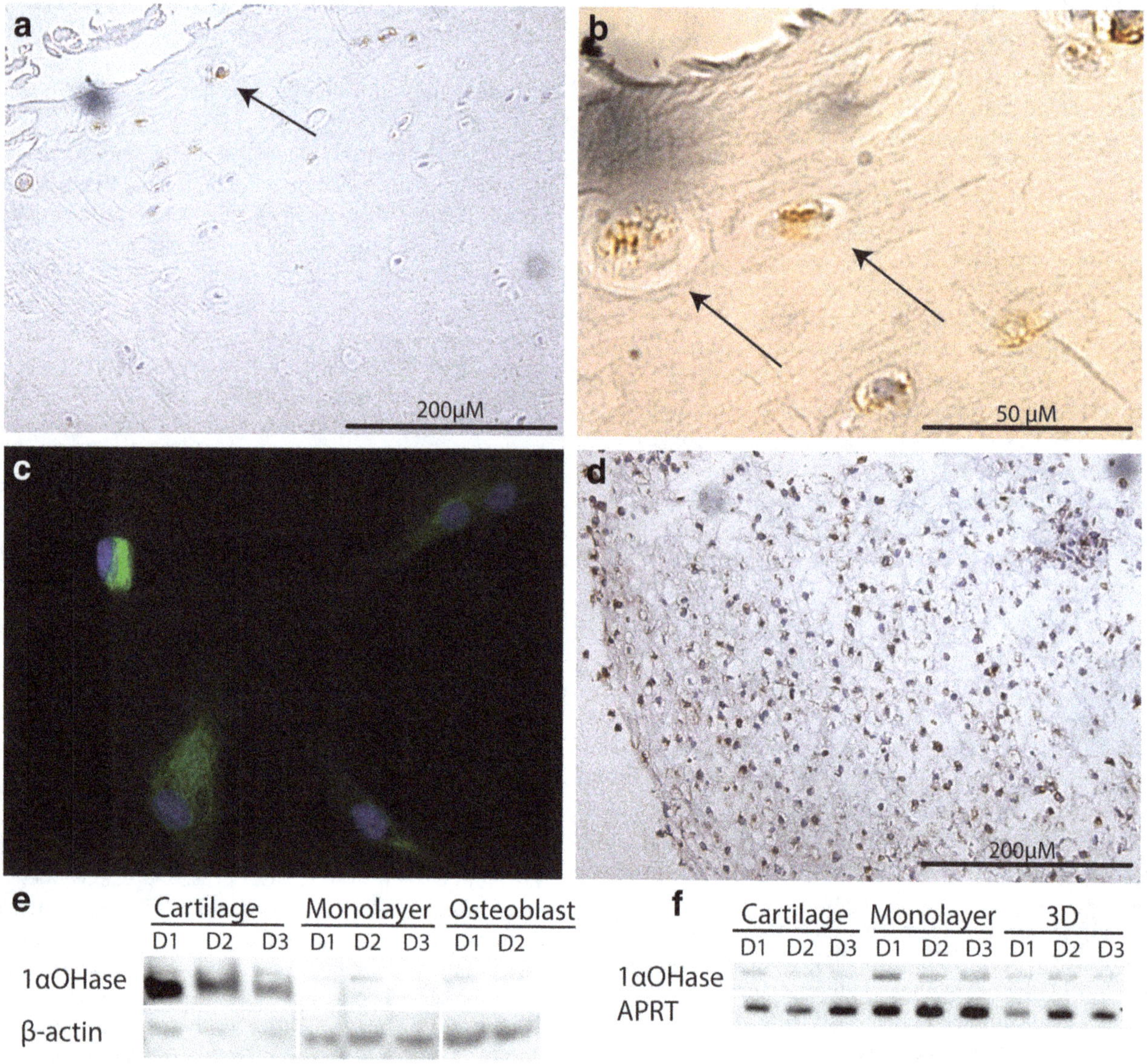

Fig. 1 Cartilage at 100 × (**a**) and 400 × (**b**) magnification, arrows indicate chondrocytes labelled with 1α-hydroxylase antibody and corresponding green labelling of cultured chondrocytes (**c**). In the two-week spheroids (**d**, 100×) brown staining of chondrocytes indicate the presence of 1α-hydroxylase. Western blot (**e**) of cartilage, monolayer chondrocytes and osteoblasts labelled with 1α-hydroxylase antibody (58 kD) and β-actin (45 kD, loading control). PCR (**f**) of cartilage, monolayer chondrocyte and spheroids (3D) using primers targeting 1α-hydroxylase (521 bp) and APRT (300 bp, quality control). Images represent the outcome of investigation of cells and tissues from three different donors

control. The expression of Collagen type I (COL1A1) and SOX9 were not affected by 25(OH)D_3 nor 1α,25(OH)$_2D_3$ treatment. Expression of Collagen type II remained undetectable in both treated and untreated samples.

On the other hand, we found that both 25(OH)D_3 and 1α,25(OH)$_2D_3$ had a positive impact on cell proliferation, both inducing a slight increase in the growth rate compared to vehicle (Fig. 6e). The three donors included in the study exhibited different growth rates, obscuring any significant differences.

Discussion

Osteoarthritis (OA) is a disease of the entire joint affecting cartilage, subchondral bone, the synovial membrane and ligaments. Clinically, the disease is characterized by joint space narrowing, osteophyte formation and sclerosis. At a microscopic level, OA is characterized by a loss of extracellular matrix, chondrocyte hypertrophy, cell proliferation and calcification [29]. The role of Vitamin D in the OA context remains controversial. Synoviocytes secrete inflammatory mediators into the synovial fluid, and it appears

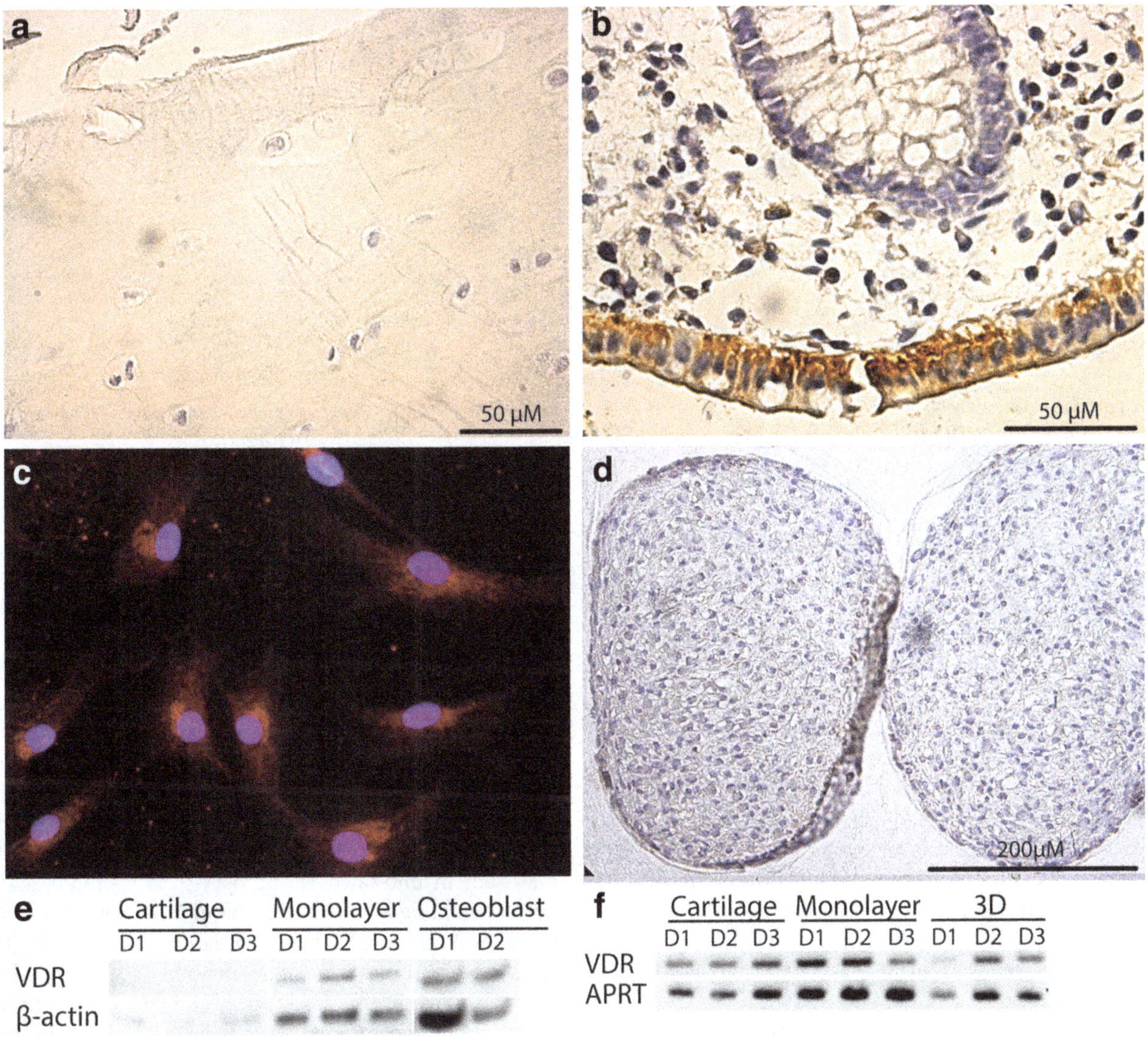

Fig. 2 Cartilage (**a**, 400×), normal colon (**b**, 400×), cultured chondrocytes (**c**) and two-day spheroids (**d**, 100×) labelled with a VDR antibody. In normal colon the brown staining of the cytoplasm represent VDR labelling and in cultured chondrocytes the VDR is correspondingly visualised by red staining, while in cartilage and two-week spheroids there is no labelling of VDR. Western blot (**e**) of cartilage, monolayer chondrocytes and osteoblasts labelled with VDR antibody (53 kD) and β-actin (45 kD). PCR (**f**) of cartilage, monolayer chondrocytes and spheroids (3D) using primers targeting VDR (336 bp) and APRT (300 bp). Images represent the outcome of investigation of cells and tissues from three different donors

that elevated levels of $1\alpha,25(OH)_2D_3$ may increase the OPG/RANKL ratio, along with a reduced IL-6 production that together contributes to a dampened inflammation [30]. In contrast, it was reported that in human articular chondrocytes, $1\alpha,25(OH)_2D_3$ induced MMPs and calcification that are usually considered detrimental events [11, 13]. The picture becomes more entangled after considering the studies that have investigated VDR expression in human cartilage. An early study from the 80's claimed that VDR is absent in resident cartilage cells, but acquires VDR during ex-vivo cultivation, i.e. cells considered as dedifferentiated [10]. A more recent report argues that VDR is inconsistently expressed in healthy human cartilage (donor dependent), but enhanced in OA cartilage [11]. Because of the existing dubiety, we pursued studying VDR expression in cartilage tissue and cells by different means. Preceded by the measurement of $25(OH)D_3$ in synovial fluid from patients with rheumatoid arthritis (mean 11,0 nM, results not shown), it was importunate to question whether the congeneric $1\alpha,25(OH)_2D_3$ hormone could be produced locally in the joint by chondrocytes. This would require the recognition that chondrocytes express 1α-hydroxylase.

In line with previous publications [10, 31], VDR transcripts were detected in cartilage tissue and monolayers, while in our hands detecting VDR protein in native

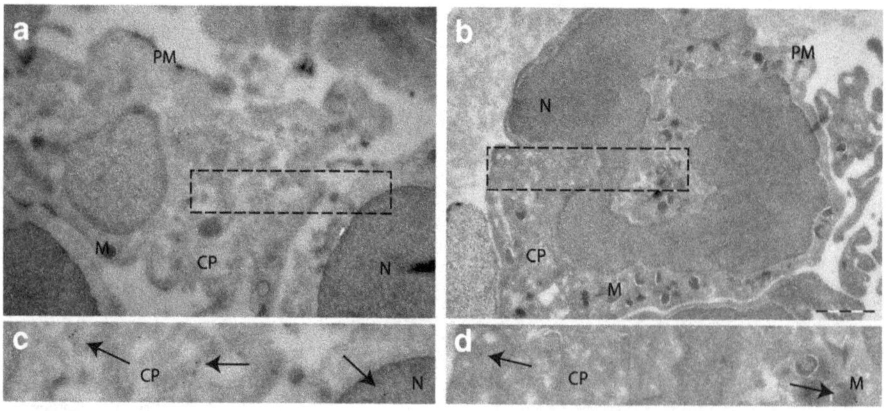

Fig. 3 Subcellular distribution of VDR (**a**) and 1α-hydroxylase (**b**) in chondrocytes assessed by immunoelectron microscopy. Panels **c** and **d** are magnifications of **a** and **b** respectively. Gold particles are marked with arrowheads. N = nucleus, M = mitochondria, PM = plasma membrane, CP = cytoplasm

cartilage by immunohistochemistry and Western blot was less evident. The expected VDR band is hardly recognizable in Fig. 2e (cartilage D1, the D2 and D3 are judged negative). Of note, the β-actin protein band from cartilage samples was also weak even though equal amount of proteins were loaded in wells. This may reflect a very low concentration of cell associated proteins compared to ECM proteins in samples prepared by short enzymatic digestion. In Fig. 5a, corresponding to the Western blot of suspension cells phenotypically similar to native cells and devoid of matrix proteins, it is more evident that the VDR protein is present in the samples. No previous publication could be recovered for a comparison on the Western blot subject, and our judgment is that VDR is expressed by resident cells in cartilage, although at very low levels.

Through immunolabelling it has previously been demonstrated that chondrocytes express the VDR protein in OA cartilage and monolayer cells [11]. The latter was confirmed here (Fig. 2c), though no signal was recorded by histological immunolabelling (Fig. 2a). It has been claimed that many VDR antibodies not only bind VDR, but also possess non-specific interactions with other unidentified proteins, determined by both immunoblotting and histochemistry [15]. These authors recommended using the antibody applied in the present study for both purposes. The questioned utility of different antibodies could explain the current divergent findings. All in all, despite the failure to detect the VDR protein in cartilage tissue by immunohistochemistry, the results from protein and transcript detection in suspension cell cultures represent an evidence that differentiated chondrocytes express VDR, which is also in agreement with both the previous report and reports on enhanced expression in OA cartilage and rheumatoid lesions [31]. In line with what we observed in tissue, a negative immunolabelling of redifferentiated cells, i.e. those in spheroids was recorded. Although VDR transcripts were detected, no or an insufficient amount of protein in spheroids enabled VDR detection.

After entering the cell, 1α,25(OH)$_2$D$_3$ binds the VDR, and the VDR-ligand complex translocates to the nucleus where it triggers a tissue-specific change in gene-transcription, resulting in altered growth, differentiation or functional activity [32]. In adherent chondrocytes, receptor translocation is evident in Fig. 4 a-d where the immunostaining shifts from a mixed nuclear/cytoplasmic stain in untreated chondrocytes, to a predominant nuclear staining after the addition of 1α,25(OH)$_2$D$_3$. This provides evidence of the internalization of 1α,25(OH)$_2$D$_3$ and subsequent receptor engagement.

An objective in this study was to investigate a putative alteration of receptor or enzyme expression during an inflammatory condition arranged by treating cells with cytokine or hormone. Cells in both suspension and monolayers were subjected to either IL-1β or 1α,25(OH)$_2$D$_3$ treatment, and relative amounts of VDR protein were recorded by Western blot. In monolayer samples, the VDR was significantly upregulated upon treatment with IL-1β (Fig. 5b), while this effect could not be detected in a suspension culture condition (Fig. 5a). The upregulation detected in monolayer cultures is in agreement with previous publications reporting upregulated VDR expression during various inflammatory conditions and could be associated to the elevated receptor expression reported in OA cartilage samples [31].

In osteoclasts, there has been observed an upregulation of VDR transcripts upon 1α,25(OH)$_2$D$_3$ stimulation at 10^{-7} M, but not at a 10^{-8} M level [33]. In the present study, 10^{-8} M was used to resemble the amounts found in the synovial fluid, yet it appeared insufficient to affect VDR expression at the protein level (Fig. 5). This indicates

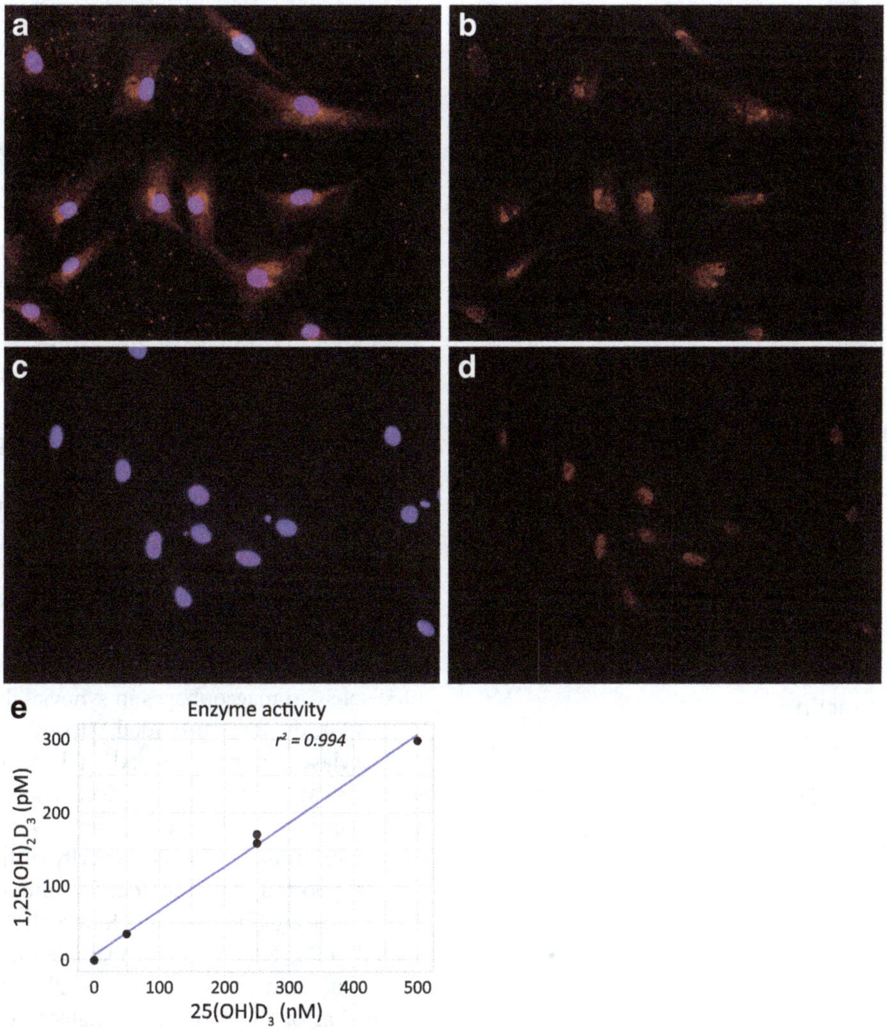

Fig. 4 Cultured chondrocytes labelled with VDR antibody (**b** and **d**) and merged image of DAPI and VDR labelling (**a** and **c**). Cells in **a** and **b** are untreated, while **c** and **d** are treated with 1α,25(OH)$_2$D$_3$ for 2 h. Cultured chondrocytes treated with 50, 250 or 500 nM 25(OH)D$_3$ for 24 h compared to level of 1α,25(OH)$_2$D$_3$ measured in the supernatant (**e**), results represent the experiment on cells from one donor

that a supplementary local hormone production is required [34], or that osteoblasts and chondrocytes are unrelated cells on this subject.

It is claimed that in general 1α,25(OH)$_2$D$_3$ has an anabolic effect on tissues [35]. In studies of proliferation, the mutual potency of 25(OH)D$_3$ and 1α,25(OH)$_2$D$_3$ was proven by the changes observed with each of the compounds. A similar pattern was seen in three donors, indicating enhanced proliferation after 25(OH)D$_3$ or 1α,25(OH)$_2$D$_3$ treatment (Fig. 5e). Chondrocyte proliferation is frequently observed in OA cartilage [29], possibly as an attempt of cells to repair the damaged cartilage or to compensate the catabolic processes established in the joint.

Moreover, from the spheroid model that investigates chondrogenic potential, a corresponding effect was observed resulting in a significant loss of matrix production (Fig. 6 a-d) during treatment with 25(OH)D$_3$ or 1α,25(OH)$_2$D$_3$, but only after applying the assay to chondrocytes that also were expanded in the presence of 25(OH)D$_3$ or 1α,25(OH)$_2$D$_3$. Spheroids prepared from chondrocytes propagated in standard growth medium were indifferent to the presence of 1α,25(OH)$_2$D$_3$ during 3D culture (data not shown), underpinning that chondrocytes in 3D cultures rapidly repress VDR expression.

The gene expression profile of cultured cells exposed to 25(OH)D$_3$ and 1α,25(OH)$_2$D$_3$ indicated an unfavourable effect on proteoglycan transcripts ACAN and VCAN, while the expression of VDR, COL1A1 and SOX9 was unchanged. This outcome is in accordance with the lower expression of proteoglycans observed by Alcian blue staining of treated spheroids. Interestingly, the CYP24A1, that was included as a positive control of 1α,25(OH)$_2$D$_3$ effects, showed increased expression also

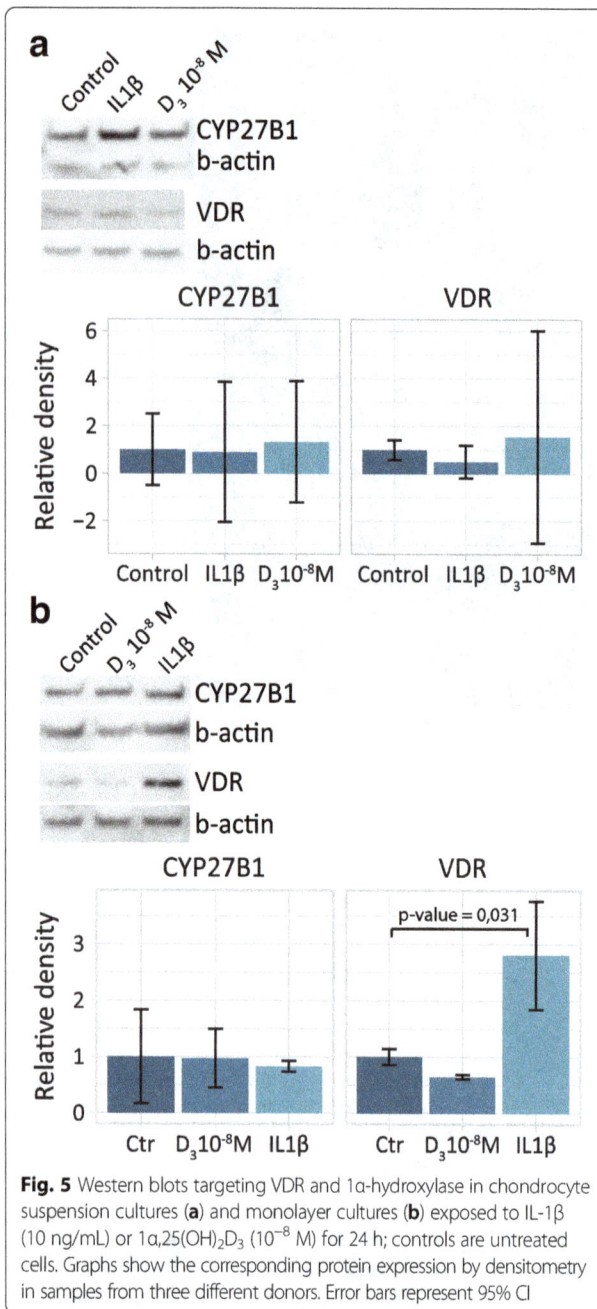

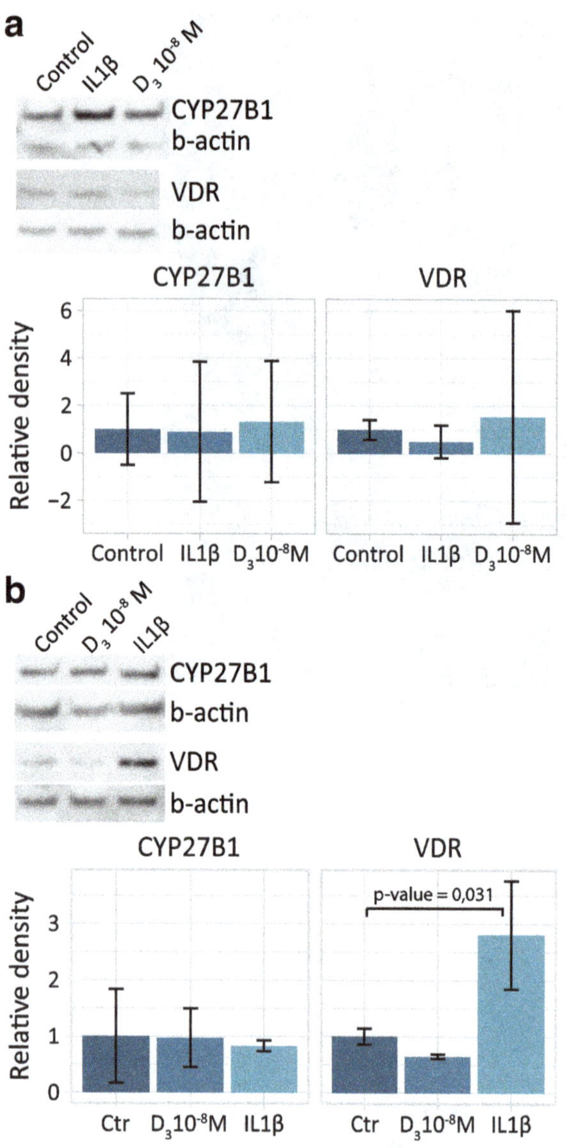

Fig. 5 Western blots targeting VDR and 1α-hydroxylase in chondrocyte suspension cultures (**a**) and monolayer cultures (**b**) exposed to IL-1β (10 ng/mL) or 1α,25(OH)$_2$D$_3$ (10^{-8} M) for 24 h; controls are untreated cells. Graphs show the corresponding protein expression by densitometry in samples from three different donors. Error bars represent 95% CI

upon 25(OH)D$_3$ treatment (Fig. 6 f), supporting the notion that chondrocytes endogenously express 1α-hydroxylase.

Striking and novel findings in this study were the expression of transcripts for the enzyme 1α-hydroxylase and the presence of the encoded protein in human osteoarthritic articular cartilage, in suspension cells, in monolayers and 3D spheroid cultures (Fig. 1). The expression in all these conditions could indicate a constitutive expression pattern. No evidence for 1α-hydroxylase regulation by IL-1β or 1α,25(OH)$_2$D$_3$ in differentiated suspension cells or dedifferentiated monolayer cells was recorded, which is in line with previous studies on osteoblasts [33]. Previously, the enzyme was detected in rat growth plate chondrocytes [36], but to the best of our knowledge there are no reports on its presence in human articular cartilage or chondrocytes. Expression of 1α-hydroxylase in cartilage from healthy donors remains to be determined.

The level of 25(OH)D$_3$ and 1α,25(OH)$_2$D$_3$ in the synovial fluid of inflamed joints in patients with rheumatoid arthritis has been measured to 20 nM and 25 pM, respectively [4]. After oral administration of vitamin D, the level of 1α,25(OH)$_2$D$_3$ in synovial fluid has been measured to up to 100 nM [37]. Based on these measurements, and to meet the sensitivity of the assay, chondrocytes were challenged with 50, 250 and 500 nM 25(OH)D$_3$, resulting in a conversion to 50, 150 and 300 pM 1α,25(OH)$_2$D$_3$, respectively (Fig. 4e). Since cell-free controls were subtracted to account for spontaneous 1α-hydroxylation, the results imply that the chondrocyte exhibits 1α-hydroxylase activity that may contribute to the pool of 1α,25(OH)$_2$D$_3$ in synovial fluid, an action that has previously been attributed solely to macrophages in synovial fluid [4, 38].

This study has provided strong evidence for 1α-hydroxylase being expressed in human articular chondrocytes, at least in OA-derived chondrocytes, whereas evidence for a VDR expression is weaker, except in culture-expanded cells. The activity of the 1α-hydroxylase was supported by the conversion of 25(OH)D$_3$ to 1α,25(OH)$_2$D$_3$ (Fig. 4e) and indirectly by the assays presented in Fig. 6 showing comparable outcomes from treatment with 25(OH)D$_3$ and 1α,25(OH)$_2$D$_3$. Hence, the co-expression of these proteins enables auto- and paracrine cell activity, exemplified here by impaired matrix production, augmented cell proliferation and shifted ACAN/VCAN expression after the application of either 1α,25(OH)$_2$D$_3$ or 25(OH)D$_3$ (Fig. 6). These changes in chondrocyte activity are indeed associated with OA progression [39], however since the functional experiments were conducted on dedifferentiated cells, some caution is advised in extrapolating these results to in vivo conditions. On the other hand, as a result of the increased expression of VDR during inflammatory conditions reported by us and others [31], some of the actions described in Fig. 6 may be part of the picture during OA and RA pathology.

The extent and types of effects 1α,25(OH)$_2$D$_3$ have on resident cells in healthy cartilage remains to be uncovered, yet a probable paracrine action affecting neighbouring cells and tissues is apparent. However, the numerous VDR responsive elements in DNA and VDR's capability to additionally engage several intracellular signalling systems, such as protein kinase C and phosphatidyl-inositol-3′ kinase reviewed in [40], vouch for a plethora of biological readouts beyond the

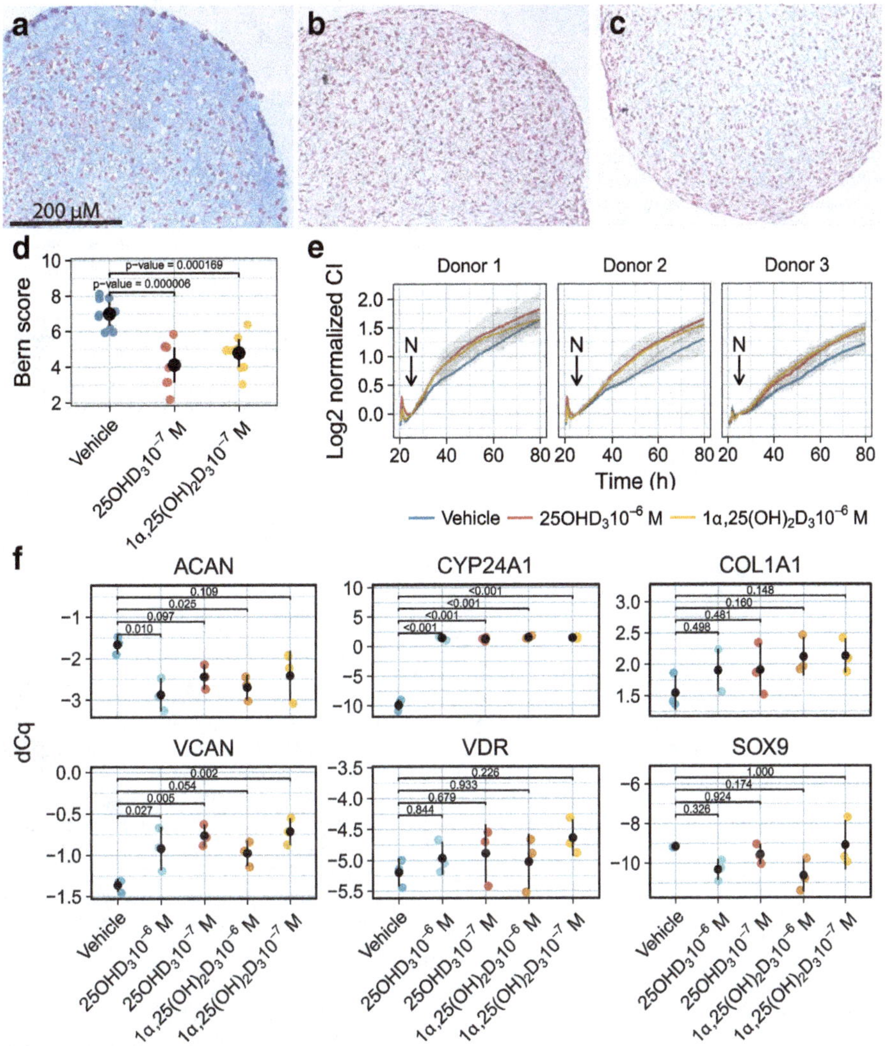

Fig. 6 Alcian blue staining of spheroids maintained in control medium (**a**) 25(OH)D$_3$ (**b**) or 1α,25(OH)$_2$D$_3$ at 10^{-7} M (**c**) for 2 weeks. Treated and untreated spheroids from three different donors histologically evaluated by Bern Score (**d**). Proliferation (**e**) of monolayer chondrocytes under continuous stimulation with 25(OH)D$_3$, 1α,25(OH)$_2$D$_3$ or vehicle for 80 h in three donors. Ribbons represent 95% confidence interval and N indicates the time of normalization. Cartilage signature gene expression in monolayer cultures from three donors (**f**). Error bars represent one standard deviation, while horizontal bars and values represent *p*-values resulting from the comparison of means of the treated samples to the mean of the vehicle samples

scope of this study to be investigated. Thus, this study does not rule out any anti-inflammatory effects of vitamin D on the joint as a whole.

Conclusion

To conclude, we report here a novel finding on the vitamin D converting enzyme, 1α-hydroxylase, in human articular chondrocytes along with compelling evidence of the enzyme facilitating the conversion of 25(OH)D$_3$ to the active hormone, 1α,25(OH)$_2$D$_3$. The expression of the vitamin D receptor is more elusive and reproducible experiments are limited to monolayer conditions where the expression of the VDR is more evident. The overall effect of both 25(OH)D$_3$ and 1α,25(OH)$_2$D$_3$ include diminished matrix production, enhanced proliferation and inversed expression of ACAN and VCAN, all pointing to an unfavourable effect of vitamin D on matrix synthesis.

Additional file

Additional file 1: Figure S1. qPCR. Relative expression of cartilage signature genes in donor matched suspension- and monolayer culture samples from three donors. Suspension cultures samples were challenged with vehicle, 1α,25(OH)$_2$D$_2$ or 1α,25(OH)$_2$D$_3$ at 10^{-8} M for 24 hours. The qPCR reaction was setup as described in material and methods. Collagen type IX alpha 1 chain (COL9A1, Hs00932129_m1) and collagen typeX alpha 1 chain (COL10A1, Hs00166657_m1) hydrolysis probes (Life Technologies by Fisher Scientific) were included in addtion to probes listed previously. The dCq was calculated by subtracting the reference gene from the gene of interest so that a higher dCq value represents an upregulation and vice versa. Delta Cq values were mean-centred and autoscaled, and normalized to a suspension culture control sample to obtain ddCq [1]. A Dunnett's test was used to compare the treated suspension cultures samples and the untreated monolayer samples to the suspension culture control sample. Error bars represent 95 % confidence intervals. References 1. Willems E, Leyns L, Vandesompele J. Standardization of real-time PCR gene expression data from independent biological replicates. Anal Biochem. 2008;379:127–9. doi:10.1016/j.ab.2008.04.036. (EPS 912 kb)

Abbreviations

1α,25(OH)$_2$D$_3$: 1α,25-dihydroxy vitamin D$_3$ – Calcitriol; 25(OH)D$_3$: 25-hydroxy D$_3$; ECM: Extracellular matrix; OA: Osteoarthritis; OPG/RANKL: Osteoprotegerin/receptor activator of nuclear factor kappa-B ligand; RA: Rheumatoid arthritis; VDR: Vitamin D receptor

Acknowledgements

Thanks to Gunnar Knutsen and Geir Tore Abrahamsen, who provided the cartilage biopsies, and to Kirsti Rønne and Ashraful Islam for technical assistance.

Funding

The study was supported by the Northern Norway Regional Health Authority. The publication charges for this article have been funded by a grant from the publication fund of UiT The Arctic University of Norway.

Authors' contributions

The experiments were performed by AKH and IZM, The manuscript was drafted by AKH and revised by IZM and YF. All authors read and approved the final manuscript.

Competing interests

The authors declare that they have no competing interests.

Author details

[1]Department of Orthopaedic Surgery, University Hospital of North Norway, Tromsø, Norway. [2]Bone and joint research group, Institute of Clinical Medicine, Faculty of Health Sciences, University of Tromsø, Tromsø, Norway. [3]Department of Laboratory Medicine, University Hospital of North Norway, Tromsø, Norway. [4]Endocrinology Research Group, Institute of Clinical Medicine, Faculty of Health Sciences, University of Tromsø, Tromsø, Norway. [5]Department of Medical Biology, Faculty of Health Sciences, University of Tromsø, Tromsø, Norway.

References

1. Chaganti RK, Lane NE. Risk factors for incident osteoarthritis of the hip and knee. Curr Rev Musculoskelet Med. 2011;4:99–104. 10.1007/s12178-011-9088-5.
2. Rahmati M, Mobasheri A, Mozafari M. Inflammatory mediators in osteoarthritis: a critical review of the state-of-the-art, current prospects, and future challenges. Bone. 2016;85:81–90. 10.1016/j.bone.2016.01.019.
3. Mabey T, Honsawek S. Role of vitamin D in osteoarthritis: molecular, cellular, and clinical perspectives. Int J Endocrinol. 2015;2015:383918. 10.1155/2015/383918.
4. Mawer EB, Hayes ME, Still PE, Davies M, Lumb GA, Palit J, et al. Evidence for nonrenal synthesis of 1,25-dihydroxyvitamin D in patients with inflammatory arthritis. J Bone Min Res. 1991;6:733–9. 10.1002/jbmr.5650060711.
5. Morris HA, Anderson PH. Autocrine and paracrine actions of vitamin d. Clin Biochem Rev. 2010;31:129–38. http://www.ncbi.nlm.nih.gov/entrez/query.fcgi?cmd=Retrieve&db=PubMed&dopt=Citation&list_uids=21170259
6. Wang Y, Zhu J, DeLuca HF. Where is the vitamin D receptor? Arch Biochem Biophys. 2012;523:123–33. 10.1016/j.abb.2012.04.001.
7. Zhang FF, Driban JB, Lo GH, Price LL, Booth S, Eaton CB, et al. Vitamin D deficiency is associated with progression of knee osteoarthritis. J Nutr. 2014; 144:2002–8. 10.3945/jn.114.193227.
8. Jin X, Jones G, Cicuttini F, Wluka A, Zhu Z, Han W, et al. Effect of vitamin D supplementation on Tibial cartilage volume and knee pain among patients with symptomatic knee osteoarthritis: a randomized clinical trial. JAMA. 2016;315:1005–13. 10.1001/jama.2016.1961.
9. Tetlow LC, Woolley DE. The effects of 1 alpha,25-dihydroxyvitamin D(3) on matrix metalloproteinase and prostaglandin E(2) production by cells of the rheumatoid lesion. Arthritis Res. 1999;1:63–70. 10.1186/ar12.
10. Bhalla AK, Wojno WC, Goldring MB. Human articular chondrocytes acquire 1,25-(OH)2 vitamin D-3 receptors in culture. Biochim Biophys Acta. 1987;931:26–32.
11. Tetlow LC, Woolley DE. Expression of vitamin D receptors and matrix metalloproteinases in osteoarthritic cartilage and human articular chondrocytes in vitro. Osteoarthr Cartil. 2001;9:423–31. 10.1053/joca.2000.0408.
12. Chen D, Li Y, Dai X, Zhou X, Tian W, Zhou Y, et al. 1,25-Dihydroxyvitamin D3 activates MMP13 gene expression in chondrocytes through p38 MARK pathway. Int J Biol Sci. 2013;9:649–55. 10.7150/ijbs.6726.
13. Orfanidou T, Malizos KN, Varitimidis S, Tsezou A. 1,25-Dihydroxyvitamin D(3) and extracellular inorganic phosphate activate mitogen-activated protein kinase pathway through fibroblast growth factor 23 contributing to hypertrophy and mineralization in osteoarthritic chondrocytes. Exp Biol Med. 2012;237:241–53. 10.1258/ebm.2011.011301.
14. Martinez I, Elvenes J, Olsen R, Bertheussen K, Johansen O. Redifferentiation of in vitro expanded adult articular chondrocytes by combining the hanging-drop cultivation method with hypoxic environment. Cell Transpl. 2008;17:987–96. http://www.ncbi.nlm.nih.gov/pubmed/19069640
15. Wang Y, Becklund BR, DeLuca HF. Identification of a highly specific and versatile vitamin D receptor antibody. Arch Biochem Biophys. 2010;494:166–77. 10.1016/j.abb.2009.11.029.
16. A Islam, AK Hansen, C Mennan, I Martinez-Zubiaurre. Mesenchymal stromal cells from human umbilical cords display poor chondrogenic potential in scaffold-free three dimensional cultures. European Cells and Materials. 2016; 31:407-424
17. Grogan SP, Barbero A, Winkelmann V, Rieser F, Fitzsimmons JS, O'Driscoll S, et al. Visual histological grading system for the evaluation of in vitro-generated neocartilage. Tissue Eng. 2006;12:2141–9. 10.1089/ten.2006.12.2141.
18. Witzel F, Fritsche-Guenther R, Lehmann N, Sieber A, Blüthgen N. Analysis of impedance-based cellular growth assays. Bioinformatics. 2015;31:2705–12. 10.1093/bioinformatics/btv216.
19. Tokuyasu KT. Application of cryoultramicrotomy to immunocytochemistry. J Microsc. 1986;143(Pt 2):139–49. http://www.ncbi.nlm.nih.gov/pubmed/3531524
20. RStudio Team. RStudio: integrated development for R. 2016. http://www.rstudio.com/.
21. Wickham H. tidyr: Easily Tidy Data with 'spread()' and 'gather()' Functions. 2016. https://cran.r-project.org/package=tidyr.
22. Wickham H, Francois R. Dplyr: a grammar of data manipulation. 2016. https://cran.r-project.org/package=dplyr.
23. Robinson D. broom: Convert Statistical Analysis Objects into Tidy Data Frames. 2017. https://cran.r-project.org/package=broom.
24. Dowle M, Srinivasan A. data.table: Extension of 'data.frame'. 2017. https://cran.r-project.org/package=data.table.
25. Wickham H. purrr: Functional Programming Tools. 2016. https://cran.r-project.org/package=purrr.
26. Wickham H. ggplot2: Elegant Graphics for Data Analysis. 2009. http://ggplot2.org.
27. Arnold JB. ggthemes: Extra Themes, Scales and Geoms for "ggplot2." 2017. https://cran.r-project.org/package=ggthemes.
28. Wickham H. The split-apply-combine strategy for data analysis. J Stat Softw. 2011;40:1–29.
29. Goldring MB, Marcu KB. Cartilage homeostasis in health and rheumatic diseases. Arthritis Res Ther. 2009;11:224. 10.1186/ar2592.
30. Feng X, Lv C, Wang F, Gan K, Zhang M, Tan W. Modulatory effect of 1,25-dihydroxyvitamin D 3 on IL1 β -induced RANKL, OPG, TNF α, and IL-6 expression in human rheumatoid synoviocyte MH7A. Clin Dev Immunol. 2013;2013:160123. 10.1155/2013/160123.

31. Tetlow LC, Smith SJ, Mawer EB, Woolley DE. Vitamin D receptors in the rheumatoid lesion: expression by chondrocytes, macrophages, and synoviocytes. Ann Rheum Dis. 1999;58:118–21. http://ard.bmj.com/content/58/2/118.full.pdf
32. Pike JW, Meyer MB. The vitamin D receptor: new paradigms for the regulation of gene expression by 1,25-Dihydroxyvitamin D3. Endocrinol Metab. 2010;39:255–69.
33. van der Meijden K, Lips P, van Driel M, Heijboer AC, Schulten EAJM, den HM, et al. Primary human Osteoblasts in response to 25-Hydroxyvitamin D3, 1,25-Dihydroxyvitamin D3 and 24R,25-Dihydroxyvitamin D3. PLoS One. 2014;9:e110283. 10.1371/journal.pone.0110283.
34. van Driel M, Koedam M, Buurman CJ, Hewison M, Chiba H, Uitterlinden AG, et al. Evidence for auto/paracrine actions of vitamin D in bone: 1alpha-hydroxylase expression and activity in human bone cells. FASEB J. 2006;20:2417–9.
35. Goltzman D, Hendy GN, White JH. Vitamin D and its receptor during late development. Biochim Biophys Acta - Gene Regul Mech. 2015;1849:171–80. 10.1016/j.bbagrm.2014.05.026.
36. Weber L, Hügel U, Reichrath J, Sieverts H, Mehls O, Klaus G. Cultured rat growth plate chondrocytes express low levels of 1alpha-hydroxylase. Recent Results Cancer Res. 2003;164:147–9. http://www.ncbi.nlm.nih.gov/entrez/query.fcgi?cmd=Retrieve&db=PubMed&dopt=Citation&list_uids=12899519
37. Smith SJ, Hayes ME, Selby PL, Mawer EB. Autocrine control of vitamin D metabolism in synovial cells from arthritic patients. Ann Rheum Dis. 1999;58:372–8. http://www.ncbi.nlm.nih.gov/pubmed/10340962. Accessed 20 Jan 2017
38. Hayes ME, Denton J, Freemont AJ, Mawer EB. Synthesis of the active metabolite of vitamin D, 1,25(OH)2D3, by synovial fluid macrophages in arthritic diseases. Ann Rheum Dis. 1989;48:723–9. http://www.ncbi.nlm.nih.gov/pubmed/2802793
39. Goldring MB, Goldring SR. Osteoarthritis. J Cell Physiol. 2007;213:626–34. 10.1002/jcp.21258.
40. Norman AW. Vitamin D receptor: new assignments for an already busy receptor. Endocrinology. 2006;147:5542–8. 10.1210/en.2006-0946.

18

Quantitative evaluation of subchondral bone microarchitecture in knee osteoarthritis using 3T MRI

Chenglei Liu[1†], Chang Liu[2†], Xvhua Ren[2], Liping Si[1], Hao Shen[3], Qian Wang[2] and Weiwu Yao[1*]

Abstract

Background: Osteoarthritis (OA) is now increasingly recognized as being related to the whole joint instead of the cartilage alone. In particular, the importance of subchondral bone in OA pathogenesis has drawn a lot of interest. The aim of this study is to investigate subchondral bone microstructural features in two femoral condyles of human knee osteoarthritis.

Methods: Eighty subjects were enrolled in our study and divided into three groups: without OA (group 0), mild OA (group 1), and severe OA (group 2). Sagittal 3D Balanced Fast Field Echo (3D–FFE) images were obtained by 3T MRI to quantify trabecular bone structure, and sagittal FatSat 3D Fast Field Echo (3D–FFE) images were acquired to assess cartilage thickness. Trabecular bone parameters, including bone volume fraction (BVF), erosion index (EI) and the trabecular plate-to-rod ratio (SCR), and trabecular thickness were evaluated using digital topological analysis. Subchondral bone and cartilage parameters between different groups and different locations were compared, and their correlations were analyzed.

Results: Within two femoral condyles, subchondral bone structure was deteriorated in mild OA, showing a lower BVF (−0.011 to −0.014 $P < 0.001$), a higher EI (0.346 to 0.310 $P < 0.001$), a lower SCR (−0.581 to −0.542 $P < 0.001$)) and lower trabecular thickness (−6.588 to −4.759 $P < 0.05$). In severe OA, BVF was further decreased, but EI, SCR and trabecular thickness showed no significant difference than mild OA($P > 0.05$). Moreover, there was a lower BVF, SCR and higher EI in the medial femoral condyle in each group. Interestingly, cartilage attrition mainly occurred in the medial femoral condyle. Medial cartilage thickness was not only positively correlated with the ipsilateral femoral BVF ($r = 0.321$ $P = 0.004$) but also with the opposite femoral BVF ($r = 0.270$ $P = 0.015$).

Conclusions: Our results indicated that deterioration in the trabecular bone structure in both femoral condyles could more sensitively reveal early OA, and BVF could be a better biomarker to evaluate OA severity.

Keywords: Magnetic resonance imaging (MRI), Osteoarthritis, Subchondral bone, Knee

Background

Osteoarthritis (OA) is a degenerative joint disease that causes joint pain, stiffness and loss of independence. Currently, the structures that initiate disease onset and progression are unclear, and no definitive cure for osteoarthritis is available. The only treatment options include pain control and ultimately joint replacement [1]. Generally, the hallmark of OA has been accepted as articular cartilage loss, and the involvement of subchondral bone was secondary to cartilage attrition. However, recent findings showed that changes in subchondral bone appeared in early-stage osteoarthritis, preceding cartilage deterioration [2]. In models of rat OA, an attenuated subchondral bone plate, decreased trabecular thickness and increased trabecular separation were detected using micro-CT as early as 2 weeks after inducing OA [3, 4]. MRI studies for osteoarthritic knees have also shown that subchondral bone marrow edema-like lesions (BMLs) were associated with pain and increased cartilage loss in the same region in early OA [5].

* Correspondence: yaoweiwuhuan@163.com
†Equal contributors
[1]Department of Radiology, Shanghai Jiao Tong University Affiliated Sixth People's Hospital, Shanghai, China
Full list of author information is available at the end of the article

Moreover, subchondral bone and cartilage form a unit in anatomic regions to sustain mechanical forces. When either of these is altered, increased loads will be transmitted from one surface to the other [6]. Increasing evidence suggests that cartilage and subchondral bone interact and that chondrocytes and bone cells are intimately interconnected in the course of disease [7]. On one hand, chondrocytes could transdifferentiate into osteoblasts in the growth plate [8]. On the other hand, various cytokines produced by subchondral bone were able to regulate cartilage metabolism [9]. In addition, pharmacological studies have shown that bone remodeling inhibitor drugs could improve clinical symptoms and reduce structural progression [10, 11]. Therefore, the assessment of bone structure, except for cartilage, is very critical for the elucidation of OA pathogenesis.

Unfortunately, in recent human osteoarthritis studies, most studies have focused on end-stage subchondral bone changes, and these results were mainly derived from analyses of tibia plateaus after joint replacement using micro-CT or histopathology. Most of the knowledge about early subchondral bone changes has come from animal OA models. Moreover, in the knee joint, in contrast to tibia plateaus, more loading forces are concentrated in the two femoral condyles [12]. Very little information is available in the literature on changes in the subchondral bone structure in these locations during OA. In recent years, with improved MRI resolution and post-processing algorithms, a few relevant studies have been performed, but the results failed to reach a conclusion. The initial MRI study demonstrated significant variations in the trabecular bone structure of the femur and tibia based on very few subjects [12]. Afterwards, Chiba K et al. noted that with OA progression, the trabecular bone structure showed osteoporotic changes in the lateral joint and sclerotic changes in the medial joint [13]. Recently, Chang G et al. used 7 T MRI to display deterioration in the subchondral bone microstructure of the distal femur in patients with mild OA [14]. However, in clinical practice, 7 T MRI is not commonly available, and its application is limited due to increased chemical shift variations, radiofrequency power deposition and magnetic field inhomogeneity [15]. Given this, we used 3T MRI to perform a cross-sectional quantitative analysis of the trabecular bone structure and cartilage to further investigate alterations in the subchondral bone microstructure during the course of OA.

Methods

Subjects

Our prospective study was approved by the hospital institutional review board (Shanghai No. 6 People's Hospital), and written informed consent was obtained from all patients. Between September 2016 and march 2017, 80 subjects were recruited by one orthopedic surgeon with 15 years of experience (SH), and diagnosis was based on a clinical examination and an anterior-posterior weight-bearing knee radiograph. The OA subjects were further divided into two groups based on the Kellgrene-Lawrence (KL) classification [16]. Thirty-three patients with KL scores of 1–2 were classified as mild OA (group 1) (17men and 16 women, age = 45.64 ± 9.09 years, body mass index (BMI) = 24.51 ± 3.32 kg/m^2). Sixteen patients with KL scores of 3–4 were categorized as severe OA (group 2) (7 men and 9 women, age = 58.19 ± 6.34 years, BMI = 24.71 ± 3.19 kg/m^2). In addition, thirty-one healthy subjects without knee impairment or radiographic signs of OA were classified as control subjects (group 0) (11 men and 20 women, age = 30.23 ± 9.34 years, BMI = 23.51 ± 1.22 kg/m^2). All subjects were performed a standardized WOMAC questionnaire (Western Ontario and McMaster Universities Arthritis Index) of pain, functional impairment and stiffness [17]. The detailed clinical data for both control and OA groups were summarized in Table 1. We excluded patients with a history of obesity, knee injury or surgery, inflammatory arthritis, osteonecrosis, or other disease that affects bone structure.

Imaging modality

Radiographs of the knee were performed on a DR (Siemens, Germany), and all patients were asked to stand with the patella facing forward in weight-bearing position while a standard plain X-ray in the anteroposterior plane was taken.

MR imaging of the knee (affected knee in OA subjects, nondominant knee in control subjects) was performed on a 3.0-T superconducting MR scanner (Koninklijke Philips NV, Amsterdam, the Netherlands) with an eight-channel knee coil. The knee flexion angle was adjusted 15°, and a dedicated holder was used to reduce motion artifacts at the time of imaging. The MR imaging protocol included two pulse sequences. The imaging sequences and parameters of each examination were as follows: Sagittal 3D Balanced Fast Field Echo Sequence (3D B-FFE) (TR/TE 19/9.7, FOV 10 cm, matrix 558 × 554, 80 slices, section thickness 1 mm, flip angle 40°, acquisition time 9 min 18 s, in-plane spatial resolution 0.18 × 0.18 mm^2) to image the subchondral bone microarchitecture, and Sagittal FatSat3D Fast Field Echo Sequence (3D–FFE) (TR/TE 25/4.8, FOV 15 cm, matrix 500 × 499, 80 slices, section thickness 1 mm, flip angle 30°, acquisition time 9 min 12 s, in-plane spatial resolution 0.30 × 0.30 mm^2) to image the cartilage.

Image analysis

A 3D measurement of the subchondral bone microstructure and cartilage was performed in the sagittal plane using an in-house program created with MATLAB (Math Works, Natick, MA). Five successive slices within the center of the medial and lateral joints were separately selected

Table 1 Clinical data for the three subject groups divided according to the degree of osteoarthritis (OA)

	Total ($n = 80$)	Control ($n = 31$)	Mild OA($n = 33$)	Severe OA($n = 16$)	P value
Age	42.18 ± 13.68	30.23 ± 9.34	45.64 ± 9.09†	58.19 ± 6.34†	0.000*
Gender					
Male	35(43.75%)	11(35.48%)	17(51.51%)	7(43.75%)	0.434
Female	45(56.25%)	20(64.52%)	16(48.49%)	9(56.25%)	
Knee joint					
Left	30(37.50%)	8(25.81%)	16(48.49%)	6(37.5%)	0.173
Right	50(62.50%)	23(74.19%)	17(51.51%)	10(62.5%)	
weight	66.01 ± 9.56	63.94 ± 6.39	68.03 ± 11.73	65.88 ± 9.38	0.233
BMI	24.17 ± 2.69	23.51 ± 1.22	24.51 ± 3.32	24.71 ± 3.19	0.222
WOMAC OA index					
Pain	4.84 ± 5.39	0.00 ± 0.00	5.30 ± 2.76	13.25 ± 3.55	0.000*
stiffness	0.96 ± 1.97	0.00 ± 0.00	1.00 ± 1.71	2.75 ± 3.00	0.000*
Function	9.16 ± 12.57	0.00 ± 0.00	9.61 ± 9.29	26.00 ± 13.14	0.000*

Data compared with ANOVA for continuous variables, Chi-squared test for categorical variables
*Statistical significance, $p < 0.05$
†Significantly different compared with normal group as determined using Scheffe's test

by a musculoskeletal radiologist (CLL). Prior to the quantitative analysis of the subchondral bone microstructure, N4 correction and a non-local means denoising approach were applied to correct signal intensity variations and image artifacts [18]. The region of interest (ROI) for subchondral bone was 5 mm wide below the subchondral bone plate covered by cartilage in each slice (Fig. 1). The ROI was established semi-automatically by a single biomedical engineer (CL). Then, the 3D interpolations function and the local thresholding algorithm were used to yield a 3D binary volume. For each VOI, a bone volume fraction (BVF) map was created by scaling voxel signal intensities from 0 to 100 (0 = pure marrow, 100 = pure bone). We utilized the digital topological analysis (DTA) to determine subchondral bone networks and compute topological classes for each ROI [19]. The measured parameters included BVF, trabecular network osteoclastic resorption (erosion index, EI), and the trabecular plate-to-rod ratio (SCR). The Fuzzy distance transform method was used for trabecular thickness measurements [20]. The cartilage was segmented using ITK-SNAP. The radiologist (CLL) manually delineated the cartilage using a graphics cursor. The cartilage region of each femoral condyle corresponded to the ROI for the trabecular bone analysis, and cartilage thickness was separately calculated (Fig. 1).

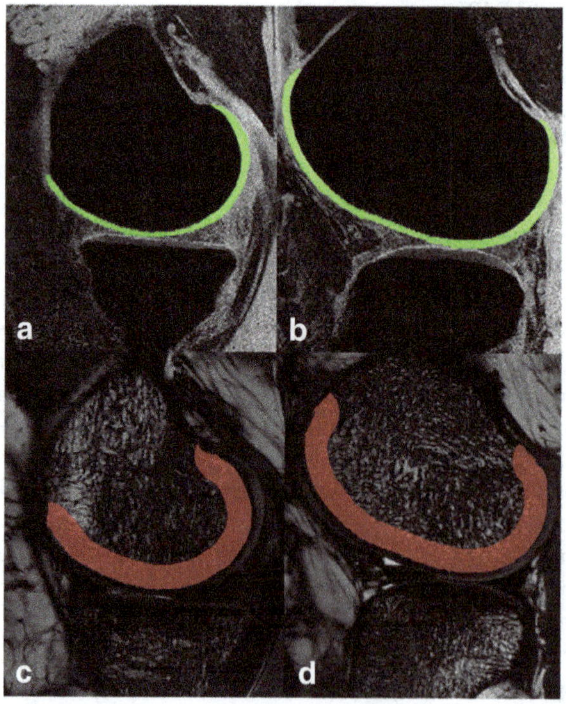

Fig. 1 Images of the regions of interest acquired by 3T MRI. Analysis of the cartilage region in the center of the medial femoral condyle (**a**) and the lateral femoral condyle (**b**) by 3D FFE imaging and the analysis of the subchondral bone region in the center of the medial femoral condyle (**c**) and the lateral femoral condyle (**d**) by 3D BFFE imaging

Statistical analysis

A statistical software package (SPSS 16.0, SPSS, Chicago, III) was used to perform the statistical analysis. The mean value and standard deviation were computed for each trabecular parameter and cartilage thickness in each femoral condyle. The significance of the observed differences between the medial and lateral femoral condyles was established using Student's paired t test. The subchondral bone and cartilage parameters between the groups were compared using an analysis of covariance (ANCOVA) with an adjustment for age. The correlation between cartilage thickness and subchondral bone parameters were analyzed by Pearson's correlation coefficient test; $P < 0.05$ was considered statistically significant.

Results

Trabecular bone structure and cartilage image processing

The data processing steps for the trabecular bone analysis are shown in Fig. 2. MR image intensity inhomogeneity was corrected and image artifacts were dropped. The MR image and BVF map clearly depict trabecular orientation and spatial distribution in the medial and lateral femoral condyles. Representative 3D BVF maps for the subchondral bone microstructures of control subjects, mild OA subjects and severe OA subjects are shown in Fig. 3 (a-c). Compared to the control subjects, the osteoarthritis subjects demonstrated sparse trabeculae and heterogeneous distribution in both femoral condyles and as the degree of OA increased, deterioration in the trabecular bone microarchitecture became further aggravated.

Representative cartilage segmentation images for varying degrees of OA are shown in Fig. 3 (d-f). There was an elaborate fitting in the inner and outer boundaries of the cartilage. Within the medial femoral condyle, compared to the control subjects, cartilage thickness did not significantly change in mild OA subjects. However, in severe OA, the cartilage was obviously thinning.

Quantitative analysis of topological parameters in the subchondral bone structure and cartilage thickness

Medial-lateral differences of trabecular structure and cartilage thickness in the femoral condyles

The descriptive statistics for bone and cartilage measurements by group were summarized in Table 2, and the mean medial-lateral differences in the femoral condyle for each group were shown in Table 3. For each group, significant differences were observed in the BVF, EI and SCR between medial and lateral femoral condyle. The BVF and SCR values were higher and the EI was lower in the lateral femoral condyle. However, no significant difference was observed in trabecular thickness between both femoral condyles. For cartilage thickness, no significant difference was observed between the two femoral condyles in the control subjects, but in the mild OA and severe OA subjects, the differences arrived at

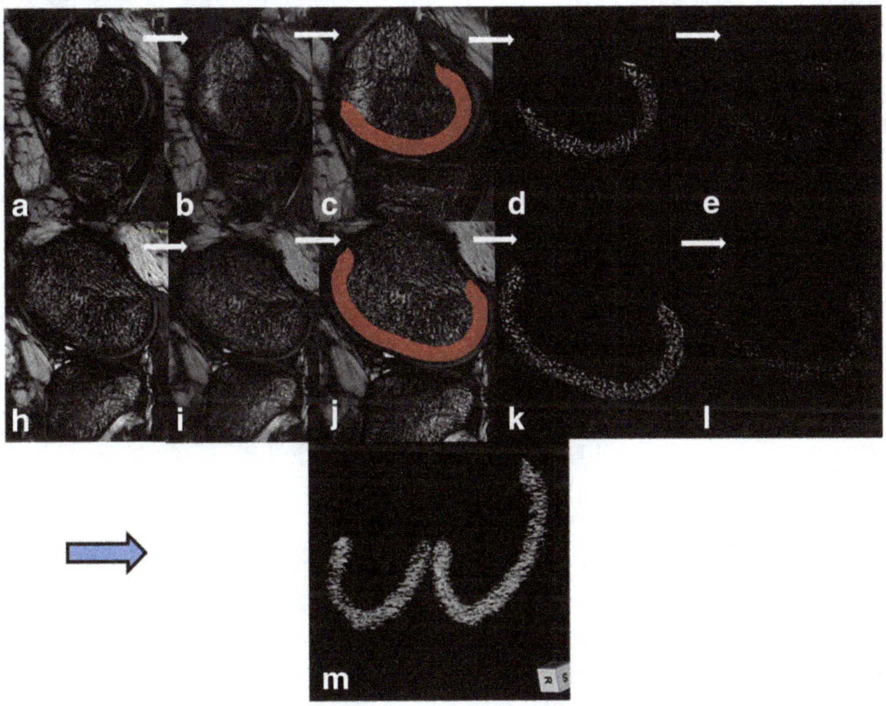

Fig. 2 Image processing steps. 1). In vivo raw MR sagittal images in the center of the medial knee joint (**a**) and the lateral knee joint (**h**). 2). Correction of signal intensity variations and image artifacts (**b**, **i**). 3). Establishment of the ROI of subchondral bone (**c**, **j**). 4). Generation of the bone volume fraction map of a single slice (**d**, **k**). 5). Image thinning for the topological analysis (**e**, **l**). 6) Generation of a 3D BVF map (**m**)

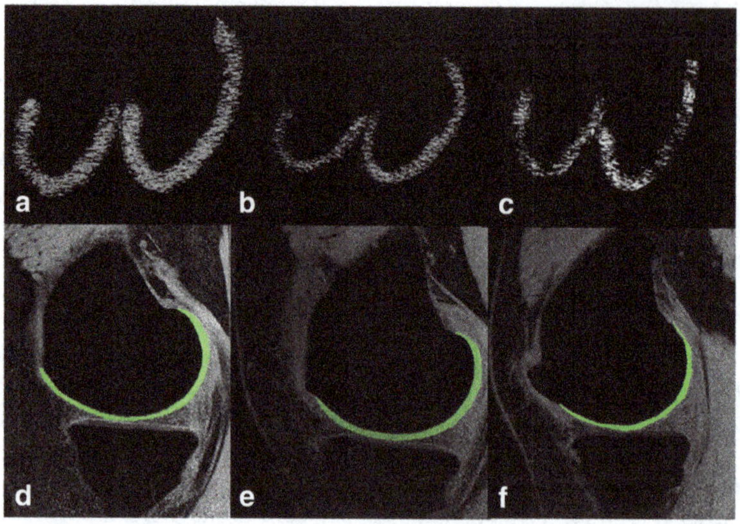

Fig. 3 Representative images of the subchondral bone and cartilage between varying stages of OA. For the analysis of the trabecular bone microstructure (**a-c**), compared to healthy control subjects (**a**), microstructural deterioration was observed in the medial and lateral femoral condyles of patients with mild OA (**b**). With disease progression, the degree of deterioration was further aggravated (**c**). For the analysis of the cartilage, there were no significant changes in cartilage thickness or volume in the medial condyle in mild OA subjects (**e**) compared with control subjects (**d**), but in the patients with severe OA (**f**), cartilage thickness was significant thinner than in mild OA and control subjects

statistical significance ($P < 0,05$). Cartilage attrition mainly occurred in area that lower bone topological parameter (medial femoral condyle), which was an interesting finding.

Differences in trabecular structure and cartilage thickness between controls and patients with OA

The trends in subchondral bone parameters and cartilage thickness in both femoral condyles between different OA subjects are shown in Fig. 4. As shown in Fig. 4, within the medial femoral condyle, compared to control subjects, the BVF, SCR and trabecular thickness showed marked decreases, and the EI rise sharply in the mild OA subjects. In the severe OA subjects, the BVF appeared to decrease further, the EI increased slightly, the SCR decreased slightly, and trabecular thickness increased slightly. Within the lateral femoral condyle, a similar trend was apparent during the course of OA. Within the medial femoral condyle, compared to control subjects, cartilage thickness slightly decreased in mild OA subjects. However, in severe

Table 2 Mean bone and cartilage parameter values for both femoral condyles between different groups of subjects

	Control ($n = 31$)	Mild OA($n = 33$)	Severe OA($n = 16$)
Medial femoral condyle			
BVF	0.145 ± 0.002	0.129 ± 0.002[a]	0.115 ± 0.003[a, b]
EI	2.086 ± 0.060	2.433 ± 0.045[a]	2.599 ± 0.082[a]
SCR	5.842 ± 0.115	5.261 ± 0.087[a]	5.168 ± 0.158[a]
Trabecular Thickness(um)	174.412 ± 1.690	167.823 ± 1.278[a]	170.817 ± 2.315
Cartilage Thickness (mm)	1.361 ± 0.051	1.199 ± 0.038	0.789 ± 0.069[a, b]
Lateral femoral condyle			
BVF	0.154 ± 0.002	0.139 ± 0.002[a]	0.124 ± 0.003[a,b]
EI	1.985 ± 0.054	2.296 ± 0.041[a]	2.478 ± 0.074[a]
SCR	5.531 ± 0.120	4.989 ± 0.091[a]	4.935 ± 0.164[a]
Trabecular Thickness(um)	173.337 ± 1.381	168.578 ± 1.044[a]	169.695 ± 1.892
Cartilage Thickness (mm)	1.365 ± 0.053	1.315 ± 0.041	1.207 ± 0.073

Data are mean ± standard error. The significance between groups is shown based on ANCOVA with adjustment for age
[a]$P < 0.01$ in comparison with control subjects
[b]$p < 0.01$ in comparison between mild OA and severe OA

Table 3 Mean medial - lateral differences in cartilage and bone parameter values between different groups of subjects

Group	BVF	EI	SCR	Trabecular Thickness(um)	Cartilage Thickness (mm)
0(n = 31)	−0.011 ± 0.007**	0.099 ± 0.047**	0.322 ± 0.149**	1.481 ± 4.661	−0.058 ± 0.161
1(n = 33)	−0.010 ± 0.010**	0.137 ± 0.104**	0.268 ± 0.197**	−0.872 ± 6.726	−0.100 ± 0.137**
2(n = 16)	−0.007 ± 0.011*	0.122 ± 0.101**	0.217 ± 0.316*	0.576 ± 9.706	−0.345 ± 0.224**

Data are mean ± standard deviation. The Mean medial - lateral differences in cartilage and bone parameter values between different groups of subjects is shown based on Student's paired t test. * = $p < 0.05$, ** = $P < 0.001$. Group0 = control subjects, Group1 = mild OA subjects, Group2 = severe OA subjects

OA, the cartilage markedly decreased. Within the lateral femoral condyle, cartilage thickness only slightly decreased during OA.

To evaluate the magnitude of these differences, the absolute value of each parameter for each OA group in the medial and lateral femoral condyles was calculated and summarized into Table 4. As illustrated in Table 4, in the comparison of control subjects and mild OA subjects, the absolute values for the BVF, EI, SCR and trabecular thickness showed significant differences in both the medial and lateral femoral condyles ($P < 0.05$). In the comparison of control subjects and severe OA subjects, significant differences were also seen in each parameter, except for trabecular thickness ($P < 0.05$). However, in the comparison of mild OA and severe OA subjects, a significant difference was seen only in BVF, and the other parameters did not show significant differences. For cartilage thickness, no significant difference was observed between the control subjects and mild OA subjects in the medial femoral condyle. However, in the comparison of mild OA and severe OA subjects, a significant difference was seen. Within the lateral femoral condyle, cartilage thickness only slightly decreased, but a significant difference was not found between the different OA groups.

Correlations between the subchondral bone parameters and cartilage thickness

To further identify the dynamics between cartilage degeneration and subchondral bone structure, we investigated the interrelationship between trabecular topological parameters and cartilage thickness in both femoral condyles. As shown in Fig. 5, medial cartilage thickness was not only positively correlated with the medial BVF ($r = 0.321$ $P = 0.004$) but also positively correlated with the lateral BVF ($r = 0.270$, $P = 0.15$). Correlations between other trabecular topological parameters and medial cartilage thickness were not found. Moreover, the relationships between lateral cartilage thickness and trabecular parameters showed no significant correlations ($P > 0.05$).

Discussion

Our current findings showed that within two femoral condyles, subchondral bone structure was deteriorated in mild OA, and in the severe OA, osteoporotic changes

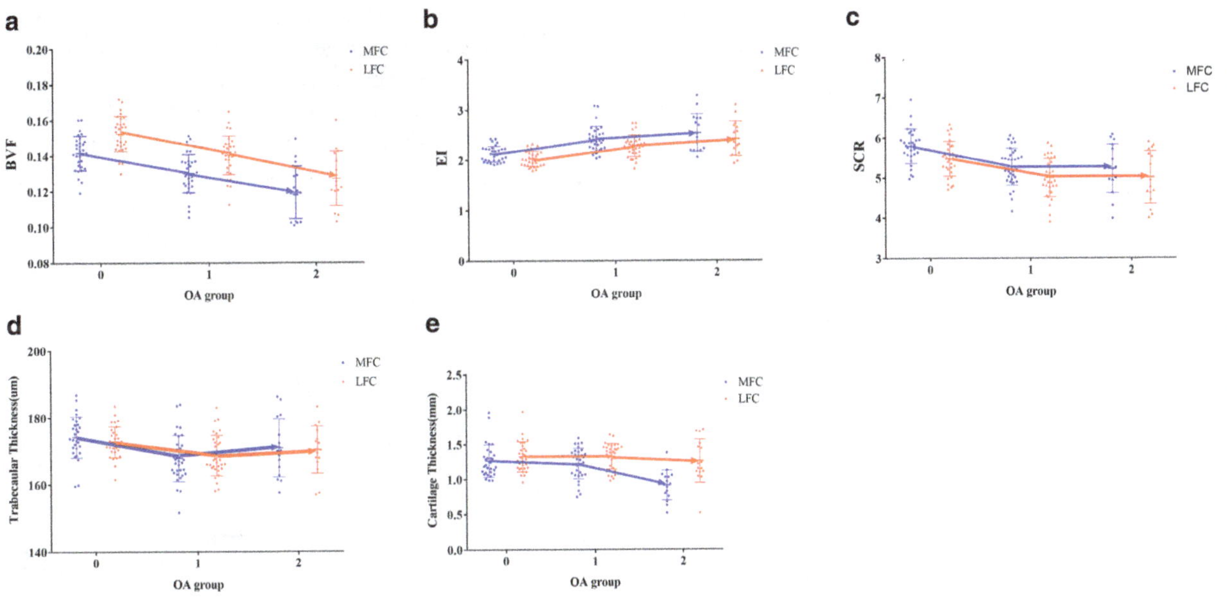

Fig. 4 The trends in subchondral bone parameters and cartilage thickness for the medial and lateral femoral condyles between different OA subjects. Group 0 = healthy control subjects; Group 1 = patients with mild OA; Group 2 = patients with severe OA. BVF = bone volume fraction. EI = Erosion Index. SCR = trabecular plate-to-rod ratio. MFC = Medial femoral condyle, LFC = lateral femoral condyle

Table 4 Mean differences in the cartilage and bone parameters for both femoral condyles between different groups of subjects

Region, group	BVF	EI	SCR	Trabecular Thickness(um)	Cartilage Thickness(mm)
MFC					
0 and 1	0.011 ± 0.003*	−0.346 ± 0.081*	0.581 ± 0.156*	6.588 ± 2.281*	0.161 ± 0.068
1 and 2	0.014 ± 1.06*	−0.166 ± 0.087	0.092 ± 0.168	−2.993 ± 2.457	0.411 ± 0.073*
0 and 2	0.029 ± 0.005*	−0.512 ± 0.120*	0.673 ± 0.232*	3.595 ± 3.392	0.571 ± 0.101*
LFC					
0 and 1	0.014 ± 0.003*	−0.310 ± 0.073*	0.542 ± 0.162*	4.759 ± 1.864*	−0.050 ± 0.071
1 and 2	0.015 ± 0.004*	−0.182 ± 0.078	−0.053 ± 0.175	−1.117 ± 2.009	0.108 ± 0.077
0 and 2	0.029 ± 0.005*	−0.492 ± 0.108*	0.596 ± 0.241*	3.642 ± 2.773	0.158 ± 0.107

Data are mean ± standard error The significance between groups is shown based on ANCOVA with adjustment for age. The differences are based on group0-group1, group1-group2 and group0-group2. * = $p < 0.05$. Group0 = control subjects, Group1 = mild OA subjects, Group2 = severe OA subjects. MFC = medial femoral condyle, LFC = lateral femoral condyle

in the trabecular bone were further aggravated. Moreover, the trabecular bone structure showed significant variations in the medial and lateral femoral condyles. Cartilage attrition mainly occurred in area that lower bone topological parameter (medial femoral condyle). In addition, our findings further confirmed that cartilage degeneration was accompanied by changes in the subchondral bone structure.

In mild OA, our findings showed that the BVF, SCR, and trabecular thickness significantly decreased and the EI significantly increased, indicating subchondral bone quality deterioration. These results were consistent with those of prior animal OA studies that showed subchondral bone plate thinning, increased porosity and BVF loss in early OA [21, 22]. In contrast, cartilage thickness loss was not significant, indicating that deterioration of the trabecular bone structure may more easily reveal early OA. Moreover, our finding was also similar to that of Chang G et al. reported using 7 T MRI. Although the spatial resolution of 3T MRI was limited, we came to consistent conclusions relative to trabecular structure changes in mild OA. In addition, in our study, sample size and disease stages increased, sagittal imaging was performed to evaluate subchondral bone and cartilage simultaneously. Increasing evidences showed that weaker subchondral bone quality alters stress-distributing and load-absorbing on cartilage, causing physical damage to the cartilage. In turn, cartilage loss also increases biomechanical loading on the subchondral bone plate and promotes subchondral bone remodeling [23, 24].

In severe OA, the BVF further decreased in both femoral condyles, which was inconsistent with previous studies that noted bone sclerosis with an increased BVF in advanced OA. These results may be due to subchondral bone cyst formation and disuse atrophy in both femoral condyles. Subchondral cysts represent a process of osteoclast-mediated bone resorption, showing decreased trabecular bone mineralization with interruptions and holes [25]. In addition, in the end-stage of OA, deceased activity may also cause osteoporotic changes in the trabecular bone structure. However, compared with mild OA, the EI slightly increased and trabecular thickness was greater, which may indicate that trabecular resorption slowed down. These findings may be related to subchondral bone marrow

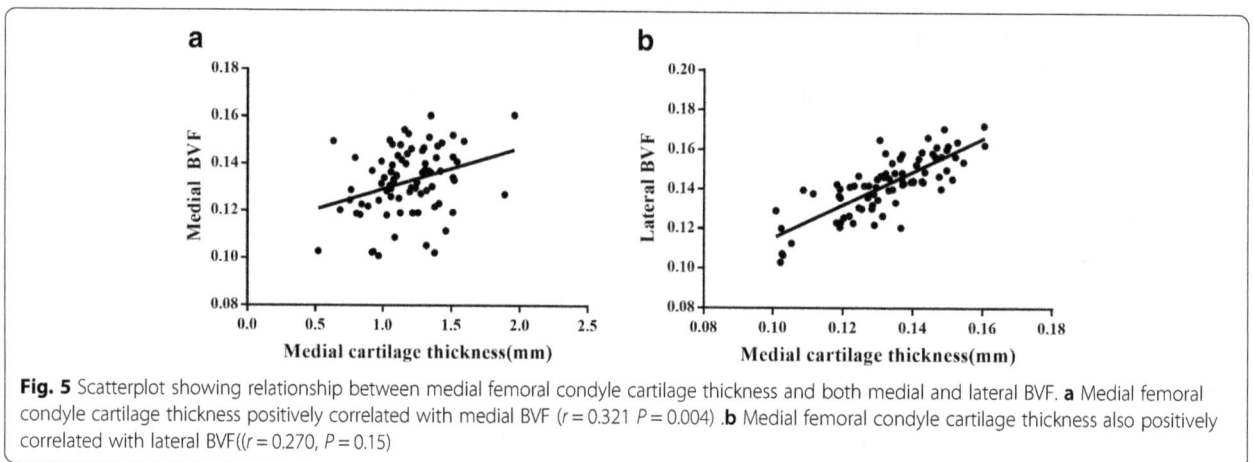

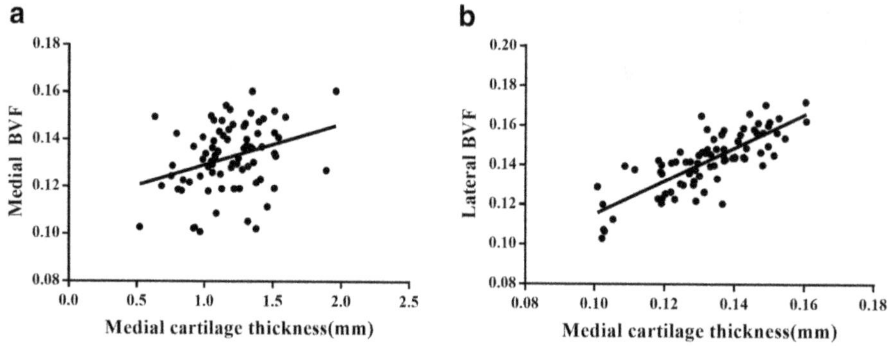

Fig. 5 Scatterplot showing relationship between medial femoral condyle cartilage thickness and both medial and lateral BVF. **a** Medial femoral condyle cartilage thickness positively correlated with medial BVF ($r = 0.321$ $P = 0.004$) .**b** Medial femoral condyle cartilage thickness also positively correlated with lateral BVF(($r = 0.270$, $P = 0.15$)

edema-like lesions (BMLs) and bone formation. Studies have shown that BMLs reflected increased bone remodeling that corresponded to trabecular bone microfractures and bone marrow fibrosis. BMLs showed higher BVF values, trabecular numbers, and thickness [26, 27]. In advanced OA, the subchondral bone microstructure was relatively heterogeneous and microscopic changes varied across the joint surface. These may partially account for this phenomenon. Using synchrotron radiation computed tomography imaging in end-stage OA, Chiba et al. also showed bone sclerosis and bone cysts mixed in the subchondral bone microstructure [25].

Moreover, our study found higher BVF, SCR and lower EI in the lateral femoral condyle when compared with the medial condyle from same group, which may be due to differences in anatomical structures and loading functions. On the sagittal plane, the lateral condyle had a wider loading surface and the loading force was more concentrated in the lateral condyle [12]. Wolff J also stated that subchondral bone remolding depends on the forces placed upon it [28]. Interestingly, cartilage attrition mainly occurred in areas that lower BVF and SCR (medial femoral condyle). This indicated cartilage degeneration was influenced by the remodeling of the underlying subchondral bone. In the future, the prevention of OA progression may be achieved through modifications of biomechanical loading and gait.

Furthermore, our findings further confirmed that medial cartilage degeneration was not accompanied by deterioration in the ipsilateral compartment but with loss in the opposite compartment. As the medial cartilage thickness loss, in the medial femoral condyle, BVF decreased, which may be due to a loading force shift from femur to tibia. Ding and Bobinac et al., using micro-CT reported BVF and trabecular thickness increased in the medial tibia and showed bone sclerosis in knee OA patients [29, 30]. In the lateral femoral condyle, BVF also decreased, which may be attributed to loading force from the lateral joint to the medial joint. Compared with BVF, correlations between other trabecular topological parameters and cartilage thickness loss were not found, which indicated BVF may be a more sensitive biomarker for evaluating OA severity. In the future, it may be used to monitor the efficacy of an osteoarthritis intervention.

In this study, we focused on a digital topological analysis, which has been validated and has shown its relative immunity to partial volume blurring and noise [31]. It has been used to quantify the architecture of human trabecular bone in MR images acquired from cadavers and in vivo [14, 32]. Our results further validated its availability and practicability.

There are several potential limitations in our study. First, lack of age-matched control groups was our primary limitation. Second, in our study, we acquired images in the sagittal direction to evaluate subchondral bone and cartilage simultaneously. This may have increased the partial volume effect in slice dimensions. Third, we conducted a cross-sectional study based on a relatively small number of subjects, so a potential selection bias or unknown confounding factors may be present. In the future, we will perform a longitudinal study of OA subjects to further investigate the temporal sequence of changes in the subchondral bone microstructure and cartilage. Finally, the image acquisition and data processing time was relatively long. Image processing and analysis algorithms should be further optimized.

Conclusions

In conclusion, the present results indicated that, with limited spatial resolution, 3T MRI coupled with image processing could simultaneously evaluate the three-dimensional trabecular bone microarchitecture and cartilage morphology in living patients with OA. In the mild OA subchondral bone microstructure was deteriorated in both femoral condyles, and as increased severity of OA, osteoporotic changes in the subchondral bone were further aggravated. In addition, medial cartilage thickness was positively correlated with both medial BVF and lateral BVF. These results indicated that MRI derived structure parameter could be a potential marker for evaluating OA severity. Overall, our results further confirmed the concept that poor subchondral bone quality was associated with OA, and may serve as a new potential therapeutic target in osteoarthritis. In the future, this technique could be used to monitor the efficacy of treatments targeting the subchondral bone tissue.

Abbreviations

BMI: Body mass index; BVF: Bone volume fraction; DTA: Digital topological analysis; EI: Erosion index; MRI: Magnetic resonance imaging; OA: Osteoarthritis; ROI: Region of interest; SCR: Trabecular plate-to-rod ratio

Acknowledgements

The manuscript had been edited by American Journal Experts.

Funding

This study was supported by Shanghai Scientific Research Plan Project (No. 16511101100, No. 16511101101), and the National Natural Science Foundation of China (No. 81771790).

Authors' contributions

Seven authors accomplished this publication. WY was communication of the paper and was in response of this study. This article was approved by all authors. All authors or institutions had no conflicts of interest. This article was not submitted to any other journal. CLL, LPS, and HS are responsible for data acquisition. XHR and CL performed data analysis. WY and QW are responsible for the conception and design of the study. CLL drafted the article, and revised it critically for important intellectual content. All authors have participated actively in carrying out and improving the study and all have approved the submission of this article.

Competing interests
The authors declare that they have no competing interest.

Author details
[1]Department of Radiology, Shanghai Jiao Tong University Affiliated Sixth People's Hospital, Shanghai, China. [2]Med-X Research Institute, School of Biomedical Engineering, Shanghai Jiao Tong University, Shanghai, China. [3]Department of Joint Surgery, Shanghai Jiao Tong University Affiliated Sixth People's Hospital, Shanghai, China.

References

1. Hunter DJ. Pharmacologic therapy for osteoarthritis–the era of disease modification. Nature reviews. Rheumatology. 2011;7(1):13–22.
2. Funck-Brentano T, Cohen-Solal M. Subchondral bone and osteoarthritis. Curr Opin Rheumatol. 2015;27(4):420–6.
3. Mohan G, Perilli E, Parkinson IH, Humphries JM, Fazzalari NL, Kuliwaba JS. Pre-emptive, early, and delayed alendronate treatment in a rat model of knee osteoarthritis: effect on subchondral trabecular bone microarchitecture and cartilage degradation of the tibia, bone/cartilage turnover, and joint discomfort. Osteoarthritis Cartilage. 2013;21(10):1595–604.
4. Zhen G, Wen C, Jia X, Li Y, Crane JL, Mears SC, Askin FB, Frassica FJ, Chang W, Yao J, Carrino JA, Cosgarea A, Artemov D, Chen Q, Zhao Z, Zhou X, et al. Inhibition of TGF-beta signaling in mesenchymal stem cells of subchondral bone attenuates osteoarthritis. Nat Med. 2013;19(6):704–12.
5. Roemer FW, Guermazi A, Javaid MK, Lynch JA, Niu J, Zhang Y, Felson DT, Lewis CE, Torner J, Nevitt MC. Change in MRI-detected subchondral bone marrow lesions is associated with cartilage loss: the MOST study. A longitudinal multicentre study of knee osteoarthritis. Ann Rheum Dis. 2009; 68(9):1461–5.
6. Zhang LZ, Zheng HA, Jiang Y, Tu YH, Jiang PH, Yang AL. Mechanical and biologic link between cartilage and subchondral bone in osteoarthritis. Arthritis Care Res (Hoboken). 2012;64(7):960–7.
7. Findlay DM, Atkins GJ. Osteoblast-chondrocyte interactions in osteoarthritis. Curr Osteoporos Rep. 2014;12(1):127–34.
8. Zhou X, von der Mark K, Henry S, Norton W, Adams H, de Crombrugghe B. Chondrocytes transdifferentiate into osteoblasts in endochondral bone during development, postnatal growth and fracture healing in mice. PLoS Genet. 2014;10(12):e1004820.
9. Karsdal MA, Bay-Jensen AC, Lories RJ, Abramson S, Spector T, Pastoureau P, Christiansen C, Attur M, Henriksen K, Goldring SR, Kraus V. The coupling of bone and cartilage turnover in osteoarthritis: opportunities for bone antiresorptives and anabolics as potential treatments? Ann Rheum Dis. 2014;73(2):336–48.
10. Pelletier JP, Roubille C, Raynauld JP, Abram F, Dorais M, Delorme P, Martel-Pelletier J. Disease-modifying effect of strontium ranelate in a subset of patients from the phase III knee osteoarthritis study SEKOIA using quantitative MRI: reduction in bone marrow lesions protects against cartilage loss. Ann Rheum Dis. 2015;74(2):422–9.
11. Bertuglia A, Lacourt M, Girard C, Beauchamp G, Richard H, Laverty S. Osteoclasts are recruited to the subchondral bone in naturally occurring post-traumatic equine carpal osteoarthritis and may contribute to cartilage degradation. Osteoarthritis Cartilage. 2016;24(3):555–66.
12. Beuf O, Ghosh S, Newitt DC, Link TM, Steinbach L, Ries M, Lane N, Majumdar S. Magnetic resonance imaging of normal and osteoarthritic trabecular bone structure in the human knee. Arthritis Rheum. 2002;46(2):385–93.
13. Chiba K, Uetani M, Kido Y, Ito M, Okazaki N, Taguchi K, Shindo H. Osteoporotic changes of subchondral trabecular bone in osteoarthritis of the knee: a 3-T MRI study. Osteoporos Int. 2012;23(2):589–97.
14. Chang G, Xia D, Chen C, Madelin G, Abramson SB, Babb JS, Saha PK, Regatte RR. 7T MRI detects deterioration in subchondral bone microarchitecture in subjects with mild knee osteoarthritis as compared with healthy controls. J Magn Reson Imaging. 2015;41(5):1311–7.
15. Zuo J, Bolbos R, Hammond K, Li X, Majumdar S. Reproducibility of the quantitative assessment of cartilage morphology and trabecular bone structure with magnetic resonance imaging at 7 T. Magn Reson Imaging. 2008;26(4):560–6.
16. Kellgren JH, Lawrence JS. Radiological assessment of osteo-arthrosis. Ann Rheum Dis. 1957;16(4):494–502.
17. Bellamy N, Buchanan WW, Goldsmith CH, Campbell J, Stitt LW. Validation study of WOMAC: a health status instrument for measuring clinically important patient relevant outcomes to antirheumatic drug therapy in patients with osteoarthritis of the hip or knee. J Rheumatol. 1988;15(12): 1833–40.
18. Vasilic B, Wehrli FWA. Novel local thresholding algorithm for trabecular bone volume fraction mapping in the limited spatial resolution regime of in vivo MRI. IEEE Trans Med Imaging. 2005;24(12):1574–85.
19. Gomberg BR, Saha PK, Song HK, Hwang SN, Wehrli FW. Topological analysis of trabecular bone MR images. IEEE Trans Med Imaging. 2000;19(3):166–74.
20. Saha PK, Wehrli FW. Measurement of trabecular bone thickness in the limited resolution regime of in vivo MRI by fuzzy distance transform. IEEE Trans Med Imaging. 2004;23(1):53–62.
21. Sniekers YH, Intema F, Lafeber FP, van Osch GJ, van Leeuwen JP, Weinans H, Mastbergen SCA. Role for subchondral bone changes in the process of osteoarthritis; a micro-CT study of two canine models. BMC Musculoskelet Disord. 2008;9:20.
22. Maerz T, Kurdziel M, Newton MD, Altman P, Anderson K, Matthew HW, Baker KC. Subchondral and epiphyseal bone remodeling following surgical transection and noninvasive rupture of the anterior cruciate ligament as models of post-traumatic osteoarthritis. Osteoarthritis Cartilage. 2016;24(4): 698–708.
23. Yuan XL, Meng HY, Wang YC, Peng J, Guo QY, Wang AY, Bone-cartilage LSB. Interface crosstalk in osteoarthritis: potential pathways and future therapeutic strategies. Osteoarthritis Cartilage. 2014;22(8):1077–89.
24. Burr DB, Gallant MA. Bone remodelling in osteoarthritis. Nature reviews. Rheumatology. 2012;8(11):665–73.
25. Chiba K, Nango N, Kubota S, Okazaki N, Taguchi K, Osaki M, Ito M. Relationship between microstructure and degree of mineralization in subchondral bone of osteoarthritis: a synchrotron radiation microCT study. J Bone Miner Res. 2012;27(7):1511–7.
26. Hunter DJ, Gerstenfeld L, Bishop G, Davis AD, Mason ZD, Einhorn TA, Maciewicz RA, Newham P, Foster M, Jackson S, Morgan EF. Bone marrow lesions from osteoarthritis knees are characterized by sclerotic bone that is less well mineralized. Arthritis Res Ther. 2009;11(1):R11.
27. Driban JB, Tassinari A, Lo GH, Price LL, Schneider E, Lynch JA, Eaton CB, McAlindon TE. Bone marrow lesions are associated with altered trabecular morphometry. Osteoarthritis Cartilage. 2012;20(12):1519–26.
28. Wolff J. The classic: on the significance of the architecture of the spongy substance for the question of bone growth: a preliminary publication. 1869. Clin Orthop Relat Res. 2011;469(11):3077–8.
29. Ding M, Odgaard A, Hvid I. Changes in the three-dimensional microstructure of human tibial cancellous bone in early osteoarthritis. J Bone Joint Surg Br. 2003;85(6):906–12.
30. Bobinac D, Spanjol J, Zoricic S, Maric I. Changes in articular cartilage and subchondral bone histomorphometry in osteoarthritic knee joints in humans. Bone. 2003;32(3):284–90.
31. Magland JF, Wehrli FW. Trabecular bone structure analysis in the limited spatial resolution regime of in vivo MRI. Acad Radiol. 2008;15(12):1482–93.
32. Gomberg BR, Saha PK, Wehrli FW. Topology-based orientation analysis of trabecular bone networks. Med Phys. 2003;30(2):158–68.

19

Quantifying bone marrow inflammatory edema in the spine and sacroiliac joints with thresholding

Ioanna Chronaiou[1*], Ruth S. Thomsen[2], Else M. Huuse[3], Leslie R. Euceda[1], Susanne J. Pedersen[4], Mari Hoff[2,5] and Beathe Sitter[1]

Abstract

Background: Psoriatic Arthritis (PsA) is a chronic inflammatory arthritis that develops in patients with psoriasis. Inflammatory edema in the spine may reflect subclinical disease activity and be a predictor of radiographic progression. A semi-quantitative method established by the spondyloarthritis research consortium of Canada (SPARCC) is commonly used to assess the disease activity in MR images of the spine. This study aims to evaluate thresholding for quantification of subtle bone marrow inflammation in the spine and the sacroiliac (SI) joints of patients with PsA and compare it with the SPARCC scoring system.

Methods: Short tau inversion recovery (STIR) MR images of the spine ($N = 85$) and the SI joints ($N = 95$) of patients with PsA ($N = 41$) were analyzed. A threshold was applied to visible bone marrow in order to mask areas with higher signal intensity, which are consistent with inflammation. These areas were considered as inflammatory lesions. The volume and relative signal intensity of the lesions were calculated. Results from thresholding were compared to SPARCC scores using linear mixed-effects models. The specificity and sensitivity of thresholding were also calculated.

Results: A significant positive correlation between the volumes and mean relative signal intensities, which were calculated by thresholding analysis, and the SPARCC scores was detected for both spine ($p < 0.001$) and SI joints ($p < 0.001$). For the spine, thresholding had sensitivity and specificity of 83% and 76% respectively, while for the SI joints the values were 51% and 88% respectively.

Conclusions: Thresholding allows quantification of subtle bone marrow inflammatory edema in patients with psoriatic arthritis, and could support SPARCC scoring of the spine. Improved image processing and inclusion of automatic segmentation are required for thresholding of STIR images to become a rapid and reliable method for quantitative measures of inflammation.

Trial registration: NCT02995460 (December 14, 2016) – Retrospectively registered.

Keywords: Psoriatic arthritis, MRI, Image processing, SPARCC, Bone marrow inflammatory edema

* Correspondence: ioanna.chronaiou@ntnu.no
[1]Department of Circulation and Medical Imaging, Faculty of Medicine and Health Sciences, NTNU – Norwegian University of Science and Technology, 7491 Trondheim, Norway, Trondheim, Norway
Full list of author information is available at the end of the article

Background

Psoriatic Arthritis (PsA) is a chronic inflammatory joint disease associated with psoriasis [1] that manifests with inflammation in peripheral joints, axial skeleton, enthesitis and dactylitis [2]. Magnetic resonance imaging (MRI) allows visualization of inflammation and damage in all structures involved in PsA [3] and has been found to be more sensitive to inflammatory changes than clinical examination [4]. The prevalence of PsA ranges from 20 to 420 per 100,000 population in all countries except Japan, where prevalence is lower [5].

The prevalence of axial PsA varies from 25% to 75% of PsA patients depending on the criteria used [6, 7]. In a subgroup of patients with axial PsA, there is subclinical inflammation in the absence of clinical symptoms. Detecting radiographic involvement of the spine and the sacroiliac (SI) joints in these patients is important for diagnosis and classification. Accurate quantification of small inflammatory lesions in the spine and SI joints is important as it may reflect subclinical disease activity [3] and be a predictor of radiographic progression [8, 9]. Additionally, an accurate method that can detect minor changes will be able to assess the effect of treatment or intervention. A semi-quantitative method established by the spondyloarthritis research consortium of Canada (SPARCC) can be used in order to assess the disease activity in MR images of the spine and SI joints. This scoring method is reliable and sensitive to changes [10], but it requires a trained reader and is labor-intensive. A computer-aided and potentially automatic method for the quantification of bone marrow inflammation is thus a possible time-efficient alternative.

Manual methods for image analysis rely on human vision, which is very sensitive, but are reader-dependent and prone to subjective errors and variation. Automatic methods offer advantages over manual methods of analysis. They are standardized and reproducible and have a consistent accuracy. Moreover, automatic methods follow a systematic approach, thus are highly repeatable. Once established, the procedure can easily be consistently applied in a large number of images, is objective and less time-consuming.

Thresholding has been used in a previous study to quantify inflammation in the SI joints of patients with chronic lower back pain originating in the SI joints [11]. Application of this approach is based on the fact that inflammatory lesions have higher signal intensity than normal bone marrow in short tau inversion recovery (STIR) images [11], which are typically used for imaging of bone marrow inflammation. The proposed method is potentially faster, easier and more robust than SPARCC and more importantly, eliminates the need of a trained reader. Another advantage of thresholding compared to SPARCC is that the former uses all images in the image set, while in the latter only a selection of slices is scored. Altogether, thresholding could be an alternative to SPARCC for quantification of subtle bone marrow inflammation in the spine and SI joints of patients with psoriatic arthritis. However, the validity of thresholding in this setting has not yet been tested.

This study aims to validate thresholding as a method suitable for accurate quantification of subtle bone marrow inflammation in patients with PsA and compare it with the SPARCC scoring system.

Methods

Patients

Patients diagnosed with PsA ($N = 43$) were recruited to the study, all being under optimal treatment at the time. Eligible patients were participating in a randomized clinical trial with high intensity interval training as intervention. Trial participants fulfilled the CASPAR-criteria for PsA, were between 18 and 65 years old and were able to exercise. Exclusion criteria were unstable PsA, unstable ischemic vascular disease, severe pulmonary disease, pregnancy, breastfeeding and drug or alcohol addictions. Two patients were excluded due to conditions that could influence the MR image analysis, one due to incidental findings (lymphoma) and one due to anomaly in the SI joints. Thus, 13 men with a mean age of 48 years (range: 30–64 years) and 28 women with a mean age of 48 years (range: 23–65 years) were included ($N = 41$). All patients have signed informed consent and the Norwegian Regional Committee for Medical and Health Research Ethics has approved the study. Patients were randomized into a control and an intervention group as part of a separate study. Effects of intervention are out of the scope of this study. Clinical evaluation at baseline, patient global assessment [mean ± standard deviation (SD): 42 ± 23 mm], disease activity score of 28 joints (mean ± SD: 2.9 ± 1.1), Bath ankylosing spondylitis disease activity index (mean ± SD: 3.4 ± 1.8), quality of life questionnaire, and high-sensitivity C-reactive protein (*hs-CRP*, median: 4.2 mg/L, range: 0.1 to 28.7 mg/L) provided patient health status.

MRI

All patients underwent MRI examinations of the spine and the SI joints based on standardized protocols [12, 13]. Examinations were performed on two 1.5 T scanners (Scanner 1: Syngo MR B17 upgraded during the study to B19, Scanner 2: Syngo MR D13, Avanto, Siemens Healthcare, Germany). An inversion recovery based sequence (STIR) was used for the examination of the SI joints and the spine in two stations (Table 1). The protocol also included T1 and T2 weighted sequences for anatomical reference. American College of Radiology phantom tests were performed on both scanners as image

Table 1 Acquisition parameters

	Spine	SI joints
Orientation	Sagittal	Semi-coronal
TR (msec)	4250	3700
TE (msec)	51 (for lower spine) 52 (for upper spine)	52
TI (msec)	145	145
Slice thickness (mm)	4 (for lower spine) 3 (for upper spine)	4
Gap	10%	10%
Number of slices	Minimum of 16	15

TR time to recovery, *TE* time to echo, *TI* time to inversion

quality control [14]. The effect of using different MR scanners was assessed with statistical analysis.

Clinical evaluation and MRI of the spine and SI joints were performed at one ($N = 4$), two ($N = 20$) and three time-points ($N = 17$). A total of 95 scans of the spine and the SI joints were acquired. Ten image sets of the spine were excluded from the analysis due to human error during the acquisition that resulted in altered protocol and different image weighting. A total of 85 scans of the spine and 95 scans of the SI joints were thus included in image analyses.

Acquisition parameters of short-tau inversion recovery (STIR) sequence used for the examination of the spine and the SI joints. Orientation, time to recovery (TR), time to echo (TE), time to inversion (TI), slice thickness, gap and number of slices are presented in the table. Images of the spine we acquired in two stations (lower spine and upper spine).

SPARCC scoring

A rheumatologist (RST) trained for the SPARCC scoring methods, blindly scored the STIR images of the spine and the SI joints according to the SPARCC SI Joint and Spine Inflammation Indices [12, 13]. In short, for the spine, the six most abnormal disco-vertebral levels on the STIR sequence are selected. Three consecutive sagittal slices, that represent the most abnormal slices for each level, are chosen for scoring at that level. The total maximum SPARCC score is 108 for all six levels of the spine. In the SI joints, the six consecutive slices covering the cartilaginous part of the joints, which is the most relevant part of the SI joints when looking for inflammation, are scored. The total maximum SPARCC score is 72 for all six slices of SI joints. Cases with positive SPARCC scores were considered positive for the presence of bone marrow inflammatory edema, whereas cases with SPARCC score of 0 were considered negative.

For the spine, only a total SPARCC score per image set ($N = 85$) was provided, while for the SI joints both a total SPARCC score per image set ($N = 95$) and a SPARCC score for each chosen slice ($N = 570$) were available.

Thresholding

Image pre-processing

Histogram-matching [15] is a histogram-based intensity normalization method that transforms the histogram of an image so that it is a match to the histogram of a reference image. Histogram-matching was performed to ensure that all image sets had the same overall brightness. All spinal MR images were histogram-matched to one reference spinal image and all MR images from SI joints were histogram-matched to one reference SI joint image. The function imhistmatch in MATLAB (MathWorks, Natick, MA, USA) was used.

Segmentation of bone marrow

Bone marrow of the sacrum and the iliac bones in the SI joints and vertebral bone marrow in the spine, excluding vascular and neural structures, were manually outlined using 3D Slicer (MIT Artificial Intelligence Lab, USA).

Volume of STIR hyper-intensity

All data processing was performed in Matlab R2016b (The MathWorks Inc., Natick, MA, 2000) using in-house scripts.

A signal intensity threshold consistent with inflammation was calculated from a circular ROI (≥ 200 pixels) at a healthy vertebra in one slice of the spinal image series and at the center of the first sacral vertebra in one slice of the SI joint image series (Fig. 1a, c). The criterion for choosing the ROI placement was the absence of bone marrow inflammatory edema. The mean signal intensity in this ROI was used as reference normal bone marrow signal intensity. A threshold was defined as the sum of the mean signal intensity in the reference normal bone marrow ROI and a percentage of the SD of signal intensity in that ROI. A receiver operating characteristic (ROC) curve was used to define the optimal threshold for the spine (area under curve [AUC] = 0.81) and the SI joints (AUC = 0.70) (Fig. 2). For the spine, the optimal threshold was defined as the sum of the mean signal intensity in the reference normal bone marrow ROI and 4.15 times the SD of signal intensity in that ROI. For the SI joints, the optimal threshold was defined as the sum of the mean signal intensity in the reference normal bone marrow ROI and 2.64 times the SD of signal intensity in that ROI.

All pixels with higher signal intensity than the threshold, consistent with inflammation [11], were selected and further used for the calculation of the volume of STIR hyper-intensity ($volume_{hyper}$) in the vertebral bodies. All connected components (objects) in the resulting

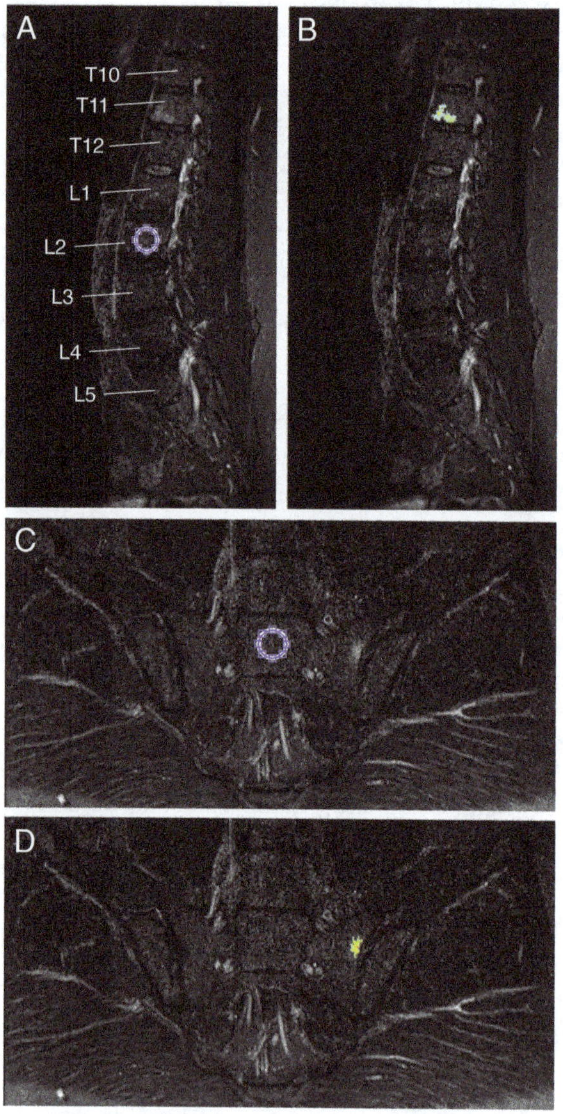

Fig. 1 Example of placement of circular region of interest (ROI, ≥ 200 pixels) at the erector spinae muscles in short-tau inversion recovery (STIR) MR images of the spine (**a**) and gluteus maximus muscle in STIR MR images of the SI joints (**c**) of psoriatic arthritis patients for the normalization to signal from muscle tissue. For the selection of reference normal bone marrow signal as part of thresholding analysis, a circular ROI (≥ 200 pixels) was placed at a healthy vertebra in one slice of spinal images (**a**) and at the center of the first sacral vertebra in one slice in sacroiliac joint images (**c**). Example of thresholding of the volume of short-tau inversion recovery (STIR) hyper-intensity in a STIR MR image of the spine (**b**) corresponding to (**a**), and of sacroiliac joints (**d**) corresponding to (**c**). Vertebrae T10-L5 can be seen in (**a**) and (**b**). Inflammation was detected in T12. Iliac bones and sacrum are visible in (**c**) and (**d**)

volumes that have fewer than 10 pixels were removed, as they were considered artefacts. $Volume_{hyper}$ was acquired by adding the volumes of all hyper-intense pixels. The number of objects per image set, which represent different lesions, was calculated.

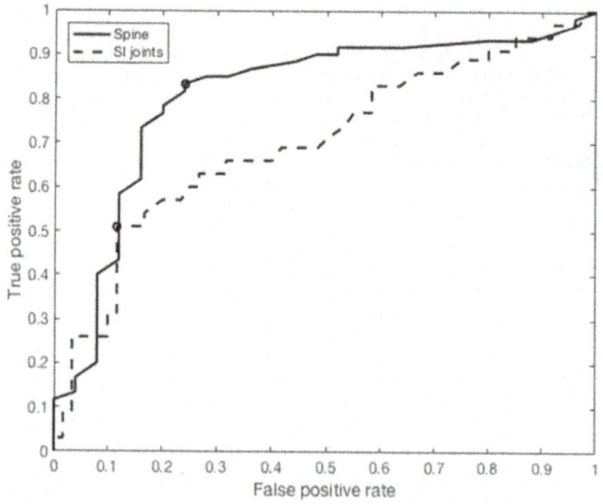

Fig. 2 A receiver operating characteristic curve for the spine (continuous line) and the sacroiliac joints (dashed line) was plotted in order to define the optimal thresholds (shown in circle)

Relative signal intensities of STIR hyper-intense pixels

All hyper-intense pixels were normalized to the mean signal intensity of normal bone marrow [11]. The relative signal intensities of STIR hyper-intense pixels ($S_{RelHyper}$) were calculated according to Eq. 1.

$$S_{RelHyper} = \left(S_{hyper} - \frac{\sum_{i=1}^{n} S_{bone,i}}{n} \right) / \frac{\sum_{i=1}^{n} S_{bone,i}}{n} \qquad (1)$$

where S_{hyper} is the signal intensity value of the respective hyper-intense pixel, S_{bone} is the signal intensity of the pixel included in the reference normal bone marrow ROI and n represents the number of pixels in the reference normal bone marrow ROI [11]. The mean ($S_{RelHyper,\ mean}$), the median ($S_{RelHyper,\ median}$), 75-percentile ($S_{RelHyper,\ 75perc}$) and 90-percentile ($S_{RelHyper,\ 90perc}$) of $S_{RelHyper}$ were calculated for all image sets.

Statistical analysis

Spearman's rank-order correlation between *SPARCC scores* and $volume_{hyper}$, $S_{RelHyper,\ mean}$, number of objects per image set and *hs-CRP* and was calculated in IBM SPSS Statistics (IBM SPSS Statistics for Macintosh, Version 22.0).

Linear mixed-effects models (LMM) [16] were built in R 3.1.1 using the function *lme* from the 'nlme' package [17] employing the method of restricted maximum likelihood. LMM incorporate two types of effects: fixed, which are systematic and controlled, and random, which encompass unsystematic differences not accounted for by the fixed effects, e.g. variation between patients. The fixed effects are essentially different explanatory variables or classification factors whose relationship with the response variable is evaluated simultaneously. LMM models were built for data from both spine and SI joints separately, including the categorical fixed effects of *intervention group* (intervention or control), *time of scan* (time-point 1, 2 or 3), and *MR scanner* (machine 1 or 2) (without interaction terms). The continuous fixed effect of *SPARCC score* was also included, while the random effect was the *patient number* and the response variables were $volume_{hyper}$, $S_{RelHyper,\ mean}$, $S_{RelHyper,\ median}$, $S_{RelHyper,\ 75perc}$, $S_{RelHyper,\ 90perc}$ or the number of objects per image set from thresholding. The latter were log10 transformed to comply with normality assumptions, confirmed by visual inspection of residual q-q plots and histograms.

We calculated sensitivity and specificity of thresholding compared to SPARCC from the proportion of patients identified with inflammatory lesions. Both for the spine ($N = 85$) and the SI joints ($N = 95$), the calculations were performed per image set including all the slices in each image set. In addition, for the SI joints, the calculations were performed per image set including only the six slices that were chosen for the SPARCC scoring method ($N = 95$) and per slice for the slices that were chosen for the SPARCC scoring method ($N = 570$).

Results

SPARCC

For the 85 image sets covering the spine, 60 were positive for inflammation using the SPARCC scoring method. For the 95 image sets covering the SI joints, 35 had a positive SPARCC score. Overall, 84 out of 570 slices of the SI joints were given a positive SPARCC score.

For the image sets with positive SPARCC scores, the mean score was 10.5 for the spine and 4.3 for the SI joints. Including all image sets, with positive or zero SPARCC scores, the mean SPARCC score for the spine was 7.4 ranging from 0 to 51 out of maximum possible score 108. The mean SPARCC score for the SI joints is 1.6, ranging from 0 to 17, out of a maximum possible score of 72.

Thresholding

Thresholding revealed inflammatory lesions in 56 out of 85 image sets of the spine and 25 out of 95 image sets of the SI joints. In the analysis of SI joints, when including only the six slices that were chosen with the SPARCC method, 25 out of 95 image sets were found positive for the presence of inflammatory lesions. In total, 92 out of 570 slices of the SI joints showed inflammation when analyzed using thresholding.

For the image sets that had inflammatory lesions, mean $volume_{hyper}$ was 2.92 cm^3 and 2.77 cm^3 for the spine and the SI joints, respectively. Including all image sets, with or without inflammatory lesions, mean $volume_{hyper}$ was 1.92 cm^3, ranging from 0 to 17.86 cm^3, in the spine and 0.73 cm^3, ranging from 0 to 19.04 cm^3, in the SI joints.

The mean and the range of $volume_{hyper}$, $S_{RelHyper,\ mean}$, $S_{RelHyper,\ median}$, $S_{RelHyper,\ 75perc}$ and $S_{RelHyper,\ 90perc}$ for the spine and the SI joints using all the slices are presented in Table 2. Examples of thresholding of the volume of STIR hyper-intensity in the SI joints and the spine are presented in Fig. 1.

Volume of short-tau inversion recovery (STIR) hyper-intense pixels ($volume_{hyper}$) and measures of lesion relative signal intensities; mean ($S_{RelHyper,\ mean}$), median ($S_{RelHyper,\ median}$), 75-percentile ($S_{RelHyper,\ 75perc}$) and 90-percentile ($S_{RelHyper,\ 90perc}$) of the relative signal intensities of STIR hyper-intense pixels for the spine and the SI joints calculated by thresholding. All values are given with standard deviations and parameter range in brackets.

Statistics

Spearman's rank-order correlation analysis revealed a significant positive correlation between SPARCC score and $volume_{hyper}$ both for the spine (correlation coefficient: 0.74, $p < 0.001$) and the SI joints (correlation coefficient: 0.52, $p < 0.001$). SPARCC score did not correlate significantly with *hs-CRP*. Correlation coefficients calculated by Spearman's rank-order correlation analysis are presented in Table 3.

Results from multilevel LMMs to simultaneously assess the relationship between $volume_{hyper}$, $S_{RelHyper,\ mean}$, $S_{RelHyper,\ median}$, $S_{RelHyper,\ 75perc}$, $S_{RelHyper,\ 90perc}$ or the number of objects per image set and the fixed effects of SPARCC score, intervention group, time of scan and MR scanner are summarized in Table 4. A significant positive correlation between $volume_{hyper}$ and SPARCC score was detected for spine (coefficient ± standard error: 0.11 ± 0.02, $p < 0.001$,) and SI joints (coefficient ± standard error: 0.31 ± 0.05, $p < 0.001$). The *intervention group*, *time of scan* (not shown) and the *MR scanner* were determined to not have a significant effect on the measurements by the thresholding method.

Table 2 Volume of short-tau inversion recovery hyper-intense pixels and measures of lesion relative signal intensities

	Spine ($N = 58$)	SI joints ($N = 36$)
$volume_{hyper}$ (cm^3)	2.92 ± 3.86 (0.04–17.86)	2.77 ± 4.18 (0.03–19.04)
$S_{RelHyper,\ mean}$	1.69 ± 0.12 (1.41–2.01)	0.66 ± 0.13 (0.45–0.92)
$S_{RelHyper,\ median}$	1.72 ± 0.23 (1.31–2.26)	0.63 ± 0.23 (0.38–1.07)
$S_{RelHyper,\ 75perc}$	2.09 ± 0.16 (1.79–2.26)	0.83 ± 0.23 (0.47–1.07)
$S_{RelHyper,\ 90perc}$	2.24 ± 0.04 (2.05–2.26)	1.00 ± 0.14 (0.57–1.07)

STIR short-tau inversion recovery, *SI* sacroiliac, $volume_{hyper}$ volume of STIR hyper-intensity, $S_{RelHyper}$ relative signal intensities of STIR hyper-intense pixels, *75perc* 75-percentile, *90perc* 95-percentile

Table 3 Spearman's rank-order correlation

	SPARCC score			
	Spine		SI joints	
	Coefficient	*p*-value	Coefficient	*p*-value
$volume_{hyper}$	0.74	< 0.001	0.52	< 0.001
$S_{RelHyper,\ mean}$	0.67	< 0.001	0.47	< 0.001
Number of lesions	0.72	< 0.001	0.52	< 0.001
hs-CRP	−0.14	0.215	0.091	0.380

SI sacroiliac, *SPARCC* spondyloarthritis research consortium of Canada, *STIR* short-tau inversion recovery, $volume_{hyper}$ volume of STIR hyper-intensity, $S_{RelHyper}$ relative signal intensities of STIR hyper-intense pixels, *hs-CRP* high-sensitivity C-reactive protein

The two methods, SPARCC and thresholding, agreed on the absence of inflammatory activity in 19 out of 85 image sets of the spine, resulting in a sensitivity of 83% and a specificity of 76%. For the SI joints, the agreement was for 53 out of 95 image sets, resulting in a sensitivity of 51% and a specificity of 88%. When comparing the scores of each slice from the whole image set of SI joints, the two methods agreed on 434 slices out of 570 showing no inflammation, resulting in a sensitivity of 48% and a specificity of 89%.

Spearman's rank-order correlation coefficients and *p*-values for the relationship of thresholding-derived metrics (volume, number of lesions and high-sensitivity C-reactive protein to spondyloarthritis research consortium of Canada.

Linear mixed-effects model (LMM) coefficients and *p*-values for the relationship of thresholding-derived metrics and number of lesions to spondyloarthritis research consortium of Canada (SPARCC) scores and MR scanner (scanner 1 or 2). The coefficients indicate how much $volume_{hyper}$, $S_{RelHyper,\ mean}$, $S_{RelHyper,\ median}$, $S_{RelHyper,\ 75perc}$ and number of lesions increase (positive coefficient) or decrease (negative coefficient) for every unit increase in the SPARCC score.

Discussion

This study evaluates thresholding as a computer-aided method for quantification of subtle bone marrow inflammation in the spine and SI joints of PsA patients. Thresholding-derived metrics ($volume_{hyper}$, $S_{RelHyper,\ mean}$, $S_{RelHyper,\ median}$, $S_{RelHyper,\ 75perc}$, $S_{RelHyper,\ 90perc}$ and number of objects per image set) correlate significantly with SPARCC scores both for the spine and the SI joints. However, the agreement on absence or presence of inflammation between the two methods was higher for the spine than for the SI joints, indicating that the proposed method of analysis performs better in the former. All metrics (mean, median, 75th-percentile and 90th-percentile) for the relative signal intensity of the hyper--intense lesions correlate with the same level of significance with the SPARCC scores. We therefore suggest that the $S_{RelHyper,\ mean}$ can be used as a standard metric for relative signal hyper-intensity of inflammatory lesions.

To validate the use of the proposed method, we compared thresholding data to SPARCC scores for 85 image sets of the spine and 95 image sets of the SI joints from 41 PsA patients. In addition, for the 570 slices from SI joints, a slice-by-slice comparison was performed on results from the two methods. There was some disagreement between the two methods. The lesions that thresholding failed to detect in the spine ($N = 10$) had a mean SPARCC score of 3.8, while correctly identified lesions ($N = 50$) had a mean SPARCC score of 11.8. The disagreement was bigger for the SI joints, where lesions that thresholding failed to detect ($N = 17$) had a mean SPARCC score of 2.5, while correctly identified lesions ($N = 18$) had a mean SPARCC score of 5.9. Sensitivity and specificity measures show that thresholding analysis is more accurate in the spine. Spearman's rank-order correlation analysis confirms higher correlation for the spine than the SI joints. Patients included in this study had little to no inflammation, especially in the SI joints, which may suggest that the method performs better in areas with higher inflammatory activity. Additionally, the examined anatomical structures in the spine are in the homogeneous image center of all slices, whereas the examined anatomical structures of the SI joints are more

Table 4 Results from linear mixed-effects model

	Spine			SI joints		
	SPARCC score		MR scanner	SPARCC score		MR scanner
	Coefficient	*p*-value	*p*-value	Coefficient	*p*-value	*p*-value
$volume_{hyper}$	0.11	< 0.001	0.467	0.31	< 0.001	0.804
$S_{RelHyper,\ mean}$	0.09	0.001	0.347	0.25	< 0.001	0.597
$S_{RelHyper,\ median}$	0.09	0.001	0.348	0.25	< 0.001	0.596
$S_{RelHyper,\ 75perc}$	0.09	0.001	0.338	0.26	< 0.001	0.560
$S_{RelHyper,\ 90perc}$	0.09	0.001	0.348	0.26	< 0.001	0.590
Number of lesions	0.13	< 0.001	0.424	0.37	< 0.001	0.672

SI sacroiliac, *SPARCC* spondyloarthritis research consortium of Canada, *STIR* short-tau inversion recovery, $volume_{hyper}$ volume of STIR hyper-intensity, $S_{RelHyper}$ relative signal intensities of STIR hyper-intense pixels, *75perc* 75-percentile, *90perc* 95-percentile

distant from the homogeneous image center, and also in varying distance through slices. This may affect the homogeneity of the acquired image. Areas that are closer to the coil appear more hyper-intense, resulting in slightly different signal intensities through an image. This issue could have been resolved using appropriate pre-processing. Anatomical differences may also contribute to lower lesion detectability in the SI joints. Additional pre-processing of the SI joint images could be used to correct for the inhomogeneities and signal intensity differences and improve the performance of thresholding in the SI joints.

Examinations were acquired using two MR scanners with different software platforms over the course of a year. During that time, one of the scanners underwent software upgrade. This should have no effect in the results of this study, and LMM also showed that different MR scanners used for imaging did not affect the measurements by the thresholding method.

The thresholding method presented here was first introduced in a previous study [11], where it was used to measure inflammatory changes in the SI joints of patients with lower back pain. However, in that study, the method was not compared to any clinical evaluation score and its validity was not tested. Additionally, the method was not tested for different threshold values to justify for the specific choice of threshold. In our study, the method is also applied in the spine.

One limitation of the thresholding method is that the ROIs of the bone marrow in the spine and the SI joints of the patients were drawn manually, in order to accurately exclude neural structures and blood vessels, but include possible inflammatory lesions. This presupposes a basic knowledge of the anatomy of SI joints. Fully automated methods for the selection of the sacrum and iliac bone ROIs should be explored. A fully automated method for the localization and segmentation of the vertebral units has been used in a previous study as part of a semi-automated framework for comparative visualization of inflammatory bone marrow lesions in MR images of the spine [18]. Combining fully automated segmentation of the spine and thresholding in such a setting could potentially assist in assessing radiological progression of patients with inflammatory lesions in the spine. Time required for SPARCC scoring depends on the experience of the reader, but also on how many lesions a patient has. A trained reader will need approximately 10 min for a patient without lesions and 30–40 min for a patient with many lesions. Time required for manual segmentation of bone marrow of a single image set is approximately 10 min. However, a fully automated segmentation of inflammation will reduce the reading time significantly and make thresholding a quantitative method feasible in the clinic.

A disadvantage of intensity-based methods for image analysis, such as thresholding, is that these methods are not able to differentiate between different pathologies that lead to increased signal intensities in the images, which is something a trained human can do easily. However, SPARCC scoring is used in patients who already have a diagnosis with a pre-investigative probability of having inflammation due to the primary diagnosis (psoriatic arthritis, spondyloarthritis, ankylosing spondylitis). Other approaches, including textural analysis, may be more beneficial in this instance. Another limitation of this study is the absence of a control group.

Overall, automatic thresholding is a novel method which performs relatively well at detecting inflammatory lesions in the spine of PsA patients, but more poorly in the SI joints. In addition to the presence or absence of inflammation, it provides volumetric information and allows localization of the lesions. The implementation of the method is generic enough to allow for application in the quantification of bone marrow inflammation in other types of spondyloarthritis. Fully automated implementation of the thresholding method should be explored.

Conclusion

Thresholding allows quantification of subtle bone marrow inflammation in PsA patients with low SPARCC scores for inflammatory activity. The significant correlation for low inflammatory scores suggests that this method can provide reliable and sensitive quantitative measures for the presence of subtle inflammation in bone marrow. With further studies, automatic segmentation and technique optimization, it is possible that automatic thresholding may eventually be an alternative or supplement to SPARCC scoring.

Abbreviations

75perc: 75-percentile; 90perc: 95-percentile; AUC: Area under curve; *hs-CRP*: High-sensitivity C-reactive protein; LMM: Linear mixed-effects models; MRI: Magnetic resonance imaging; PsA: Psoriatic arthritis; ROC: Receiver operating characteristic; ROI: Region of interest; S_{bone}: Signal intensity of pixel included in reference normal bone marrow ROI; SD: Standard deviation; S_{hyper}: Signal intensity value of hyper-intense pixel; SI: Sacroiliac; SPARCC: Spondyloarthritis research consortium of Canada; $S_{RelHyper}$: Relative signal intensities of STIR hyper-intense pixels; STIR: Short tau inversion recovery; $volume_{hyper}$: Volume of STIR hyper-intensity

Acknowledgements

Not applicable

Funding

This study was funded by Sør-Trøndelag University college (HiST) / Norwegian University of Science and Technology (NTNU). The funding body had no involvement in the conduct of the research and preparation of the article.

Authors' contributions
IC, RST, EMH, MH and BS made substantial contributions to conception and design of the study. RST, SJP, LRE and IC acquired and analysed the data. All authors were involved in the interpretation of the data. IC, LRE and RST drafted the manuscript. All authors were involved in revising the manuscript. All authors gave final approval of the version to be published and agreed to be accountable for all aspects of the work in ensuring that questions related to the accuracy or integrity of any part of the work are appropriately investigated and resolved.

Competing interests
The authors declare that they have no competing interests.

Author details
[1]Department of Circulation and Medical Imaging, Faculty of Medicine and Health Sciences, NTNU – Norwegian University of Science and Technology, 7491 Trondheim, Norway, Trondheim, Norway. [2]Department of Public Health and Nursing, Faculty of Medicine and Health Sciences, NTNU – Norwegian University of Science and Technology, Trondheim, Norway. [3]Department of Radiology and Nuclear Medicine, St Olav's Hospital, University Hospital in Trondheim, Trondheim, Norway. [4]Copenhagen Center for Arthritis Research, Center for Rheumatology and Spine Diseases, Rigshospitalet - Glostrup, Copenhagen, Denmark. [5]Department of Rheumatology, St Olav's Hospital, University Hospital in Trondheim, Trondheim, Norway.

References
1. Kalkan G, Karadag AS. Psoriatic arthritis epidemiology. East J Med. 2014;19(1):1–7.
2. Østergaard M, Glinatsi D, Pedersen SJ, Sørensen IJ. Utility in clinical trials of magnetic resonance imaging for psoriatic arthritis: a report from the GRAPPA 2014 annual meeting. J Rheumatol. 2015;42(6):1044–7.
3. Poggenborg R, Sørensen I, Pedersen S, Østergaard M. Magnetic resonance imaging for diagnosing, monitoring and prognostication in psoriatic arthritis. Clin Exp Rheumatol. 2015;33(5 Suppl 93):66.
4. Wiell C, Szkudlarek M, Hasselquist M, Møller JM, Vestergaard A, Nørregaard J, Terslev L, Østergaard M. Ultrasonography, magnetic resonance imaging, radiography, and clinical assessment of inflammatory and destructive changes in fingers and toes of patients with psoriatic arthritis. Arthritis Res Ther. 2007;9(6):R119.
5. Dhir V, Aggarwal A. Psoriatic arthritis: a critical review. Clin Rev Allerg Immu. 2013;44(2):141–8.
6. Baraliakos X, Coates LC, Braun J. The involvement of the spine in psoriatic arthritis. Clin Exp Rheumatol. 2015;33(5 Suppl 93):S31–5.
7. Gladman DD. Axial disease in psoriatic arthritis. Curr Rheumatol Rep. 2007;9(6):455–60.
8. Savnik A, Malmskov H, Thomsen HS, Graff LB, Nielsen H, Danneskiold-Samsøe B, Boesen J, Bliddal H. MRI of the wrist and finger joints in inflammatory joint diseases at 1-year interval: MRI features to predict bone erosions. Eur Radiol. 2002;12(5):1203–10.
9. Bond SJ, Farewell VT, Schentag CT, Gladman DD. Predictors for radiological damage in psoriatic arthritis: results from a single centre. Ann Rheum Dis. 2007;66(3):370–6.
10. LandewÉ RB, Hermann K-GA, van der Heijde DM, Baraliakos X, Jurik A-G, Lambert RG, Østergaard M, Rudwaleit M, Salonen DC, Braun J. Scoring sacroiliac joints by magnetic resonance imaging. A multiple-reader reliability experiment. J Rheumatol. 2005;32(10):2050–5.
11. Fritz J, Henes JC, Thomas C, Clasen S, Fenchel M, Claussen CD, Lewin JS, Pereira PL. Diagnostic and interventional MRI of the sacroiliac joints using a 1.5-T open-bore magnet: a one-stop-shopping approach. AJR Am J Roentgenol. 2008;191(6):1717–24.
12. Maksymowych WP, Inman RD, Salonen D, Dhillon SS, Krishnananthan R, Stone M, Conner-Spady B, Palsat J, Lambert RG. Spondyloarthritis research consortium of Canada magnetic resonance imaging index for assessment of spinal inflammation in ankylosing spondylitis. Arthritis Care Res. 2005;53(4):502–9.
13. Maksymowych WP, Inman RD, Salonen D, Dhillon SS, Williams M, Stone M, Conner-spady B, Palsat J, Lambert RG. Spondyloarthritis research consortium of Canada magnetic resonance imaging index for assessment of sacroiliac joint inflammation in ankylosing spondylitis. Arthritis Care Res. 2005;53(5):703–9.
14. Chen C-C, Wan Y-L, Wai Y-Y, Liu H-L. Quality Assurance of Clinical MRI scanners using ACR MRI phantom: preliminary results. J Digit Imaging. 2004;17(4):279–84.
15. Manjón JV. MRI preprocessing. In: Martí-Bonmatí L, Alberich-Bayarri A, editors. Imaging biomarkers: development and clinical integration. Switzerland: Springer International Publishing; 2017. p. 53–63.
16. Pinheiro J, Bates D. Linear mixed-effects models: basic concepts and examples. Mixed-effects models in S and S-PLUS. New York, NY, USA. New York: Springer; 2000.
17. Pinheiro J, Bates D, DebRoy S, Sarkar D, R Core Team: Nlme: linear and nonlinear mixed effects models. R package version 3.1–117. 2014.
18. Griffith JF, Wang D, Shi L, Yeung DK, Lee R, Shan TL. Computer-aided assessment of spinal inflammation on magnetic resonance images in patients with Spondyloarthritis. Arthritis Rheumatol. 2015;67(7):1789–97.

20

Expression of adiponectin in the subchondral bone of lumbar facet joints with different degrees of degeneration

Qi Lai[1,2†], Yuan Liu[1,2†], Leitao Huang[1,2†], Xuqiang Liu[1,2], Xionglong Yu[1,2], Qiang Wang[1,2], Runsheng Guo[1,2], Jianghao Zhu[1,2], Hanxiong Cheng[1,2], Min Dai[1,2*] and Bin Zhang[1,2*]

Abstract

Background: Osteoarthritis research has been most commonly performed in the setting of the articular cartilage of the knee. To the best of our knowledge, no studies have evaluated the role of adiponectin in osteoarthritis of the lumbar facet joint (FJOA). Therefore, in this study, we explored whether adiponectin was expressed in the lumbar facet joints and evaluated the role of adiponectin in FJOA.

Methods: We enrolled patients who underwent lumbar computed tomography (CT) and magnetic resonance imaging (MRI) at the Orthopedic Department of the First Affiliated Hospital of Nanchang from May 2015 to June 2016. Lumbar facet joints were obtained from 135 patients at the time of lumbar fusion surgery and divided into three groups according to the Weishaupt grade. Cytokine levels in the subchondral bones were evaluated by enzyme-linked immunosorbent assays (ELISAs), and adiponectin levels were determined by immunohistochemistry, western blotting, and quantitative polymerase chain reaction (qPCR).

Results: By ELISA, adiponectin levels were examined in the subchondral bone for lumbar facet joint, and adiponectin was found to be negatively correlated with BMI in 52 patients ($p < 0.001$, $r = -0.861$). By immunohistochemistry analysis, adiponectin was found to be expressed in the subchondral bone of the lumbar facet, whereas the cartilage area was negative for adiponectin expression. Immunostaining intensity and area was related to the degeneration of the lumbar facet joint, and, in our research, considerably decreased staining intensity and area were observed in more severely degenerated lumbar facet joints. Furthermore, the expression of adiponectin was also reduced in degenerated lumbar facet joints, and the level of decline corresponded to degeneration detected by western blotting and qPCR analysis ($n = 27$, $p < 0.0001$).

Conclusions: Adiponectin expression was observed in the subchondral bone of the lumbar facet joint and decreased as the degree of degeneration increased. Thus, the results of this study provide new insights into the relationship between adiponectin and osteoarthritis.

Keywords: Adiponectin, Facet joint, Osteoarthritis, Subchondral bone, Cartilage, Bone degeneration

* Correspondence: 15879177108@163.com; acker11@126.com
†Equal contributors
[1]Department of Orthopedics, The First Affiliated Hospital of Nanchang University, 17 Yongwai Street, Nangchang, Jiangxi 330006, China
Full list of author information is available at the end of the article

Background

Lumbar facet joint osteoarthritis (FJOA) is present in approximately 40% of patients with low back pain [1–3]. Therefore, in addition to studies on disc degeneration, studies of FJOA are essential for the prevention of low back pain. The lumbar facet joint is a synovial joint composed of cartilage, synovium, and an articular capsule, and its characteristics are similar to those of other synovial joints, such as the knee [4–6]. However, most studies of osteoarthritis (OA) have focused on the knee joint [7–10]. Some studies have shown that knee OA may be a disease of the entire joint, including articular cartilage, subchondral bone, meniscus, ligament, and neuromuscular groups [11, 12]. Moreover, the subchondral bone plays a major role in knee joint degeneration. However, few studies have evaluated lumbar facet OA or the subchondral bone by basic research, with scholars instead focusing more on clinical research areas [13, 14].

In 2015, we reported a predictive experiment involving cytokine screening in five cases of lumbar facet joint specimens by RayBio® Human Inflammation Antibody Array G3. The screening results showed that interleukin (IL)-1β, TNF α and β, leptin, adiponectin, Chemokine (CCL)-11, CCL-24, colony stimulating factor (CSF)-2, CSF-3, intercellular adhesion molecule (ICAM-1), interferon (IFNg), IL-1–16, monocyte chemotactic protein (MCP), macrophage inflammatory protein (MIP), and others were detected in five cases of lumbar facet joint specimens. The authors discovered that adiponectin showed a strong positive reaction and high expression. Adiponectin is a cytokine secreted by adipose tissue [15, 16] and is abundantly expressed in the circulation in three different molecular forms: trimer, hexamer, and high-molecular-weight (HMW) species [17]. Early studies have suggested that adiponectin plays a key role in the control of energy homeostasis because its plasma levels are inversely correlated with body mass index (BMI), intra-abdominal fat, and indices of insulin resistance [18, 19]. Therefore, adiponectin may be inversely correlated with OA because BMI is a risk factor of OA. In addition, Berner et al. [20] discovered that adiponectin and its receptors are expressed in bone-forming cells in mice and that adiponectin may affect bone metabolism. Moreover, Berner et al. [20] suggest that fatty acids have a regulatory effect on adiponectin mRNA expression, and fatty acids provide increased energy supply to cells and enhance adiponectin expression in osteoblasts. Coincidentally, Francin and Presle et al. [21] reported that the elevated level of adiponectin found in chondrocytes from patients with knee OA might contribute to matrix remodelling during OA; notably, the regulation of bone metabolism by adipokines is largely unknown, and the observed expression and secretion of adiponectin by bone-forming cells serves to add more complexity, as well as redundancy, to this intriguing issue. Therefore, the specific role of adiponectin in FJOA is still unclear and controversial.

Accordingly, in this study, we aimed to evaluate whether adiponectin was expressed in the subchondral bone of lumbar facet joints and to explore the role of adiponectin in FJOA.

Methods

Clinical samples and data

Subchondral bone was obtained from the lumbar facet joints of 135 patients (median age: 51.38 years; range: 16–77 years) at the time of lumbar fusion surgery. Additionally, BMI data of 60 of the patients (BMI: 19.4–33.8 kg/m^2; mean 23.85 kg/m^2),which were part of the 135 patients, were collected to examine the release of adiponectin from the subchondral bone of the lumbar facet joint in relation to BMI. Thirty-two normal facet joint specimens were obtained from L3-L5 vertebral fracture decompression or fusion surgeries, and 103 degenerative samples were obtained from L3-S1 single segment lumbar disc herniation fusion surgeries (60 for ELISAs, 48 for immunohistochemical analysis, and 27 for qPCR and western blotting). Samples were stored at −80 °C after surgery until use. All samples were obtained from the Orthopedic Department of the First Affiliated Hospital of Nanchang University from May 2015 to June 2016. All lumbar facet joints were grouped according to the Weishaupt [22] grade, as determined by computed tomography (CT) and magnetic resonance imaging (MRI), as follows: 0, normal; 1, slight degeneration; 2, moderate degeneration; 3, severe degeneration (Fig 1). Lumbar facet joints were divided into three groups (normal group [NG]: grade 0; degeneration group [DG]: grades 1 or 2; severe degeneration group [SDG]: grade 3) according to computed tomography (CT) and magnetic resonance imaging (MRI) results based on Weishaupt grading because of subjective interference in grades 1 and 2 [23].

Inclusion criteria were as follows: L3-L5 vertebral burst fracture or L3-S1 lumbar disc and facet joint degeneration; no history of spinal surgery; underwent lumbar CT and MRI examination. The exclusion criteria were as follows: lumbar spondylolisthesis, scoliosis, lumbar spine infection, spinal tumors and other spine-related diseases; diabetes, hypertension, and other relevant medical history; history of smoking or alcoholism; psychological disorders, mental disorders, or drug use and other history. The study protocol was approved by the Institutional Review Board of the First Affiliated Hospital of Nanchang University, and written informed consent was obtained from all study participants.

Screening of chemical factors by ELISA

Lumbar facet joint samples were obtained from 60 patients (NG, n = 11; DG, n = 34; SDG, n = 15; BMI:

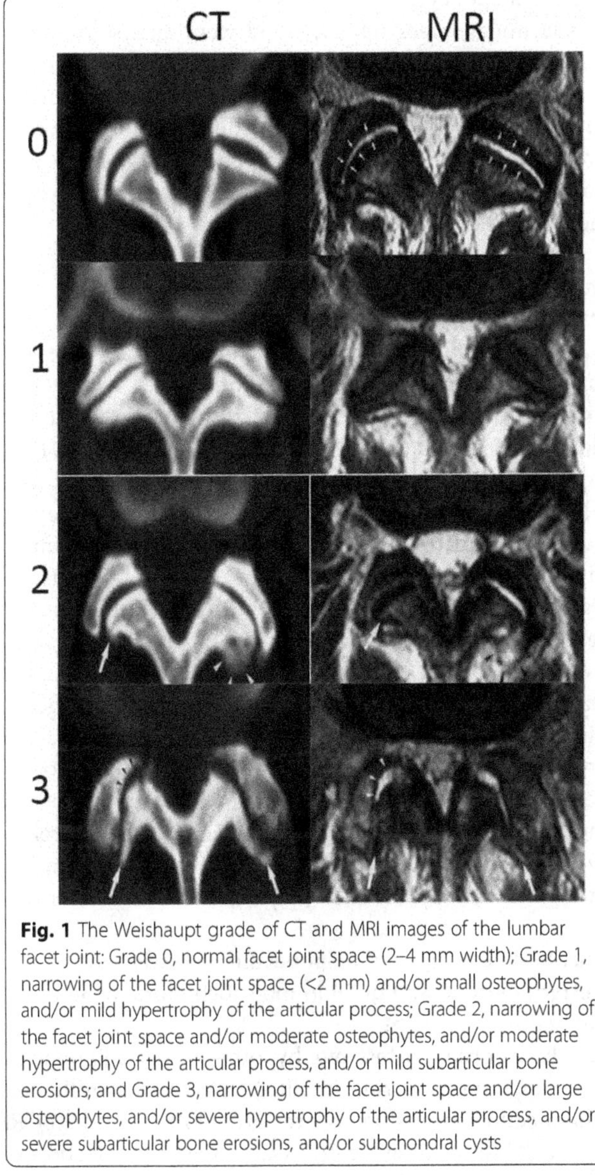

Fig. 1 The Weishaupt grade of CT and MRI images of the lumbar facet joint: Grade 0, normal facet joint space (2–4 mm width); Grade 1, narrowing of the facet joint space (<2 mm) and/or small osteophytes, and/or mild hypertrophy of the articular process; Grade 2, narrowing of the facet joint space and/or moderate osteophytes, and/or moderate hypertrophy of the articular process, and/or mild subarticular bone erosions; and Grade 3, narrowing of the facet joint space and/or large osteophytes, and/or severe hypertrophy of the articular process, and/or severe subarticular bone erosions, and/or subchondral cysts

19.4–33.8 kg/m^2; mean 23.85 kg/m^2). After washing the lumbar facet joint in sterile phosphate buffered saline (PBS), full-depth standardized subchondral bones (120 mg for each specimen) were collected using a scalpel. The subchondral bone (30 mg) was ground with liquid nitrogen into a powder, which was mixed with 1000 μL tissue lysis solution. Then, tissue debris was removed by centrifugation at 12,000×*g* at 4 °C for 15 min. In addition, 800 μL supernatant samples were obtained. ELISA kits (RayBiotech, Inc.) were used to quantify IL-1β, TNF-α, leptin, and adiponectin in supernatants after centrifugation. Briefly, eight steps were performed according to the instructions of ELISA kits. Finally, the absorbance of the sample was measured at 450 nm. The mean absorbance for each set of duplicate standards, controls, and samples was calculated, and the average zero standard optical density was subtracted. The standard curve was plotted on log-log graph paper, with the standard concentration on the x-axis and the absorbance on the y-axis.

Assessment of adiponectin expression by immunohistochemistry

The lumbar facet joint samples were obtained from 48 patients (NG, n = 12, median age: 45.56 years; DG, n = 12, median age: 47.33 years; SDG, n = 24, median age: 58.75 years) were fixed in 4% buffered paraformaldehyde for 48 h and decalcified with buffered ethylenediaminetetraacetic acid (EDTA, 20%; pH 7.4); the buffer was replaced every 3 days until the pin could be easily pierced. After dehydration and embedding in paraffin, sections were cut to a thickness of 4 μm. Samples were heated for 90 min, deparaffinized with dimethylbenzene, and dehydrated in a graded ethanol series (85%, 90%, and 100%). The sections were then subjected to antigen retrieval using microwave heating in citrate buffer (pH 6.0) for 12 min, and endogenous peroxidases were blocked with 3% H_2O_2 for 8 min. Serial sections from each case were stained with hematoxylin, hydrochloric acid alcohol, and carbonic acid aluminium and then washed three times with PBS. The sections were incubated with anti-adiponectin antibodies (1:400) or PBS alone as a control at 4 °C for 12 h, followed by washing and incubation with biotinylated secondary antibodies at 37 °C for 30 min. The immunoreaction was finally visualized with diaminobenzidine (DAB) and counterstained with hematoxylin. Human adipocyte tissue was used as a positive control. Specimens were evaluated under a light microscope by an expert pathologist and scored based on a semiquantitative approach of the percentage of positive subchondral bone (0–100%) and the staining intensity (0, negative; 1, weak; 2, moderate; 3, strong) in each subchondral bone sample.

Assessment of adiponectin expression by western blotting

Lumbar facet joint samples were collected from 27 patients (NG, n = 9, median age: 44.44 years; DG, n = 9, median age: 45.33 years; severe SDG, n = 9, median age: 57.22 years). Protease inhibitor (10 μL) and 990 μL RIPA buffer were added to the 50 mg samples, and the samples were then ground on ice and mixed on a rotator for 30 min at 4 °C. Tissue debris was removed by centrifugation at 12,000×*g* at 4 °C for 15 min, and protein concentrations were measured using a Bio-Rad Protein Assay kit (Bio-Rad, Hercules, CA, USA). Protein samples (20 μg) were subjected to sodium dodecyl sulfate polyacrylamide gel electrophoresis and electrophoretically transferred to polyvinylidene difluoride membranes. The membranes were sequentially blotted with the primary antibody (anti-adiponectin 19F1; ab22554; Abcam, Cambridge, UK) and secondary antibody and developed using enhanced chemiluminescence.

Assessment of adiponectin expression by qPCR

Subchondral bone (50 mg) was ground with liquid nitrogen into a powder, and total RNA was extracted using TRIzol reagent (Transgen Biotechnology Co., Beijing, China), per the manufacturer's instructions. Total RNA (1 μg) was employed to prepare cDNA via reverse transcription using a PrimeScript RT Reagent kit with gDNA Eraser (Perfect Real Time; DRR047A; TakaRa, Shiga, Japan). cDNA samples (2.8 μL per 20 μL reaction) were analysed for genes of interest and reference genes (h-actin and adiponectin). qPCR was performed using SYBR Premix Ex TaqTM II (Tli RNaseH Plus; DRR820A; TakaRa) with an ABI StepOnePlus system (Applied Biosystems, Inc., Foster City, CA, USA). The cycling profile was as follows: denaturation at 94 °C for 30 s; 40 -cycles of annealing at 60 °C for 15 s, primer extension at 72 °C for 60 s, and denaturation at 95 °C for 30 s; and a final extension for 2 min. The comparative RQ value method was used to determine fold changes in expression using β-actin as a control. The following primers were used: H-actin-285, F5′-AGCGAGCATCCCCCAAAGTT-3′ and R5′-GGGCACGAAGGCTCATCATT-3′; ADI POQ (214 bp), F5′-CATGCCCATTCGCTTTACCA-3′ and R5′-GGAGGCCTGGTCCACATTAT-3′. The primer sequence was selected for high match similarity to *Homo sapiens* adiponectin gene through NCBI primer blast.

Statistical analysis

Statistical analysis was conducted with GraphPad Prism 5.0 software (San Diego, California, USA). To study the release of adiponectin from the subchondral bone of the lumbar facet joint in relation to the BMI, Pearson correlation analysis was performed on adiponectin content data determined by ELISA and the BMI measurements of patients. Additionally, data analysis of the immunohistochemistry, western blotting, and qPCR experiments was performed using one-way ANOVA with post hoc examination of significant main effects using the Dunnett method. Data are presented as the mean ± SD, unless stated otherwise. A p value less than 0.05 was considered significant for differences and correlations.

Results

Expression of IL-1β, TNF-α, leptin, and adiponectin in lumbar facet joints

First, we evaluated the expression of several cytokines in lumbar facet joint specimens using ELISA. Since IL-1β, TNF-α, and leptin were detected in only a few specimens, they were not included in the statistical analysis. For the adiponectin content data, extreme values (8 case of specimens) were removed and were analysed via descriptive statistics. The result showed that adiponectin was detected in all facet joint specimens, and adiponectin content was different in the different degeneration groups (Fig. 2a). In addition, adiponectin was negatively correlated with BMI in 52 patients (correlation coefficient: $p < 0.001$, $r = -0.861$; Fig. 2b).

Qualitative analysis of adiponectin by immunohistochemistry

Next, we examined whether adiponectin was expressed in the subchondral bone of the lumbar facet joint by immunohistochemistry. We evaluated adiponectin expression in 48 specimens (NG, 12; DG, 12; SDG, 24) by immunohistochemical staining. The results showed that adiponectin was expressed in the subchondral bone but not in the cartilage (Fig 3). Compared to the percentage of immunohistochemical staining in the normal group, significant differences ($p < 0.0001$) were identified in the severe degeneration group by one-way ANOVA (Fig. 4c). Compared to the percentage of immunohistochemical staining in the normal group, a statistically significant difference ($p < 0.05$) was observed in the degeneration group by one-way ANOVA (Fig. 4c). In addition, compared to the percentage of immunohistochemical staining in the degeneration group, a significant difference ($p < 0.05$) was also found in the severe degeneration group by one-way ANOVA (Fig. 4c).

Quantitative analysis of adiponectin expression by western blotting and qPCR in the subchondral bone of the lumbar facet joint

Finally, in order to test our hypothesis that adiponectin plays an important role in FJOA, we further evaluated adiponectin expression by western blotting and qPCR. Western blot analysis demonstrated that adiponectin expression was significantly higher in the normal group than in the degenerative and severe degeneration groups by one-way ANOVA ($p < 0.0001$; Fig. 4a and b). In addition, adiponectin mRNA levels were significantly lower in the degenerative and severe degeneration groups as compared with those in the normal group when normalized to the expression of β-actin by one-way ANOVA ($p < 0.0001$; Fig. 4d).

Discussion

As a part of the three-column structure of vertebrae, facet joints play a key role in maintaining the stability of spinal motion, particularly in the lumbar area [24]. Therefore, most doctors are concerned with the biomechanical and mechanical factors affecting lumbar facet joints. However, the pathogenesis of FJOA has not been fully elucidated. Accordingly, in this study, we

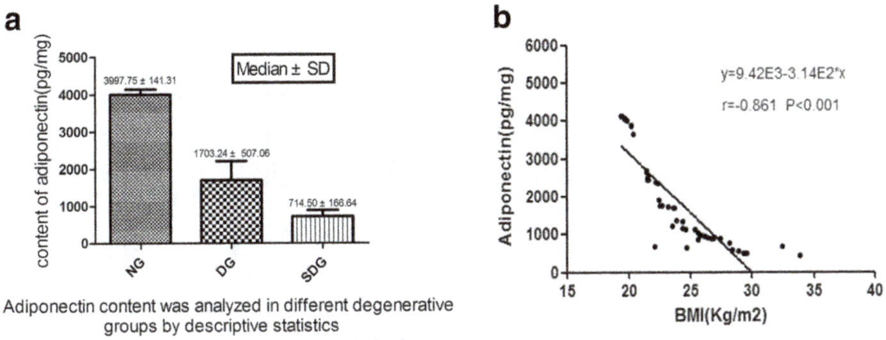

Fig. 2 **a** The mean value of the adiponectin concentration was 3997.75 ± 141.31 pg/mg in the normal group, 1703.24 ± 507.06 pg/mg in the degenerative group, and 714.50 ± 166.64 pg/mg in the severe degenerative group by descriptive statistics. **b** Adiponectin was negatively correlated with the BMI of 52 patients (8 cases having extreme values were removed), $p < 0.001$ and $r = -0.861$

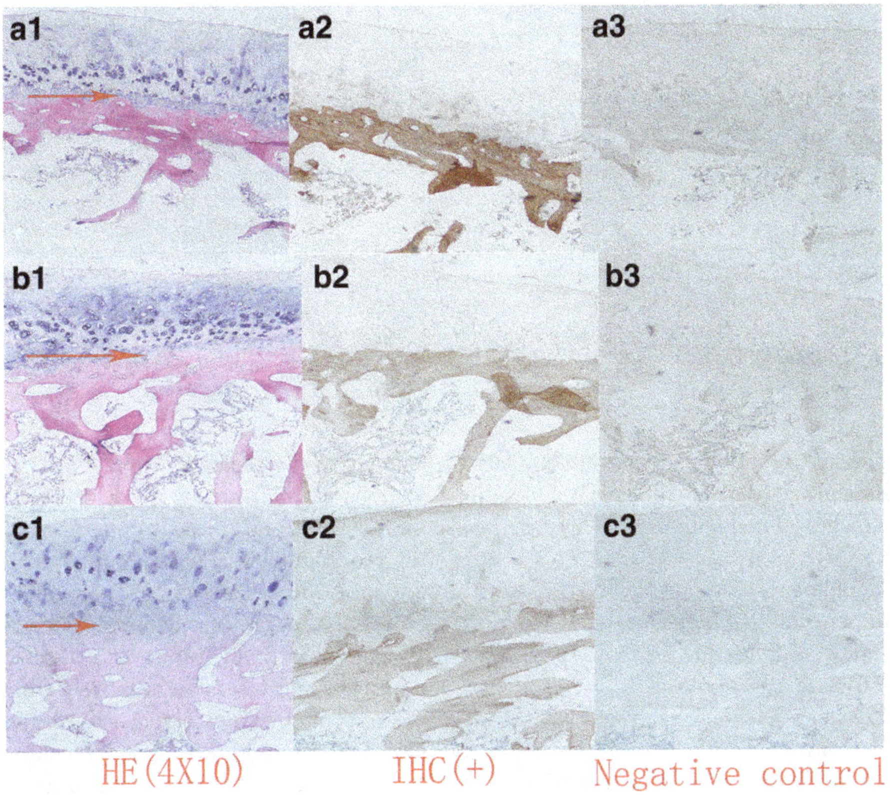

Fig. 3 **a1** Hematoxylin-eosin(HE) staining of the lumbar facet joint in the normal group showed that that the cartilage and subchondral bone boundary were clear and the chondrocyte arrangement rules (a: NG, normal group). **a2** Immunohistochemistry of the lumbar facet joint in the normal group showed strong positive staining in the subchondral bone area, whereas the cartilage area showed negative staining. **a3** PBS, instead of a primary antibody, was used as a negative control in the immunohistochemical analysis. **b1** HE staining of the lumbar facet joint in the degeneration group showed that the cartilage and the subchondral bone area had blurred boundaries and irregular chondrocyte arrangement. (b: DG, degenerative group). **b2** Immunohistochemistry of the lumbar facet joint in the degeneration group showed that the subchondral bone area stained positive, and the cartilage area stained negative. **b3** PBS, instead of a primary antibody, was used as a negative control in the immunohistochemistry. **c1** HE staining of the lumbar facet joint in the severe degeneration group showed that chondrocytes extended through the cartilage line and that chondrocytes were reduced in number and disordered (c: SDG, severe degeneration group). **c2** Immunohistochemistry of the lumbar facet joint in the severe degeneration group showed that the subchondral bone area staining was weakly positive, whereas the staining of the cartilage area was negative. **c3** PBS, instead of a primary antibody, was used as a negative control in the immunohistochemical analysis

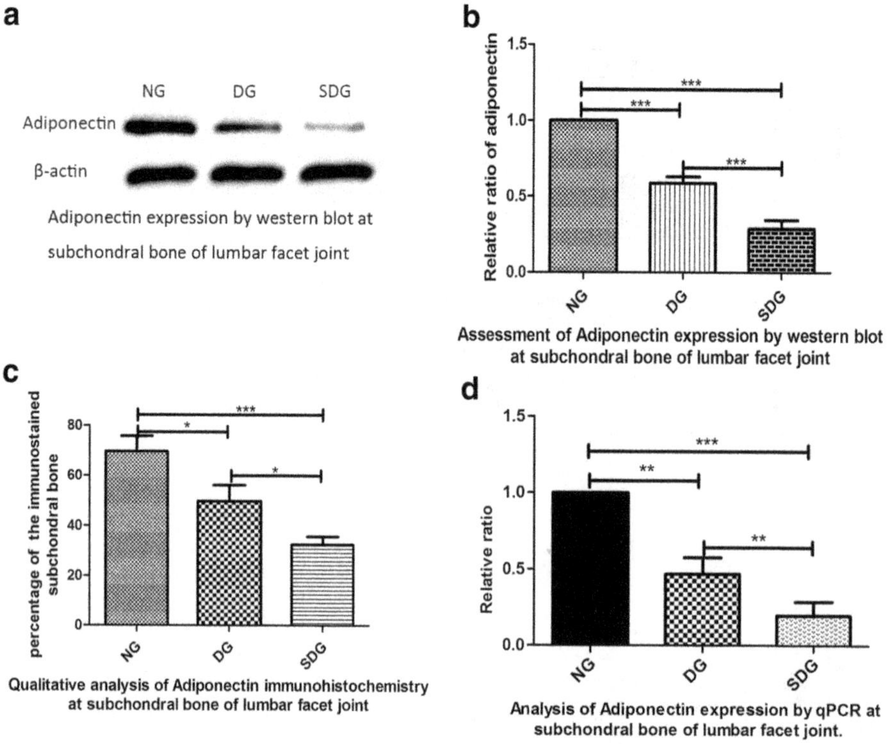

Fig. 4 **a** The expression of adiponectin in the subchondral bone area of the lumbar facet joints by western blotting. The results showed that adiponectin levels were significantly reduced in correlation with the degree of lumbar facet joint degeneration. Representative results from three experiments are shown. (NG: normal group; DG: degenerative group; SDG: severe degenerative group). **b** The grey value of the protein band was analysed by one-way ANOVA. The results showed significant differences in the three group. (NG: normal group, $n = 9$; DG: degenerative group, $n = 9$; SDG: severe degenerative group, $p < 0.0001$). **c** Determination of the immunohistochemical staining percentages was performed in the three groups by one-way ANOVA. The results showed that $p < 0.0001$ in NG compared to SDG and $p < 0.05$ in NG compared to DG and DG to SDG. **d** Adiponectin levels were significantly reduced in correlation with the degree of FJOA by qPCR. Determination of RQ values was performed by one-way ANOVA. The results showed that $p < 0.0001$ in the NG group compared to the SDG group, whereas $p < 0.001$ in NG compared to DG and DG to SDG. Additionally, * represents $p < 0.05$, ** represents $p < 0.001$, and *** represents $p < 0.0001$

evaluated the expression of adiponectin in lumbar facet joints. Our results showed that adiponectin expression was significantly downregulated with increasing degeneration of the lumbar facet joint.

Adiponectin is an adipocyte factor specifically secreted from fat cells. Adiponectin is composed of 244 amino acids; the N-terminus contains one secretory signal sequence, and the C-terminus contains a spherical egg white function threshold. Previous studies have shown that adiponectin is involved in glucose homeostasis, insulin sensitivity, and vascular inflammatory diseases [25, 26]. Adiponectin in human peripheral blood circulation has three different types of polymer, including low- molecular-weight trimers (LMW), a middle-molecular-weight hexamers (MMW), and high numbers of monomers that compose high-molecular-weight multimers (HMW). Yamauchi et al. [27] reported that the affinity of adiponectin varies between different subtypes and receptors and that the adiponectin monomer, AdipoR1, and AdipoR2 have higher affinity, while MMW and HMW are mainly associated with T-cadherin. Therefore, the biological effects of the different types of adiponectin polymers may vary considerably. In research on metabolic and cardiovascular disease, HMW adiponectin was found to induce proinflammatory cytokine production [28], whereas LMW adiponectin was shown to inhibit the release of inflammatory factors [29]. Additionally, in studies focusing on arthritis, the adiponectin monomer and OA were negatively correlated, and HMW adiponectin was not associated with the degree of OA [30]. Furthermore, Kang et al. [31] showed that adiponectin is a potential catabolic mediator of OA in vitro. Therefore, the relationship between adiponectin and OA is of considerable interest.

In this study, the results showed that adiponectin expression was significantly higher than IL-1β, TNF-α, and leptin expression in the lumbar facet joints by ELISA and that adiponectin was negatively correlated with BMI. These findings support a model in which adiponectin is negatively correlated with FJOA. Furthermore, western blotting and qPCR confirmed the down regulation of adiponectin in degenerative joints compared with that in normal joints. Therefore, our findings suggest that degeneration of the lumbar facet joint may be significantly associated with adiponectin expression. However, the specific mechanism is not clear. Berner et al. [20] found that adiponectin and its receptors are expressed in bone-forming cells of the juvenile mouse mandible and that adiponectin promotes the metabolism of osteoblasts in bone. Chen et al. [32] provided evidence for the protective role of adiponectin in knee OA. The study found that adiponectin can activate p38 mitogen-activated protein kinase (p38MAPK) pathway, involved in the pathogenesis of OA [33, 34]. However, few studies have evaluated the subchondral bone, which can play an important role in FJOA. The subchondral bone of the lumbar facet is composed of the cortical plate, trabecular bone, bone trabecula, and vascular lacuna. Small veins, small arteries, and sinusoidal ducts enter the subchondral bone area and then into the cartilage and cartilage radiation layer through the cortical plate, providing nutrients to the deeper cartilage [35, 36]. Orth and Cucchiarini [37] demonstrated that the subchondral bone functions to provide nutrients to articular cartilage, promote the synthesis of protein polysaccharides and collagen fibres, increase the contact surface area, and maintain cartilage. Taken together with the findings of this study, we hypothesize that adiponectin promotes the growth of osteoblasts via the p38 mitogen-activated protein kinase pathway in the subchondral bone of the facet joint that leads to bone remodelling, which results in delayed facet joint degeneration.

Limitations

There are some limitations in this basic experimental study. In this study, we speculated that adiponectin promotes the growth of osteoblasts via the p38 mitogen-activated protein kinase pathway in the subchondral bone of the facet joint and that this leads to bone remodelling, thereby resulting in delayed facet joint degeneration. However, we have only explored preliminary phenomenon thus far and the specific mechanism involved has not yet been fully determined. Therefore, we will further study the specific mechanism of lumbar facet OA.

Conclusions

Based on our findings in this study, we hold that adiponectin was expressed in the subchondral bone of the lumbar facet joint and that adiponectin may be inversely correlated with the degree of degeneration of the lumbar facet joint. Therefore, we hypothesize that adiponectin may play a role in protection of the lumbar facet joint degeneration via the modulation of osteoblasts and osteoclasts. Studies are currently underway in our laboratory to further investigate this hypothesis.

Abbreviations

BMI: Body mass index; CT: Computed tomography; DG: Degeneration group; ELISA: Enzyme-linked immunosorbent assay; FJOA: Osteoarthritis of the lumbar facet joint; MRI: Magnetic resonance imaging; NG: Normal group; OA: Osteoarthritis; p38 MAPK: p38 mitogen-activated protein kinase; PBS: Phosphate-buffered saline; SDG: Serious degeneration group; TNF: Tumour necrosis factor

Acknowledgements

We greatly appreciate the assistance of the company Editage in Shanghai, which provided English language editing.

Funding

All research costs were supplied by the following three project grants: Gan-Po Talents Project 555 of Jiangxi Province, Jiangxi Provincial Department of Science and Technology (20171BAB205059) and Jiangxi Province Postgraduate Innovation Special Funds(YC2016-S107).

Authors' contributions

QL, YL, BZ, and MD conceived and designed the study; QL and Lt H performed the experiments, and Xq L and Xl Y analysed the data. QL and QW wrote the paper; QL,YL, Rs G, Jh Z, Hx C, BZ, and MD reviewed and edited the manuscript. All authors read and approved the manuscript.

Competing interests

The authors declare that they have no competing interests.

Author details

[1]Department of Orthopedics, The First Affiliated Hospital of Nanchang University, 17 Yongwai Street, Nangchang, Jiangxi 330006, China. [2]Artificial Joints Engineering and Technology Research Center of Jiangxi Province, Nanchang, Jiangxi 330006, China.

References

1. Goode AP, Carey TS, Jordan JM. Low back pain and lumbar spine osteoarthritis: how are they related? Curr Rheumatol Rep. 2013;15:305–17.
2. Schwarzer AC, Aprill C, Derby R, et al. Clinical features of patients with pain stemming from the lumbar zygapophyseal joints. Is the lumbar facet syndrome a clinical entity? Spine. 1994;10:1132–7.
3. Manchkanti L, Pampati V, Fellows B, et al. Prevalence of facet joint pain in chronic low back pain. Pain Physician. 1999;2:59–64.
4. Engel R, Bogduk N. The menisci of the lumbar zygapophysial joints. J Anat. 1982;135:795–809.
5. Glover JR. Arthrography of the joints of the lumbar vertebral arches. Orthop I Clin North Am. 1977;8:37–42.
6. Giles LGF, Taylor JR. Intra-articular synovial protrusions in the lower lumbar apophyseal joints. Bull Hosp Jt Dis Orthop Inst. 1982;42:248–55.
7. Hunter DJ, Schofield D, Callander E. The individual and socioeconomic impact of osteoarthritis. Nat Rev Rheumatol. 2014;10:437–41.
8. Cheng C, Gao S, Lei G. Association of osteopontin with osteoarthritis. Rheumatol Int. 2014;34:1627–31.
9. Gao SG, Li KH, Zeng KB, et al. Elevated osteopontin level of synovial fluid and articular cartilage is associated with disease severity in knee osteoarthritis patients. Osteoarthr Cartil. 2010;18:82–7.
10. Gao SG, Zeng C, Li LJ, et al. Correlation between senescence-associated beta-galactosidase expression in articular cartilage and disease severity of patients with knee osteoarthritis. Int J Rheum Dis. 2016;19:226–32.
11. Lories RJ, Luyten FP. The bone-cartilage unit in osteoarthritis. Nat Rev Rheumatol. 2011;7:43–9.
12. Brandt KD, Radin EL, Dieppe PA, et al. Yet more evidence that osteoarthritis is not a cartilage disease. Ann Rheumat Dis. 2006;65:1261–4.
13. Netzer C, Urech K, Hugle T, Benz RM, Geurts J, Schren S. Characterization of subchondral bone histopathology of facet joint osteoarthritis in lumbar spinal stenosis. J Orthop Res. 2016;34(8):1475–80.

14. Murray KJ, Le Grande MR, Ortega de Mues A, Azari MF. Characterisation of the correlation between standing lordosis and degenerative joint disease in the lower lumbar spine in women and men: a radiographic study. BMC Musculoskelet Disord. 2017;18(1):330.
15. Maeda K, Okubo K, Shimomura I, et al. cDNA cloning and expression of a novel adipose specific collagen-like factor, apM1 (adipose most abundant gene transcript 1). Biochem Biophys Res Commun. 1996;221:286–9.
16. Scherer PE, Williams S, Fogliano M, et al. A novel serum protein similar to C1q, produced exclusively in adipocytes. J Biol Chem. 1995;270:26746–9.
17. Pajvani UB, Du X, Combs TP, et al. Structure–function studies of the adiponectin-secreted hormone Acrp30/adiponectin: implication for metabolic regulation and bioactivity. J Biol Chem. 2003;278:9073–85.
18. Arita Y, Kihara S, Ouchi N, et al. Paradoxical decrease of an adipose-specific protein, adiponectin, in obesity. Biochem Biophys Res Commun. 1999;257:79–3.
19. Cnop M, Havel PJ, Utzschneider KM, et al. Relationship of adiponectin to body fat distribution, insulin sensitivity and plasma lipoproteins: evidence for independent roles of age and sex. Diabetologia. 2003;46:459–69.
20. Berner HS, Lyngstadaas SP, Spahr A, et al. Adiponectin and its receptors and expressed in bone-forming cells. Bone. 2004;35:842–9.
21. Francin PJ, Abot A, Guillaume C, Presle N. Association between adiponectin and cartilage degradation in human osteoarthritis. Osteoarthr Cartil. 2014;22:519–26.
22. Weishaupt D, Zanetti M, Boos N, et al. MR imaging and CT in osteoarthritis of the lumbar facet joints. Skelet Radiol. 1999;28:215–9.
23. Zhou X, Liu Y, Zhou S, et al. The correlation between radiographic and pathologic grading of lumbar facet joint degeneration. BMC Med Imaging. 2016;6:27.
24. Gellhorn AC, Katz JN, Suri P. Osteoarthritis of the spine: the facet joints. Nat Rev Rheumatol. 2013;9:216–24.
25. Worf G. Adiponectin: a regulator of energy homeostasis. Nutr Rev. 2003;61:290–2.
26. Ouchi N, Kihara S, Funahashi T, et al. Obesity, adiponectin and vascular inflammatory disease. Curr Opin Lipidol. 2003;14:561–6.
27. Yamauchi T, Kamon J, Ito Y, Tsuchida A, Yokomizo T, Kita S, et al. Cloning of adiponectin receptors that mediate antidiabeticmetabolic effects. Nature. 2003;423:762–9.
28. Hangen F, Drevon CA. Activation of nuclear factor-kappaB by high molecular weight and globular adiponectin. Endocrinology. 2007;148(11):5478–86.
29. Neumeier M, Weigert J, Schfiffier A, et al. Different effects of adiponectin isoforms in human monocytic cells. J Leukoc Bio. 2006;79(4):803–8.
30. Klein-Wieringa IR, Andersen SN, Herb-van Toorn L, et al. Are baseline high molecular weight adiponectin levels associated with radiographic progression in the rheumatoid arthritis and osteoarthritis? J Rheumatol. 2014;41(5):853–8.
31. Kang EH, Lee YJ, Kim TK, et al. Adiponectin is a potential catabolic mediator in osteoarthritis cartilage. Arthritis Res Ther. 2010;12:R231.
32. Chen TH, Chen L, Hsieh MS, et al. Evidence for a protective role for adiponectin in osteoarthritis. Biochim Biophys Acta. 2006;1762:711–8.
33. Koskinen A, Juslin S, Nieminen R, et al. Adiponectin associates with markers of cartilage degradation in osteoarthritis and induces production of proinflammatory and catabolic factors through mitogen-activated protein kinase pathways. Arthritis Res Ther. 2011;13(6):184.
34. Tong KM, Chen CP, Huang KC, et al. Adiponectin increases MMP-3 expression in human chondrocytes through adiporl signaling pathway. J Cell Biochem. 2011;112:143l–40.
35. Pallante-Kichura AL, Cory E, Bugbee WD, et al. Bone cysts after osteochondral allograft repair of cartilage defects in goats suggest abnormal interaction between subchondral bone and overlying synovial joint tissues. Bone. 2013;57:259–68.
36. Yu DG, Ding HF, Mao YQ, et al. Strontium ranelate reduces cartilage degeneration and subchondral bone remodeling in rat osteoarthritis model. Acta Pharmacol Sin. 2013;34:393–402.
37. Orth P, Cucchiarini M, Zurakowski D, et al. Parathyroid hormone [1-34] improves articular cartilage surface architecture and integration and subchondral bone reconstitution in osteochondral defects in vivo. Osteoarthr Cartil. 2013;21:614–24.

21

Effects of Osteoglycin (OGN) on treating senile osteoporosis by regulating MSCs

Xia Chen[1†], Junsong Chen[2†], Dongliang Xu[3†], Shuangxia Zhao[4], Huaidong Song[4] and Yongde Peng[1*]

Abstract

Background: Significant amount of bone mass is lost during the process of aging due to an imbalance between osteoblast-mediated bone formation and osteoclast-mediated bone resorption in bone marrow microenvironment, which leads to net bone loss in the aging population, resulting in the pathogenesis of osteoporosis.

Methods: Firstly, differences in proliferative capacity of adipocyte or adipogenic differentiation in mouse mesenchymal stem cells (MMSCs) and senile mouse model-derived bone marrow mesenchymal stem cells (SMMSCs), as well as mRNA expression of OGN and PPARγ2 were observed. Secondly, osteogenic abilities of MMSCs and SMMSCs treated with rosiglitazone (a PPARγ2 agonist) to induce osteogenic changes were observed, and negative correlation of PPARγ2 with OGN was evaluated. Thirdly, the role of SMMSCs in promoting osteogenesis was examined through enhancing expression of OGN; besides, the related mechanism was investigated by means of expression of related adipocyte and osteoblast specific genes.

Results: Forced OGN expression by OGN-infected lentivirus could increase expression of Wnt5b, RUNX2, OCN, ALP and Colla1, as well as bone formation, while decreases expression of adipogenesis marker PPARγ2. It resulted in expression inhibition of adipocyte genes such as adipocytic differentiation related genes adipocyte binding protein 2 (aP2) and osteoclast differentiation factor Rankl in bone marrow, giving rise to increased bone mass.

Conclusion: OGN may plays a significant role in osteoporosis, which may also provide a potential target for therapeutic intervention of senile osteoporosis characterized by altered differentiation of BMSCs into osteoblasts and adipocytes.

Keywords: Osteoglycin, Peroxisome proliferators-activated receptor-γ 2, Senile osteoporosis, Adipogenesis, Osteoblastogenesis, Mesenchymal stromal cells

Background

Senile osteoporosis, which is defined by low bone mass and micro-architectural deterioration of bone tissue, leads to increased bone fragility and susceptibility to fracture [1, 2], thus becoming a severe societal problem threatening human health. Significant amount of bone is lost during the process of aging, which can be attributed to an imbalance between osteoblast-mediated bone formation and osteoclast-mediated bone resorption in bone marrow microenvironment. It leads to net bone loss in the aging population, resulting in the pathogenesis of osteoporosis [3, 4]. The reasons accounting for such imbalance inform us of the knowledge of senile osteoporosis.

Multiple endogenous and exogenous factors are proved to be involved in regulating bone remodeling, suggesting that both genetic and environmental factors are linked to bone mass and susceptibility to osteoporosis [5, 6]. However, the key regulating factor and the underlying mechanism of senile osteoporosis remain to be clearly defined. It is shown in a number of recent studies that deficiency in number and function of osteoblast, together with increase in marrow adipogenesis, may account for the key etiological factor of osteoporosis [7, 8]. Bone marrow-derived multipotent mesenchymal stromal cells (BMSCs) in the marrow pool are the major source of adipocytes and osteoblasts, which contribute to bone remodeling in adults. MSCs have the

* Correspondence: pengyongde0909@126.com
†Equal contributors
[1]Department of Endocrinology and Metabolism, Shanghai General Hospital of Nanjing Medical University, 100 Haining Road, Shanghai 200080, China
Full list of author information is available at the end of the article

plasticity to differentiate into either osteoblasts or adipocytes; as a result, unbalanced differentiation of MSCs into marrow adipocytes and osteoblasts can result in bone loss by the excessive accumulation of marrow adipocytes [9]. Consequently, understanding factors regulating the osteogenic differentiation of BMSCs, as well as controlling the differentiation of MSCs to stimulate osteoblastogenesis while inhibit adipogenesis marks an effective way to treat senile osteoporosis. Studies on peroxisome proliferators-activated receptor-γ (PPARγ), a master regulator of adipocyte differentiation [10], support this hypothesis at least partly due to suppression of osteogenic differentiation of MSCs. PPARγ1 is widely expressed, particularly in adipose, liver, heart, and spleen; whereas expression of PPARγ2 is largely restricted to adipocytes [11].

Osteoglycin (OGN) may be one of the muscle-derived humoral bone anabolic factors [12], the level of which together with effects of conditioned medium on OGN-modulated myoblasts is positively correlated with phenotype and mineralization of osteoblasts [13]. Therefore, OGN can be served as a common factor to regulate the directional differentiation of MSCs, and a novel target of therapy for senile osteoporosis. This research aimed to carry out an intensive study on the regulatory effect of OGN on osteoblastogenesis and adipogenesis of MSCs, influence of inhibiting the adipogensis of MSCs by OGN on the function of osteoblasts and osteoclasts, as well as the molecular mechanisms by which OGN controlled differentiation of MSCs.

Methods

Materials

Cell culture

Mouse mesenchymal stem cells (MMSCs) were derived from bone marrow of femur and humerus in C57BL/6 mice (MUBMX-01001, Cyagen Biosciences Inc., CA. US), which had the potential to develop into mature cells that produced fat, cartilage, bone, tendon, and muscle. MMSCs were cultured in OriCell Mouse Mesenchymal Stem Cell Growth Medium (Cat. No. MUXMX-90011, Cyagen Biosciences Inc. CA. US) and maintained at 37 °C in a humidified atmosphere with 5% CO_2. MMSCs have been passaged no more than 3 times. PPARγ2 selective agonist Rosiglitazone for cell culture experiments was purchased from Abcam (ab120762, USA), dissolved in DMSO to prepare the stocking solution with concentration of 40 mM, and stored at −20 °C. Part of cells received no treatment (Naïve) while the remaining cells were treated with vector (DMSO, with the final concentration of 0.1%). Relevant protein or mRNA expression and activation, as well as accumulative expression of fat droplets were analyzed 14 days after cell culture with drug treatment.

Primary bone marrow cell cultures were prepared from senescence accelerated mouse prone/6 (SAM-P6, female) of 4–5 months of age were acquired from Shanghai Tanhui Bio Co. Ltd. China. All animal studies were reviewed and approved by the Institutional Animal Care and Use Committee of Nanjing Medical University, and SAM-P6 mice were housed in a temperature-controlled (kept at 24 ± 1 °C) room with a 06.00–18.00 h light cycle. Full details of the study approval can be found under the approval ID, 20,140,871. After mice were anesthetized using isoflurane and killed by cervical dislocation, one femur and two tibiae were aseptically dissected and soft tissues were removed, and then the bone were put in phosphate buffered saline (PBS). Marrow was flushed from the femur and tibia, and was strained using a 70 μm cell strainer. Subsequently, it was suspended in MSC medium consisting of α-minimal essential medium (MEM, which contained 10% fetal bovine serum (FBV) and 100 U/ml penicillin), 100 μg/ml streptomyocin, and 0.25 μg/ml Amphotericin-B. Medium was replaced three times per week and the cells have been passaged no more than 3 times.

Osteogenic differentiation

MMSCs and primary bone marrow cells from senescence accelerated mouse model (SMMSCs) were cultured in osteogenic differentiation medium (Cyagen, Santa Clara, CA, USA) for 2 weeks, so as to induce osteogenic differentiation, with medium being replaced every 3 days. Osteogenic medium was comprised of 10% FBS (Hyclone), 100 U/ml penicillin, 100 mg/ml streptomycin, 0.1 mM dexamethasone, 0.2 mM ascorbate and 10 mM β-glycerophosphate (Sigma-Aldrich)).

Adipogenic differentiation

MMSCs and SMMSCs were cultivated in adipogenic differentiation medium consisting of DMEM-low glucose (Gibco) that was supplemented with 10% FBS (Hyclone), 1% penicillin-streptomycin, 1 mM dexamethasone, 0.5 mM methyisobutylxanthine, 100 μM indomethacin, and 10 mg/ml insulin (all Sigma-Aldrich) for the first 3 days, and the medium was replaced every 3 days. Six days later, cells were cultured in maintenance medium consisting of 10% FBS, 1% penicillin-streptomycin and 5 mg/ml insulin. Cultures were alternated weekly between differentiation medium and maintenance medium for two more weeks.

Alizarin red staining, ALP staining and quantitative assay of osteogenesis

Alizarin red staining and ALP staining on MMSCs and SMMSCs were performed according to instructions from manufacturer (2% aqueous solution, Sigma-Aldrich, St. Louis, MO, USA), so as to detect mineral deposition. Briefly, cells were rinsed and fixed in 4% formaldehyde for 30 min at 4 °C. Subsequently, cells were washed with distilled water, exposed to Alizarin red or ALP for 20 min at room temperature, and washed again with distilled water for 5 min for 4 times. Quantitative analysis was conducted after Alizarin red staining by means of optical density value at 450 nm, and discs without cells were also stained as controls. ALP activity assay was performed in accordance with instructions from manufacturer. Briefly, culture solution on 14th day of subculture was collected from the 6-well plates, and quantitative detection of ALP levels was thereby carried out using poly-biochemical analyzer. Each experiment was performed in triplicate. Eventually, cells were observed and photographed under phase-contrast microscopy.

MTT and colony formation assay

Cells at the concentration of 1×10^3/well were seeded into the 96-well culture plates for MTT assay. Cell viability was assessed using 3-(4,5-dimethylthiazol-2-yl)-2, 5-diphenyl tetrazolium bromide (MTT, Sigma) dye in accordance with the protocol and the incubation time recommended by manufacturers. Amount of MTT formazan product was analyzed using spectrophotometry at a wavelength of 490 nm (Bio-Rad). Each individual experiment was repeated for at least 3 times.

Colony formation assays were performed in the 6-well culture plates at the cell seeding density of 1000. Cells were washed with PBS and fixed with methanol at room temperature for 20 min after 14 days. Colonies were stained with 0.1% crystal violet (Sigma) and counted. The cultures were replaced twice weekly, and colonies of more than 30 cells were scored. All experiments were conducted in triplicate.

Lipid accumulation and quantitative assay of adipogenesis

Oil Red O staining (Sigma, St. Louis, MO, USA) was performed to detect lipid accumulation in adipocytes. Cultures were fixed in 10% phosphate buffered formalin for 10 min. Cells were rinsed with PBS once for 1 min, followed by 60% isopropanol for 5 min, so as to facilitate the staining of neutral lipids. Subsequently, cells were stained with an aqueous filtered solution of Oil Red O at 37 °C for 30 min in darkness. Later, cells were destained with 60% isopropanol for 10 min, and rinsed with PBS for 3 min for 3 times altogether. Cultures were magnified through light microscopy (Olympus) and photographed; in addition, lipid accumulation was quantified by Nile Red staining.

Quantitative real-time RT-PCR (qRT-PCR)

Total RNA was extracted and genomic DNA was removed with TRIzol (Invitrogen, Carlsbad, CA, USA). cDNA was synthesized by total RNA using Superscript II Reverse Transcriptase (Invitrogen) according to the recommendations from manufacturers. Quantitative RT-PCR (qRT-PCR) was performed by adopting FastStart Universal SYBR Green Master with LightCycler 2.0 real-time PCR system (Roche Germany). Validated primers were purchased from Biosystems (as was shown in Table 1). Relative transcript levels were analyzed in a 20 μL reaction system on 96-well plates using a BIORAD CFX96 real-time PCR system. The reaction conditions were shown as follows: Hot-Start activation at 95 °C for 2 min, and 40 cycles of denaturation (at 95 °C for 16 s) and annealing/extension (at 54 °C for 65 s). β-actin was used as an internal reference. Expression levels of PCR products of interest relative to those in the naïve cultures (control groups) were calculated on the basis of relative quantitative method ($2^{\Delta\Delta CT}$), and the data were expressed as "Relative expression Vs. day 0". All reactions were conducted in duplicate, and all experiments were repeated for at least 3 times.

Lentivirus production

Human cDNA of OGN was subcloned into the pLJM1-EGFP lentiviral vector (Plasmid #1931, Addgene diagnostic digest). Viral vector, the expression of which was highly cell specific (target gene), was transfected into HEK293T cells in accordance with the instructions from

Table 1 Primers of genes

Gene (mouse)		DNA sequence (forward/reverse, 5'-3')
PPARγ2	Forward	ATGGGTGAAACTCTGGGAGA
	Reverse	GAGCTGATTCCGAAGTTGGT
OGN	Forward	GGCGCTACCTGTATCAATGG
	Reverse	TCAGCCAACTCGTCACAGTC
ALP	Forward	GTGCAGTCTGTGTCTTGCCTG
	Reverse	CCTTGCCTGTATCTGGAATCCT
RUNX2	Forward	CACCGAGACCAACCGAGTCA
	Reverse	TGCTCGGATCCCAAAAGAAG
Col1a1	Forward	CAACCTGGACGCCATCAAG
	Reverse	ATCGGTCATGCTCTCTCCAAA
OCN	Forward	AGCTTAACCCTGCTTGTGACG
	Reverse	GGAGGATCAAGTCCCGGAGA
Rankl	Forward	CACCATCAGCTGAAGATAGT
	Reverse	CCAAGATCTCTAACATGACG
aP2	Forward	CACCGCAGACGACAGGAAG
	Reverse	GCACCTGCACCAGGGC
Wnt5b	Forward	CTGCTGTTTTGAGGGGATTC
	Reverse	CGCACTGAGCAATTAAGCAG
β-actin	Forward	GTTGTCGACGACGAGCG
	Reverse	GCACAGAGCCTCGCCTT

manufacturers (Addgene). Viral supernatants were collected after 48 h, centrifuged at 1500×*g* for 5 min, filtered with a 0.45 μm filter, aliquoted, and stored at −80 °C. Viral titer was determined by serial dilution and infection of SMMSCs. SMMSCs, which were isolated from SAM-P6 mouse, were infected with empty control vector pLJM1-EGFP for 8 h, respectively. Cells were screened out by puromycin for 8 days after 2 days of infection, the resistant clones of which were pooled and confirmed as OGN-positive SMMSCs by Western blotting and EmGFP for easy determination of lentiviral titer by flow cytometry (data not shown).

Western blot analysis

Cell lysates containing 30 μg of protein were separated by SDS-PAGE and transferred to activate PVDF membranes (Millipore Corp, Bedford, MA) that were blocked in defatted milk (5% in Tris-buffered saline with TWEEN-20 buffer) for 1 h and incubated with antibodies. These antibodies were shown as below: anti-OGN (Osteoglycin Antibody (K-14), sc-47,277, Santa Cruz Biotechnology, Inc., CA); anti-PPAR gamma EP4394(N) (ab191407, abcam, US); anti-RUNX2 (EPR3099, ab92336, abcam, US); anti-aP2/Fabp4 (2120S, Cell Signaling Technology, US); anti-Rankl (ab45039, abcam, US); anti-Wnt5b (ab93134, abcam, US); anti-Osteocalcin (ab13420, abcam, US); anti-Alkaline Phosphatas (ab108337, abcam, US) and anti-β-actin (ab8227, abcam, US), with the last one being served as a loading control. In the following steps, blots were incubated in horseradish peroxidase-conjugated secondary antibodies (Santa Cruz), and developed using a chemiluminescence detection system (Millipore) after washing. Protein bands were analyzed on the basis of an image analysis system (Bio-Rad).

Statistical methods

Statistical analyses in this research were performed adopting Prism 5 (GraphPad SoftwareInc., La Jolla, CA) and Student's t-test was utilized for analyzing difference between the experimental groups and control group. Besides, Bonferroni correction was also used in which multiple comparisons were made. Differences were considered as statistically significant when P values were less than 0.05. Data were expressed as means ± standard deviation.

Results

Compared with MMSCs in vitro, proliferation and osteogenic differentiation of SMMSCs were impaired, but adipogenic differentiation was enhanced

SMMSCs were isolated from SAM-P6 mouse. SMMSCs and MMSCs shared a similar fibroblast-like spindle shape, as could be seen in Fig. 1A [a, d]. Results of MTT analysis and colony formation assay indicated that cell growth rate of SMMSCs was significantly slower than that of MMSCs. Furthermore, such prominent difference persisted for 15 days of cell culture in Mesenchymal Stem Cell Medium (Fig. 1B and 1C, $p < 0.05$). It could be observed that, MMSCs and SMMSCs could undergo adipogenic differentiation and lipid accumulation in adipogenic induction medium, with adipogenic SMMSCs being more confluent than MMSCs. However, efficient osteogenic differentiation of SMMSCs could not be induced in osteogenic induction medium compared with MMSCs. Abilities of osteogenic and adipogenic differentiation of MMSCs and SMMSCs were evaluated and compared by ALP staining and Oil Red O staining in this research. It could be observed from Fig. 1A[b] and [e] that, ALP staining showed that MMSCs displayed a remarkably higher ALP level relative to SMMSCs after 14 days of subculture. In contrast, Oil Red O staining presented an enhanced ability of SMMSCs for lipid accumulation (Fig. 1A[c] and [f]). It can be found based on these results that under similar culture conditions, proliferation capacity of SMMSCs was retarded, which gave rise to their gradual loss of ability to differentiate into osteogenic lineage; however, their ability of adipogenic differentiation was still enhanced.

OGN might play a marked role in bone formation by means of osteoblasts at the well-differentiated stage [14, 15]. mRNA expression levels of OGN from 0 to 14 days after the induction of osteogenic differentiation were detected by RT-qPCR, so as to investigate expression of OGN in SMMSCs with impaired osteogenesis. Compared with MMSCs, weak expression of OGN could be seen in SMMSCs after 3 days of osteogenic differentiation. (Fig. 2a [left], $p < 0.05$).

mRNA expression level of PPARγ2 in SMMSCs was higher than that in MMSCs cultivated in adipogenic differentiation medium. Moreover, PPARγ2 might be negatively correlated with mRNA expression level of OGN

OGN could be stimulated by expression of Cbfa1 gene, which was a key gene of osteoblastogenesis [16]. PPARγ activity contributed to inhibiting osteoblastic maturation, as could be seen in changes in Runx2/Cbfa1 activity and OCN expression [17]. Expression levels of PPARγ2 and OGN in MMSCs and SMMSCs cultured in adipogenic differentiation medium were examined in this research. The results indicated that, compared with the control, expression of PPARγ2 was up-regulated for more than 12 times in SMMSCs from 0 to 14 days after the induction of adipogenic differentiation (day 0), as could be seen in Fig. 2b. However, only weak or absent expression of OGN could be seen in SMMSCs during the same time period. RT-qPCR assay in MMSCs after 0 to 14 days of induction of adipogenic differentiation also presented

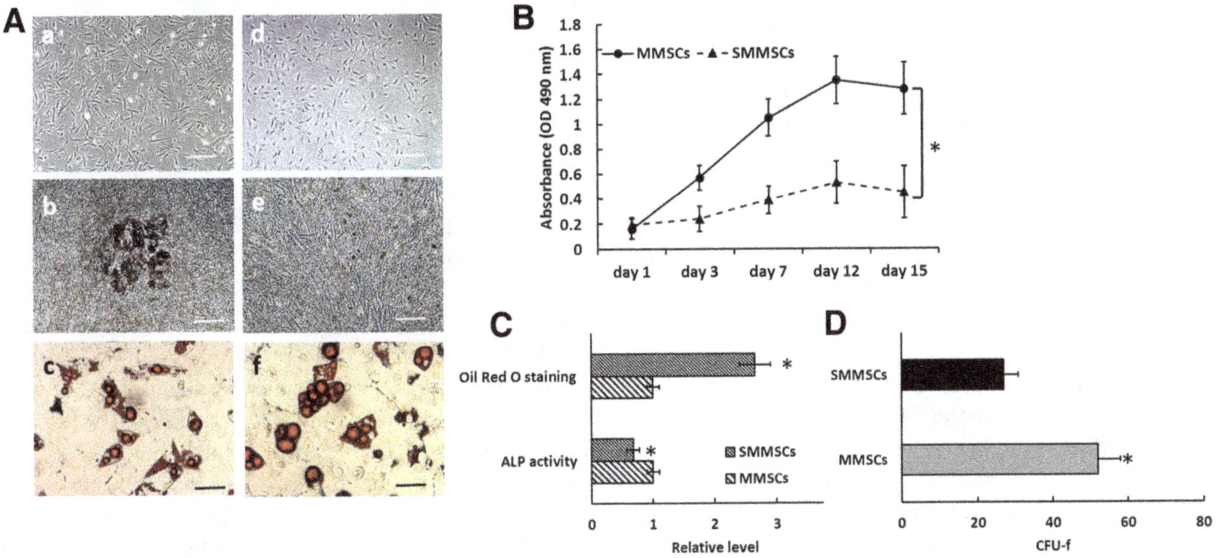

Fig. 1 Proliferation and differentiation of MMSCs and SMMSCs in vitro. **A** The MMSCs cells (A[a]) and SMMSCs (A[d]) have similar typical fibroblast-like morphology after cultured 3 days in vitro. The differentiation was induced in MMSCs and SMMSCs for 2 weeks in vitro and progress of adipogenic and osteogenic differentiation was explored by cytochemistry. Osteogenic differentiation by ALP staining (b, e). Adipogenic differentiation was detected by Oil Red O staining (c, f). In contrast to MMSCs, efficient osteogenic differentiation could not be induced in SMMSCs [compare (b) vs. (e)]. The bars extend 100 μm (a-e) and 20 μm (c, f). **B** MTT assay was performed for cell proliferation after 1, 3, 7, 12 and 15 days culture with passages 5–8 cells of MMSCs and SMMSCs. The results show the cell growth rate of SMMSCs was significantly slower than MMSCs. **C** osteogenesis and adipogenic quantitative assay in MMSCs and SMMSCs groups. **D** CFU-f numbers in MMSCs and SMMSCs groups. After 15 days cultured in Mesenchymal Stem Cell Medium, colonies were stained with crystal violet and counted. Data are expressed as mean ± SD from all experiments, as indicated * $P < 0.05$

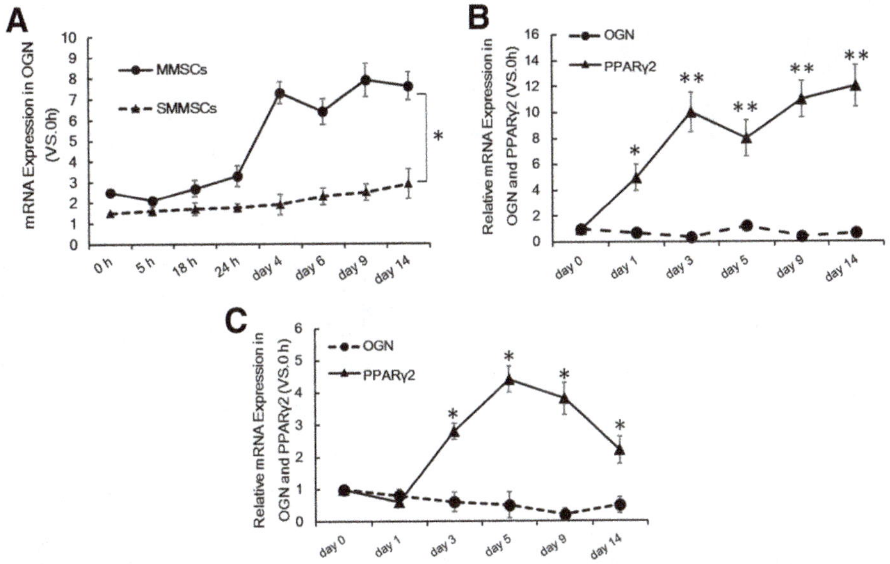

Fig. 2 The mRNA expression of PPARγ2 and OGN in osteogenic or adipogenic differentiation of MMSCs and SMMSCs in vitro. **a** To investigate PPARγ2 and OGN in gene expression following differentiation, RT-qPCR was performed from 0 h to 14 days after induction of osteogenic differentiation in MMSCs and SMMSCs. **b** From 0 to 14 days after induction of adipogenic differentiation (PPARγ2 and OGN) in SMMSCs. **c** From 0 to 14 days after induction of adipogenic differentiation in MMSCs. Before differentiation (day 0) in SMMSCs served as controls as 1. Each assay was performed in three independent experiments. Data are expressed as mean ± SD from all experiments, as indicated * $P < 0.05$ and ** $P < 0.01$

similar results, but expression of PPARγ2 was only up-regulated for 3–4 times compared with the control (day 0). mRNA expression level of OGN was quite low, which was down-regulated progressively. Conversely, mRNA expression level of PPARγ2, an adipogenic differentiation marker, had notably increased in adipogenic MMSCs (as was shown in Fig. 2b and c), indicating that the down-regulation of OGN might be involved in the functional increase in PPARγ2 expression. PPARγ2 might be negatively correlated with expression level of OGN in BMSCs during adipogenic differentiation.

Effects of rosiglitazone on adipocyte or adipogenic differentiation in MMSCs and SMMSCs

MMSCs and SMMSCs were bipotential and were capable of differentiating into both osteoblast and adipocyte. Cells could mineralize the extracellular matrix in the presence of osteogenic differentiation stimuli. In contrast, the addition of a PPAR-γ ligand, such as rosiglitazone, to the adipogenic differentiation medium could induce fat accumulation and adipocyte differentiation, while suppressed the osteoblast phenotype of these cells, which was associated with down-regulation of OGN expression. As was presented in Fig. 3A, intracellular lipid droplet accumulation could be identified visually by oil red staining. The results indicated that compared with MMSCs group, which were treated by 10 μM rosiglitazone, SMMSCs could effectively promote fat droplet accumulation after 14 days of induced adipogenic differentiation culture.

Subsequently, effects of rosiglitazone on expression of phenotype specific gene markers in MMSCs were examined. It could be observed from Fig. 3B that, rosiglitazone affected expression of adipocyte-specific marker PPARγ2 at respective concentrations (0.1 μM, 1 μM and 10 μM, while 0 μM was treated as a control). Enhanced PPARγ2 expression could only be observed when concentration of rosiglitazone was greater than 1 μM. Compared with control group, expression of PPARγ2 mRNA could be up-regulated to 10–13 times in MMSCs (Fig. 3B) and 13–22 times in SMMSCs treated with 10 μM rosiglitazone (Fig. 3C).

Rosiglitazone could also effectively inhibit mRNA expression of OGN in MMSCs and SMMSCs. mRNA expression of OGN in MMSCs was reduced by 50% compared with control group after 5 days of induced

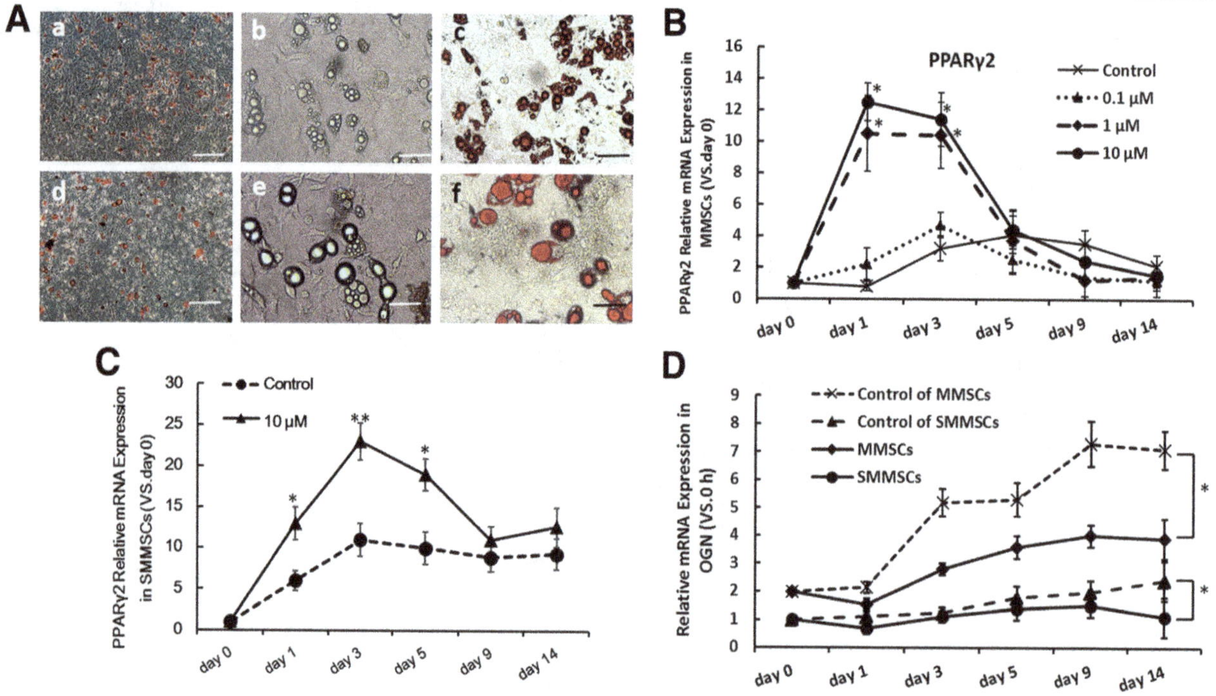

Fig. 3 Influence of rosiglitazone on cell osteogenic or adipogenic differentiation in MMSCs and SMMSCs. **A** Adipogenic differentiation of MMSCs(a-c) and SMMSCs(d-f) treated with rosiglitazone (10 μM) for 14 days were detected by Oil red-O staining(a, c, d, f) or unstaining (b, e). The bars extend 100 μm (a, d) and 20 μm (b, c, e, f). **B** The expression of PPARγ2 in MMSCs were measured by RT-qPCR from 0 to 14 days in induction of adipogenic differentiation treat with different dose of rosiglitazone (0.1 μM, 1 μM and 10 μM). 0 μM rosiglitazone as control group., **C** The expression of PPARγ2 in SMMSCs from 0 to 14 days in induction of adipogenic differentiation treat with rosiglitazone (10 μM). **D** The expression of OGN in MMSCs and SMMSCs from 0 to 14 days in induction of osteogenic differentiation treat with rosiglitazone (10 μM). 0 μM rosiglitazone as control group. Before differentiation (day 0) served as controls as 1. Each assay was performed in three independent experiments. Data are expressed as mean ± SD from all experiments, as indicated * $P < 0.05$ and ** $P < 0.01$

osteogenic differentiation and rosiglitazone treatment. In addition, mRNA expression of OGN in SMMSCs was not even improved compared with day 0 (Fig. 3D). These results suggested that SMMSCs were more susceptible to the inhibition of rosiglitazone (as a PPAR-γ agonist), which made it more difficult to differentiate into osteoblasts in osteogenic induction culture. These data had validated that SMMSCs was a reliable model in vitro to investigate the roles of PPAR-γ2 and OGN in regulating differentiation of BMSCs into osteoblasts and adipocytes in senile mouse model.

Forced OGN expression promoted osteogenic differentiation while inhibited adipocyte-specific marker expression in SMMSCs and MMSCs

Quantitative analysis of alizarin red staining in lentivirus OGN-infected SMMSCs was presented to be increased by an average of 75.6% (on day 5) and 56.8% (on day 14) in comparison with vector treatment cells (as control group) during osteogenic differentiation, as could be observed from Fig. 4A and C ($p < 0.05$).The same results were observed in MMSCs group (data not shown). In addition, the enhanced ALP staining demonstrated that infection of lentivirus OGN contributed to promoting mineralization of SMMSCs and MMSCs in the cultured osteogenic medium on day 2, 5, 9 and 14 (Fig. 4B). Quantification of ALP staining was performed by ALP activity, the results of which indicated that staining in lentivirus OGN-infected SMMSCs was increased by an average of 97.2% (on day 5) and 135% (on day 9) in comparison with the control(Fig. 4D). In MMSCs group, ALP staining was increased by an average of 56% (on day 9) and 77.8% (on day 14) in comparison with the control (Fig. 4E). All these findings revealed that OGN promoted the osteogenic differentiation of SMMSCs.

Forced OGN expression down-regulated expression of adipocyte-specific marker while promoted that of osteoblast-specific gene marker by suppressing PPARγ2 expression

Adipocyte-specific markers as downstream PPARγ2 targets such as aP2, as well as Rankl, which was a ligand for osteoprotegerin that functioned as a key factor for osteoclast differentiation and activation, were examined by western blotting and RT-qPCR. In this way, the potential mechanism underlying the osteogenic differentiation mediated by OGN could be further explored. Compared with the vector group, PPARγ2 expression in lentivirus OGN-infected SMMSCs was down-regulated by 35.8% (on day 3, $p < 0.05$) and 51.3% (on day 6, $p < 0.05$) upon the stimulation of osteogenic differentiation, which were then increased to same levels as the

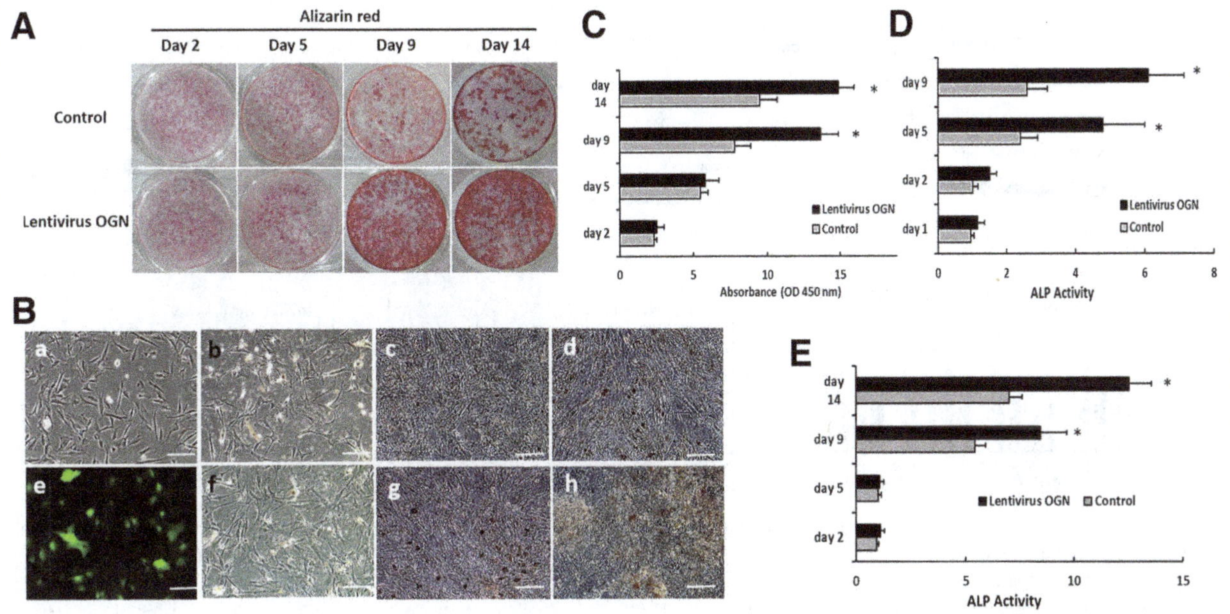

Fig. 4 Influence of Lentivirus OGN on cell osteogenic differentiation in SMMSCs and MMSCs. **A** Alizarin-Red staining after osteogenic differentiation at 2, 5, 9 and 14 days in osteogenic medium. Compared with control group (A upper line), Lentivirus OGN enhanced the mineralization ability of osteoporotic SMMSCs (A lower line). **B** The differentiation was induced in SMMSCs (as control group, C [a-d]) and infected by Lentivirus OGN (as experimental group, C [e-h]) for 12 days in osteogenic medium and progress of osteogenic differentiation was explored by ALP staining at day 2 (b, f), 5 (c, g) and 9 (d, h). **C** Quantification of A was performed by optic density (O.D.) measurement at O.D. 450 nm ($n = 3$). **D** Quantification of B was performed by ALP activity. **E** Quantification of the differentiation was induced in MMSCs infected with Lentivirus OGN by ALP staining. Each assay was performed in three independent experiments. Data are expressed as mean ± SD from all experiments, as indicated * $P < 0.05$

control group at late phase of culture (Fig. 5c). As downstream PPARγ2 targets, expression of aP2 and Rankl in lentivirus OGN-infected SMMSCs presented similar results as PPARγ2, which were reduced mRNA (Fig. 5c) and protein (Fig. 5a and b) levels after 2 days of osteogenic differentiation cultured.

In contrast, compared with the vehicle group, mRNA levels of osteogenic marker genes (which were treated as downstream OGN targets), namely, runt-related transcription factor 2 (RUNX2), osteocalcin (OCN), wingless-type MMTV integration site family, member 5B (Wnt5b) were not changed at early phase. Nevertheless, RUNX2 was up-regulated at late phase by 36.5% (on day 6) and 81% (on day 9), OCN by 34.8% (on day 6) and 62% (on day 9) (Fig. 5d, $p<0.05$), and Wnt5b by 2.7-fold (on day 6) and 3-fold (on day 9) relative to vector group (Fig. 5c, $p<0.01$). ALP was the key enzyme utilized in the standard ALP staining method to detect mineralization of the matrix by osteoblasts. Production of controllable factor of type I collagen (Colla1) was increased rapidly at the beginning of induced osteogenic differentiation in lentivirus OGN-infected SMMSCs, as was shown in Fig. 5d. It was consistent with changes in protein expression levels of these osteogenic marker genes (Fig. 5a and b). The same results were observed in MMSCs group (Fig. 5e and f). All these results indicated that PPARγ2 was a positive promoter of adipogenesis as well as a negative regulator of osteoblastogenesis. OGN might play a distinct role in the retardative osteogenesis of osteoporotic SMMSCs through mediating the functional regulation of PPARγ2 expression.

Discussion

Several conditions including senile osteoporosis are associated with bone loss, which is characterized by decreased osteoblastogenesis while increased adipogenesis in bone marrow [1, 18]. It supports the concept that various lineage-specific genes have exerted important roles during adipocyte, osteoblast and osteoclast differentiation, including RUNX2, OCN, ALP, Wnt5b, PPARγ2, aP2 and Rankl. It has been demonstrated in previous studies that PPARγ2 is up-regulated during aging, and that it is involved in adipocyte differentiation in vitro and in vivo as a key transcription factor [19].

Significant decreases in cell proliferation and osteogenic differentiation can be seen in senile osteoporotic SMMSCs; consequently, down-regulation of OGN may be associated with changes in osteoporotic SMMSCs. In addition, expression of PPARγ2 in SMMSCs and MMSCs within adipogenic differentiation medium is

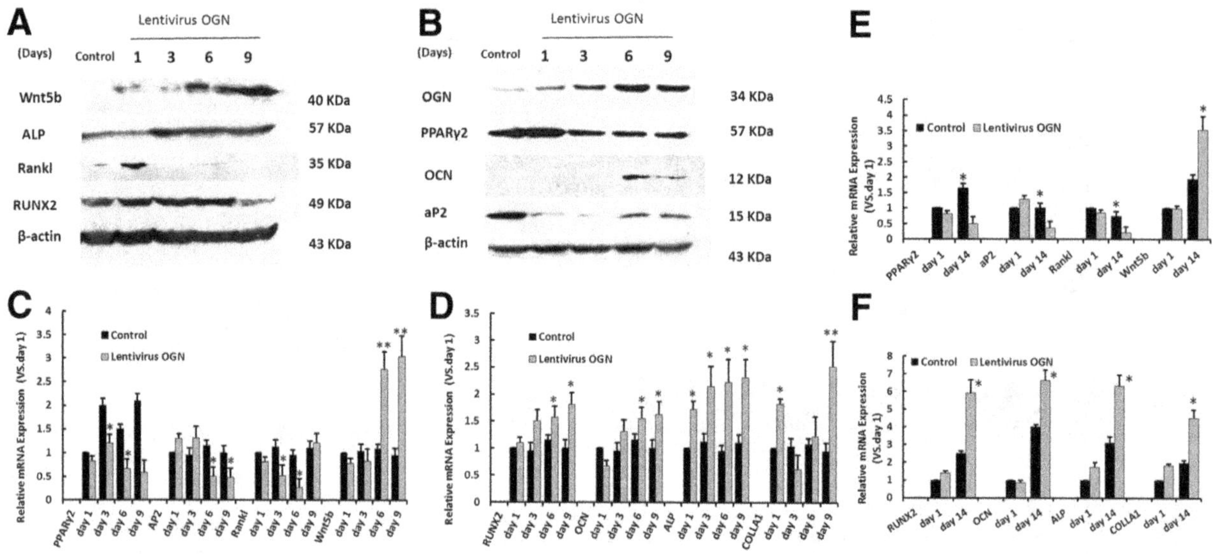

Fig. 5 The mRNA and protein expression of osteogenic or adipogenic differentiation markers of SMMSCs and MMSCs infected by Lentivirus OGN compared with control groups. **a**, **b** Western blotting were employed to examine the protein expression of osteogenic markers genes RUNX2, Ocn, ALP, Wnt5b and adipogenesis marker genes AP2, PPARγ2 of SMMSCs infected by Lentivirus OGN compared with control groups at days 1, 3, 6 and 9. **c** The quantitative expression of adipogenesis markers gene AP2 and PPARγ2 were measured by RT-qPCR at days 1, 3, 6 and 9 after induction of adipogenic differentiation in SMMSCs infected by Lentivirus OGN. Uninfected cells as control group. **d** The quantitative expression of osteogenic markers gene RUNX2, Ocn, ALP, Colla1 and Wnt5b were measured by RT-qPCR at days 1, 3, 6 and 9 after induction of adipogenic differentiation in SMMSCs infected by Lentivirus OGN. Uninfected cells as control group. After differentiation 1 day served as controls as 1. **e** The quantitative expression of adipogenesis markers gene at days 1 and 14 after induction of adipogenic differentiation in MMSCs infected by Lentivirus OGN. **f** The quantitative expression of osteogenic markers gene at days 1 and 14 after induction of adipogenic differentiation in MMSCs infected by Lentivirus OGN. Each assay was performed in three independent experiments. Data are expressed as mean ± SD from all experiments, as indicated * $P<0.05$ and ** $P<0.01$

examined in this research, the results of which suggest that expression of PPARγ2 is outstandingly enhanced in SMMSCs and MMSCs in comparison with OGN. mRNA expression level of PPARγ2 in SMMSCs is higher than that in MMSCs cultivated in adipogenic differentiation medium. SMMSCs isolated from senile mouse gradually lose the ability to differentiate into the osteogenic lineage during osteoporosis, but adipogenic differentiation is still enhanced.

It is found in the present research that rosiglitazone, a PPARγ2 agonist, can activate expression of PPARγ2 and promotes PPARγ2 activity in adipocyte cultures. PPARγ2 can induce the differentiation of MMSCs and SMMSCs into adipocyte lineages; besides, it can negatively regulate osteoblast differentiation by means of suppressing expression of osteoblast specific transcription factor OGN. As is indicated in our findings, up-regulation of PPARγ2 is involved in inhibiting expression of osteogenic-related marker (such as OGN) in senile osteoporosis. SMMSCs are more susceptible to the inhibition of rosiglitazone, which adds to the difficulties to differentiate into osteoblasts in osteogenic induction culture.

Consequently, it is presumed that OGN may be of great significance to the retardative osteogenesis of senile osteoporotic SMMSCs through regulating expression of osteogenesis specific genes such as RUNX2, OCN, ALP and Wnt5b. Lentiviral vectors are applied to restore OGN expression in osteoporotic SMMSCs, so as to determine the effect of OGN on regulating osteogenic differentiation. It is found that the over-expression of OGN can up-regulate expression of osteogenesis-related markers (RUNX2, OCN, ALP and Wnt5b), while down-regulates that of genes characterizing phenotype of adipocyte (such as aP2 and PPARγ2), thus promoting osteogenic differentiation in osteoporotic SMMSCs. These results indicated that OGN-mediated signaling may plays an important role in regulating osteoblast differentiation and physiopathology of senile osteoporosis.

To gain further insight into the potential underlying mechanism of OGN, protein expression of these genes is investigated, including osteogenic marker genes RUNX2, OCN, ALP and Wnt5b as well as adipogenesis marker gene aP2 and osteoclast differentiation factor Rankl. Results of western blotting present that expression levels of osteogenic marker genes ALP, Wnt5b and OCN (the late stage osteogenic marker, which indicates bone formation [20]) are remarkably up-regulated in lentivirus OGN-infected SMMSCs at late stage of induced osteogenic differentiation (from day 3 to 9). Expression of another osteogenic marker gene RUNX2 is up-regulated rapidly at the beginning of osteogenic differentiation (from day 1 to 6), which is down-regulated on day 9. ALP is the key enzyme utilized in standard ALP staining method to detect matrix mineralization by osteoblasts, and ALP staining (Fig. 4c) supports the results of western blotting. As a member of the Wnt signaling pathway and Wnt receptor-ligand complex, Wnt5b has also been found to modulate different stages of osteogenic differentiation of hMSC when it is chemically induced in osteogenic differentiation [21]. In contrast, expression levels of adipogenesis marker genes aP2 and osteoclast differentiation factor Rankl are notably down-regulated in lentivirus OGN-infected SMMSCs compared with the control group, as is shown by results of western blotting. Besides, OGN is proved to inhibit expression of adipogenesis and osteoclast differentiation specific genes as well as lipid accumulation, thus preventing the transformation of BMSCs into adipocytes induced by the cultured differentiation. The same results were observed in MMSCs group. Taken together, these data suggest that OGN regulates the balance between adipogenesis and osteoblastogenesis in vitro in the manner of regulating Runx2. Furthermore, expression of OCN and ALP may be regulated through the Wnt5b/Wnt signaling pathway. Forced OGN expression by lentivirus-infected OGN contributes to increasing expression levels of RUNX2, OCN, ALP and Wnt5b expression, as well as bone formation, while decreasing expression of adipogenesis marker PPARγ2. It results in expression inhibition of adipocyte genes, such as adipogenesis-related genes aP2 and lipoprotein lipase (LPL) in the bone marrow, leading to increased bone mass. Therefore, PPARγ2 shows negative correlation with protein or mRNA expression levels of OGN. It can be found on the basis of these findings that PPARγ2 positively promotes adipogenesis while negatively regulates differentiation of BMSCs into osteoblast in vivo, implying that PPARγ2 is a negative regulator of bone mass. As a PPARγ2 antagonist, OGN helps to correct the imbalance between osteoblastogenesis and adipogenesis and displays a positive effect on bone mass, as compared with the up-regulated expression of osteogenic specific genes and osteoblast differentiation induced. In next steps, we will do further study on the appropriate manipulation of PPARγ2 expression by regulating OGN in senescence accelerated mouse prone/6 (SAM-P6), which is to the benefit of preventing bone loss in senile osteoporosis.

Conclusion

In summary, PPARγ2 plays an important role in controlling the differentiation of marrow stromal cells into osteoblasts or adipocytes in senile osteoporosis, as is indicated in existing evidences. It is demonstrated in the present research that SAM-P6 mouse derived SMMSCs have a weakened capacity of osteogenic differentiation, which can be attributed to down-regulation of OGN. In addition, over-expression of OGN contributes to reversing the reduced capacity of osteogenic differentiation of

SMMSCs. Furthermore, OGN can inhibit expression of adipogenesis marker gene aP2 and osteoclast differentiation factor Rankl by decreasing that of adipogenesis marker PPARγ2, which thereby promotes expression of osteogenic marker genes Wnt5b, RUNX2, OCN, ALP and Colla1, leading to osteoblast differentiation, as is suggested in a mechanistic analysis. Taken together, it is indicated by our findings that OGN may plays an important role in senile osteoporosis by regulate expression of osteogenic and adipogenesis genes, which may provide a potential target for therapeutic intervention for senile osteoporosis characterized by altered differentiation of BMSCs into osteoblasts and adipocytes.

Abbreviations

BMSCs: Bone marrow-derived multipotent mesenchymal stromal cells; Colla1: Type I collagen; LPL: Lipoprotein lipase; MMSCs: Mouse mesenchymal stem cells; OCN: Osteocalcin; OGN: Osteoglycin; PPARγ: Peroxisome proliferators-activated receptor-γ; RUNX2: Runt-related transcription factor 2; SAM-P6: Senescence accelerated mouse prone/6; SMMSCs: Senescence accelerated mouse mesenchymal stem cells; Wnt5b: Wingless-type MMTV integration site family, member 5B

Acknowledgements

Not applicable.

Funding

This study was funded by National Natural Science Foundation of China. (No. 30900503).

Authors' contributions

Authors XC and YDPeng were involved in overall study design and funding. Authors XC and JSC designed and wrote the analysis plan for the current paper. Author DLX undertook the statistical analyses. Author JSC wrote the first draft of the manuscript. Data was collected by SXZ and HDS analyzed the data. All authors critically read the manuscript to improve intellectual content. All authors have approved the final manuscript in its present form.

Competing interests

The authors declare that they have no competing interests.

Author details

[1]Department of Endocrinology and Metabolism, Shanghai General Hospital of Nanjing Medical University, 100 Haining Road, Shanghai 200080, China. [2]Key Laboratory of Systems Biomedicine(Ministry of Education), Shanghai Center for Systems Biomedicine, Shanghai Jiao Tong University, 800 Dongchuan Road, Shanghai 200240, China. [3]Department of Urology, Shanghai General Hospital, Shanghai Jiao Tong University School of Medicine, 100 Haining Road, Shanghai, Shanghai 200080, China. [4]Shanghai Ninth People's Hospital, Shanghai Jiaotong University School of Medicine, No. 639 zhizaoju Road, Shanghai, China.

References

1. Herrera A, Lobo-Escolar A, Mateo J, Gil J, Ibarz E, Gracia L. Male osteoporosis: a review. World J Orthop. 2012;3(12):223–34.
2. Tan J, Xu X, Tong Z, Lin J, Yu Q, Lin Y, Kuang W. Decreased osteogenesis of adult mesenchymal stem cells by reactive oxygen species under cyclic stretch: a possible mechanism of age related osteoporosis. Bone Res. 2015;3:15003. Published online 2015 Mar 17. doi:10.1038/boneres.2015.3.
3. Karsenty G. The complexities of skeletal biology. Nature. 2003;423:316–8.
4. Chen H, Zhou X, Fujita H, Onozuka M, Kubo K-Y. Age-related changes in Trabecular and cortical bone microstructure. Int J Endocrinol. 2013;2013:213234. Published online 2013 Mar 18. doi:10.1155/2013/213234c.
5. Kling JM, Clarke BL, Sandhu NP. Osteoporosis prevention, screening, and treatment: a review. J Women's Health (Larchmt). 2014;23(7):563–72.
6. Manolagas SC. Wnt signaling and osteoporosis. Maturitas. 2014;78(3):233–7.
7. Gao B, Yang L, Luo Z-J. Transdifferentiation between bone and fat on bone metabolism. Int J Clin Exp Pathol. 2014;7(5):1834–41.
8. Yang F, Yuan P, Hao Y-Q, Lu Z-M. Emodin enhances osteogenesis and inhibits adipogenesis. BMC Complement Altern Med. 2014;14:74. doi:10.1186/1472-6882-14-74.
9. Wang C, Meng H, Wang X, Zhao C, Peng J, Wang Y. Differentiation of bone marrow Mesenchymal stem cells in Osteoblasts and Adipocytes and its role in treatment of osteoporosis. Medical Science Monitor: International Medical Journal of Experimental and Clinical Research. 2016;22:226–33. doi:10.12659/MSM.897044.
10. Akune T, Ohba S, Kamekura S, Yamaguchi M, Chung UI, et al. PPARgamma insufficiency enhances osteogenesis through osteoblast formation from bone marrow progenitors. J Clin Invest. 2004;113:846–55.
11. Feige JN, Gelman L, Rossi D, Zoete V, Metivier R, Tudor C, et al. The endocrine disruptor monoethyl-hexyl-phthalate is a selective peroxisome proliferator-activated receptor gamma modulator that promotes adipogenesis. J Biol Chem. 2007;282:19152–66.
12. Kaji H. Interaction between muscle and bone. Journal of Bone Metabolism. 2014;21(1):29–40. 10.11005/jbm.2014.21.1.29.
13. Tanaka K, Matsumoto E, Higashimaki Y, et al. Role of osteoglycin in the linkage between muscle and bone. J Biol Chem. 2012;287:11616–28.
14. Chan CY, Masui O, Krakovska O, Belozerov VE, Voisin S, Ghanny S, et al. Identification of differentially regulated secretome components during skeletal myogenesis. Mol Cell Proteomics. 2011;10:M110.004804.
15. Patel MJ, Liu W, Sykes MC, Ward NE, Risin SA, Risin D, et al. Identification of mechanosensitive genes in osteoblasts by comparative microarray studies using the rotating wall vessel and the random positioning machine. J Cell Biochem. 2007;101:587–99.
16. Zambotti A, Makhluf H, Shen J, Ducy P. Characterization of an osteoblast-specific enhancer element in the CBFA1 gene. J Biol Chem. 2002;277(44):41497–506.
17. Kawaguchi H, Akune T, Yamaguchi M, Ohba S, Ogata N, Chung UI, Kubota N, Terauchi Y, Kadowaki T, Nakamura K. Distinct effects of PPARgamma insufficiency on bone marrow cells, osteoblasts, and osteoclastic cells. J Bone Miner Metab. 2005;23(4):275–9.
18. Meunier P, Aaron J, Edouard C, Vignon G. Osteoporosis and the replacement of cell populations of the marrow by adipose tissue. A quantitative study of 84 iliac bone biopsies. Clin Orthop Relat Res. 1971;80:147–54.
19. Tontonoz P, Hu E, Spiegelman BM. Regulation of adipocyte gene expression and differentiation by peroxisome proliferator activated receptor γ. Curr Opin Genet Dev. 1995;5(5):571–6.
20. Kyllönen L, Haimi S, Mannerström B, Huhtala H, Rajala KM, Skottman H, et al. Effects of different serum conditions on osteogenic differentiation of human adipose stem cells in vitro. Stem Cell Res Ther. 2013;4(1):17.
21. Granchi D, Ochoa G, Leonardi E, Devescovi V, Baglio SR, Osaba L, et al. Gene expression patterns related to osteogenic differentiation of bone marrow-derived mesenchymal stem cells during ex vivo expansion. Tissue Eng Part C Methods. 2009;16:511.

22

The likelihood of total knee arthroplasty following arthroscopic surgery for osteoarthritis

Amelia R. Winter[1], Jamie E. Collins[1,3] and Jeffrey N. Katz[1,2,3,4*]

Abstract

Background: Arthroscopic surgery is a common treatment for knee osteoarthritis (OA), particularly for symptomatic meniscal tear. Many patients with knee OA who have arthroscopies go on to have total knee arthroplasty (TKA). Several individual studies have investigated the interval between knee arthroscopy and TKA. Our objective was to summarize published literature on the risk of TKA following knee arthroscopy, the duration between arthroscopy and TKA, and risk factors for TKA following knee arthroscopy.

Methods: We searched PubMed, Embase, and Web of Science for English language manuscripts reporting TKA following arthroscopy for knee OA. We identified 511 manuscripts, of which 20 met the inclusion criteria and were used for analysis. We compared the cumulative incidence of TKA following arthroscopy in each study arm, stratifying by type of data source (registry vs. clinical), and whether the study was limited to older patients (≥ 50) or those with more severe radiographic OA. We estimated cumulative incidence of TKA following arthroscopy by dividing the number of TKAs among persons who underwent arthroscopy by the number of persons who underwent arthroscopy. Annual incidence was calculated by dividing cumulative incidence by the mean years of follow-up.

Results: Overall, the annual incidence of TKA after arthroscopic surgery for OA was 2.62% (95% CI 1.73–3.51%). We calculated the annual incidence of TKA following arthroscopy in four separate groups defined by data source (registry vs. clinical cohort) and whether the sample was selected for disease progression (either age or OA severity). In unselected registry studies the annual TKA incidence was 1.99% (95% CI 1.03–2.96%), compared to 3.89% (95% CI 0.69–7.09%) in registry studies of older patients. In unselected clinical cohorts the annual incidence was 2.02% (95% CI 0.67–3.36%), while in clinical cohorts with more severe OA the annual incidence was 4.13% (95% CI 1.81–6.44%). The mean and median duration between arthroscopy and TKA (years) were 3.4 and 2.0 years.

Conclusions: Clinicians and patients considering knee arthroscopy should discuss the likelihood of subsequent TKA as they weigh risks and benefits of surgery. Patients who are older or have more severe OA are at particularly high risk of TKA.

Keywords: Osteoarthritis, Total knee arthroplasty, Arthroscopic partial meniscectomy, Arthroscopy

Background

Osteoarthritis (OA) is a debilitating disease, affecting over 40 million people in the United States [1, 2]. Of those affected, approximately 14 million have symptomatic knee OA [3], which presents with pain, loss of knee joint function, and loss of valued activities. In addition, about 90% of those with symptomatic knee OA have meniscal tears (MT) documented on magnetic resonance imaging (MRI) [4]. However, no available treatments modify the structural progression associated with OA. Symptoms are generally managed with conservative therapies (e.g., nonsteroidal anti-inflammatory drugs (NSAIDs), exercise, physical therapy). Patients and their physicians often turn to surgical treatments to address progressive pain and disability, including arthroscopy and total knee arthroplasty (TKA).

Over 600,000 arthroscopic partial meniscectomies (APM) are performed each year in the United States [5],

* Correspondence: jnkatz@partners.org
[1]Orthopaedic and Arthritis Center for Outcomes Research (OrACORe), Department of Orthopedic Surgery, Boston, MA, USA
[2]Division of Rheumatology, Immunology and Allergy, Brigham and Women's Hospital, 60 Fenwood St, Suite 5016, Boston, MA 02115, USA
Full list of author information is available at the end of the article

most commonly on persons over 45 with MT [5, 6]. The benefit of arthroscopic surgery in patients with OA is uncertain and debated. Moseley et al. showed that sham surgery and arthroscopic surgery for OA had similar pain relief and functional improvement up to 2 years post-surgery [7]. Kirkley and colleagues showed that arthroscopy and a conservative exercise regimen had similar symptomatic and functional outcomes in persons with knee OA [8]. With respect to MT in the setting of OA, several trials demonstrated that surgery was not superior to nonoperative therapy or sham surgery in intention to treat analyses [9–12], while one trial showed a benefit for surgery [13]. Thus, arthroscopic surgery is felt to be ineffective for OA per se, while the effectiveness of APM in persons with MT and concomitant OA is debated [14].

Often, people who undergo arthroscopic surgery for osteoarthritis progress to TKA. While some studies suggest that up to 20% of patients undergo TKA within one year of arthroscopy [15], other studies have shown TKA rates under 5% [16]. The various studies of the rate of TKA after arthroscopy have not been summarized, to our knowledge. Such a summary of the risk of TKA following arthroscopy and the duration between arthroscopy and TKA would be helpful for clinicians to better advise patients and their families on appropriate treatments plans. Surgery is expensive – about $2 billion dollars are spent on arthroscopy for OA [17] and over $10 billion dollars are spent on TKAs each year [18]. Therefore, improved knowledge of the risk for TKA following arthroscopy could also lead to better resource allocation for OA.

We performed a systematic review of the literature on the risk of TKA following arthroscopic surgeries for OA. We expected to see older patients and those with more severe OA, progress to TKA more quickly after surgery.

Methods

Definition of search terms

A search by title was performed on PubMed, Embase, and Web of Science using the major search terms: *osteoarthritis, knee; arthroscopy; and arthroplasty* (see Additional file 1: Table S1 for search strings). The search was performed in September 2016 and titles were downloaded to EndNote. One reviewer (ARW) manually screened titles for inclusion and exclusion criteria, arriving at a final list of titles. For these titles, the reviewer assessed abstracts for inclusion and exclusion criteria. For each abstract that was not excluded, the full manuscript was read to determine ultimate inclusion in the final analysis. A second reviewer confirmed that the final selected manuscripts met inclusion criteria.

Inclusion and exclusion criteria

We sought studies investigating the rate of arthroplasty after arthroscopic knee surgery for osteoarthritis. Therefore, inclusion criteria included: English language and human studies on the risk of TKA occurring following arthroscopic procedures for knee OA. Manuscripts were excluded if they were duplicates, written in a language other than English, or conducted on animals. Studies were also excluded if they examined only arthroscopy or arthroplasty rather than the risk of arthroplasty following arthroscopy. Case studies and studies with cohorts of mean age < 40 were also excluded. Confusion regarding inclusion of a study was resolved by consulting with the senior author (JNK).

Data abstraction

From the manuscripts, the reviewer (ARW) extracted the following information (if available): author, year, title, administrative data (e.g., clinical cohort or registry), country, patient selection criteria (e.g. age, KL grade), subgroup information, size of analysis group, mean age, analysis method (e.g., cumulative incidence), duration between arthroscopy and TKA, duration of follow-up, percentage of TKA, and study arm population description. Another reviewer abstracted key data (e.g., country, administrative data, patient selection criteria, follow-up years, analysis group, and total TKA numbers) from the included studies. The results from both abstractions were compared and found to be the same.

Categorization of studies

We examined the cumulative incidence of TKA following knee arthroscopy in specific patient subgroups. These included source of data (administrative data registries vs. clinical cohort studies), OA severity, older age (e.g., selection for population ≥ 50), and country. Some of the clinical cohort studies recruited patients with advanced OA, (i.e., KL grade ≥ 3 or Outerbridge score ≥ 2). We defined these study arms as "Clinical Cohort – More Severe OA." One study (Lyu et al., 2015) was included among the "Clinical Cohort – More Severe OA" group as its patient population was over 75% KL grade 3 or higher. Some registry studies were restricted to subjects with age greater than 50. We referred to these as "Registry – Older Age." We created a final categorization combining the source of data and selection criteria: "Registry – Unselected," "Registry – Older Age," "Clinical Cohort – Unselected," and "Clinical Cohort – More Severe OA." For countries, we combined England and Scotland as "U.K."

Quality assessment

We used the Quality Assessment Tool for Observational Cohort and Cross-Sectional Studies developed by investigators at the National Heartt, Lung and Blood Intitute (NHLBI), based upon work done at the Agency for Health Care Research and Quality. (https://www.nhlbi.nih.gov/health-pro/guidelines/in-develop/cardiovascular-risk-reduction/tools/cohort) [19]. This measure includes 14 items relevant to the quality of cohort studies, with emphasis on explicit specification of sample characteristics, exposures, primary outcomes and potential confounders. Two authors performed the assessment independently and resolved any disagreements.

Analyses

For studies that did not provide cumulative incidence data, we calculated cumulative incidence using the number of TKAs divided by the number of arthroscopic patients included for follow-up analysis. We first examined the association between the type of data source – registry vs. cohort – and TKA rates. Then, we evaluated the association between study category ("Registry – Unselected," "Registry – Older Age," "Clinical Cohort – Unselected," and "Clinical Cohort – More Severe OA," as described above) and annual incidence. In secondary analyses, we evaluated the difference between TKA annual incidence in unselected study arms (clinical and registry) vs. selected study arms, regardless of registry status. We compared studies in which mean age of the study was >65 to those with mean age < 65.

We divided cumulative incidence of TKA by mean years of follow-up to obtain an annual incidence estimate. We computed exact confidence intervals for each yearly incidence value. We used a logistic random-effects model to create an overall combined estimate of annual TKA incidence across all studies and to evaluate the effect of study-level characteristics on TKA incidence. This approach allows for studies with zero cells (i.e., 0% incidence rate) without requiring an ad-hoc adjustment [20]. All analyses were conducted using SAS 9.4 (SAS Institute, Cary NC).

Results

Five hundred eleven unique articles were found using our search terms and three search engines. After screening the titles, we were left with 328 articles whose abstracts were subsequently reviewed. Over half of the articles excluded did not have arthroscopic surgery before TKA (36%) or did not report TKA (24%). Fifty-five articles underwent full article review. Thirty-five of the manuscripts were excluded from our analysis: 11 were not written in English, 2 did not report on arthroscopic procedures before TKA, 3 did not report on TKA, and 19 were excluded for other reasons, such as mixed cohort (e.g., OA and post-traumatic arthritis), secondary sources, or insufficient data on methodology.

These exclusions left 20 articles for the analysis (Fig. 1). The 20 studies contained 28 unique study arms (Table 1). The 28 study arms were reported from eight countries. The U.S.A. accounted for 15 of the 28, the U.K. for 5, Canada for 3, and Australia, Belgium, Italy, South Korea, and Taiwan for one each. The quality assessment documented relatively little variability in quality. Essentially all the studies stated the research question clearly, specified the population and defined the exposure and outcome explicitly. Only one study provided a power calculation. Rates of participation among eligible subject and rates of follow up were generally high, particularly for administrative data studies in which participation and follow-up rates are typically 100%. Some of the quality items did not apply to the studies we reviewed because all subjects in our studies were 'exposed' (had arthroscopy).

Overall, the yearly incidence for TKA after arthroscopic surgery for OA was 2.62% (95% CI 1.73–3.51%). The mean and median duration between arthroscopy and TKA (years) were 3.4 and 2.0 years. From our 28 study arms, we identified sixteen clinical cohorts and twelve registry samples. The clinical cohort studies had a yearly TKA incidence of 2.94% (95% CI 1.54–4.33%), compared to the registry studies, which had an incidence of 2.36% (95% CI 1.26–3.46%) (p = 0.5048). We examined separately the risk of TKA in four distinct subgroups: "Registry – Unselected," "Registry – Older Age," "Clinical Cohort – Unselected," and "Clinical Cohort – More Severe OA." The four subgroups are shown in Fig. 2.

Registry - unselected

A total of nine study arms were unselected registries, with a median of 6972 (range 842–159,975) patients per study arm (Table 1). Of these, the average yearly incidence for TKA was 1.99% (95% CI 1.03–2.96%) (Fig. 2).

Registry – Older age

A total of three study arms were registries using data from patients ≥50 years old, with a median of 6212 (range 3033–40,804) patients per study arm (Table 1). Of these studies, the average yearly incidence for TKA was 3.89% (95% CI 0.69–7.09%) (Fig. 2).

Clinical cohort – Unselected

A total of seven study arms were unselected clinical cohorts, with a median of 42 (range 8–183) patients per study arm (Table 1). Of these studies, the average yearly incidence for TKA was 2.02% (95% CI 0.67–3.36%) (Fig. 2).

Clinical cohort – More severe OA

A total of nine study arms were clinical cohorts selecting for patients with more severe OA on the basis of KL grade or Outerbridge score, with a median of 69 (range 68–844) patients per study arm (Table 1). Of these studies, the average yearly incidence for TKA was 4.13% (95% CI 1.81–6.44%) (Fig. 2).

Comparisons: Age and OA severity

We evaluated the association between TKA incidence and study inclusion criteria using a logistic random-effects model. We found that selected studies - those

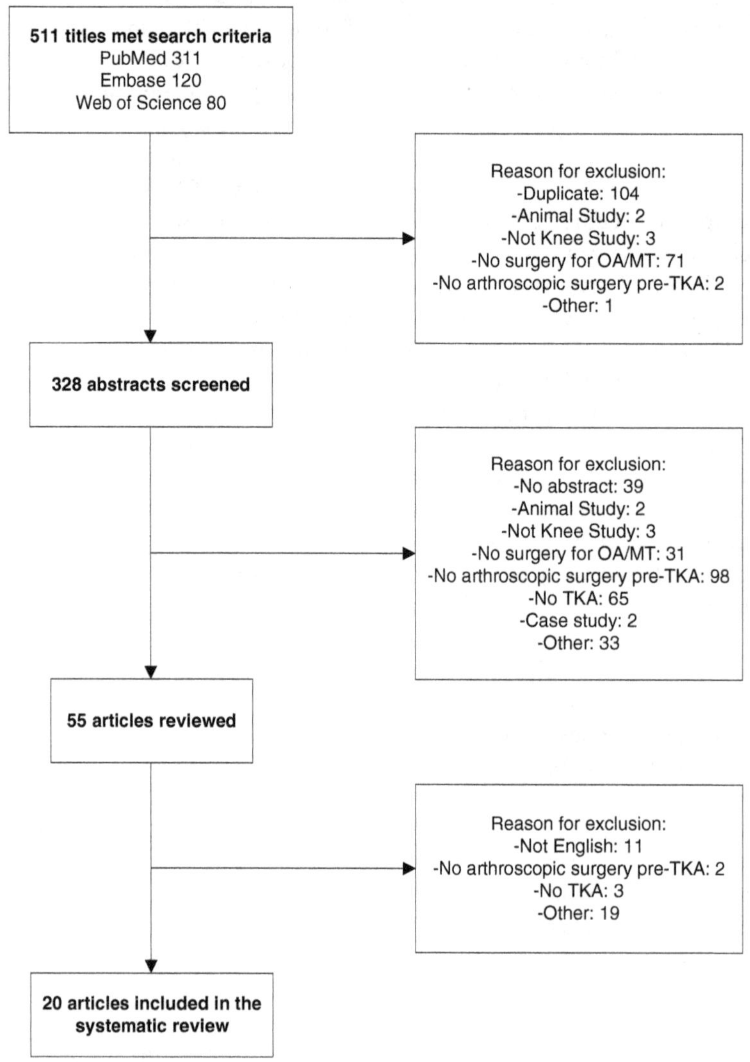

Fig. 1 Search and selection process

that selected subjects based on OA severity or age - were twice as likely to undergo TKA compared to unselected studies (4.05% compared to 2.00%; p = 0.0243). Studies of subject with a mean age of less than 65 had a yearly incidence of 1.87% (95% CI 1.16–2.57%) compared to 5.13% (95% CI 2.61–7.64%) for those with mean age over 65. This difference was statistically significant (p = 0.0027).

Discussion

We evaluated published literature on the risk of TKA in patients undergoing knee arthroscopy. A concern about the use of arthroscopic surgery in the setting of OA and OA with meniscal tear is that APM may lead to more rapid OA progression, leading to TKA more quickly [1, 15]. We found that on average the risk of TKA following arthroscopy was about 2% per year and that the mean and medican duration between arthroscopy and TKA were 3.4 and 2.0 years respectively. Further, study arms of patients who were older or had more advanced radiographic OA at the time of arthroscopy had two-fold higher risk of TKA than unselected study arms. These findings should be viewed in the context of other documented risk factors for OA progression including older age, female gender, varus and valgus malalignment and bone marrow lesions, among others [21].

Our findings are consistent with studies showing that OA severity and age are associated with TKA [22–32]. Indeed, surgeons may be reluctant to offer TKA to younger patients, because they face a risk of a revision TKA. Advanced OA is a typical indication for TKA, as embodied in guidelines such as those of the American Academy of Orthopaedic Surgeons [33].

Our study must be interpreted in the context of several limitations. The clinical cohort data provided insight into the KL grades and Outerbridge scores of patients

Table 1 Characteristics of included studies

			Author and Year	Country	Follow-Up (Years)	Mean Duration (years)	Analysis Group	Total TKA	Annual Incidence (%)	Lower 95% CI	Upper 95% CI
Clinical Cohort	Selected for More Severe OA	KL ≥ 3	Bernard et al. (2004) [22]	U.K.	5	Unknown	100	11	2.20%	1.10%	3.90%
		KL = 4	Bin et al. (2008) [34]	South Korea	4	4	68	4	1.36%	0.37%	3.43%
		Outerbridge ≥2	Koyonos et al. (2009)[a] [16]	U.S.A.	1	0.5	30	1	3.33%	0.08%	17.22%
						0	29	0	0.00%	0.00%	11.94%
		KL ≥ 3	Lyu et al. (2015) [35]	Taiwan	1	1	844	116	13.74%	11.49%	16.25%
		KL = 4	Pearse and Craig (2003) [36]	U.K.	4	4	126	39	7.14%	5.13%	9.64%
		KL ≥ 3	Rand et al. (1985) [37]	U.S.A.	2	0.5	87	2	1.15%	0.14%	4.09%
		Outerbridge ≥2	Skedros et al. (2014) [30]	U.S.A.	3	3	42	11	8.73%	4.44%	15.08%
		KL ≥ 3	Steadman et al. (2013) [31]	U.S.A.	10	4.4	69	43	6.23%	4.55%	8.30%
	Unselected					2	8	0	0.00%	0.00%	8.81%
			Jackson et al. (2003)[a] [25]	U.S.A.	5		32	0	0.00%	0.00%	2.28%
							39	3	1.54%	0.32%	4.43%
							42	12	5.71%	2.99%	9.77%
			McGinley et al. (1999) [27]	U.S.A.	13	7	91	30	2.50%	1.69%	3.55%
			Raaijmaakers et al. (2010) [28]	Belgium	3	1	183	40	6.83%	4.92%	9.18%
			Sansone et al. (2015) [29]	Italy	20	13.3	75	12	0.80%	0.41%	1.39%
Registry	Selected for Older Age	Age > 60	Dearing et al. (2010) [38]	U.K.	9	6	3033	800	2.93%	2.73%	3.14%
		Age > 65	Johanson et al. (2011) [26]	U.S.A.	10	9	40,804	13,261	3.25%	3.20%	3.30%
		Age > 50	Wai et al. (2002) [32]	Canada	3	3	6212	1146	6.15%	5.81%	6.50%
	Unselected		Adelani et al. (2016)[a] [39]	U.S.A.	4	2	6972	266	0.95%	0.84%	1.07%
							10,645	496	1.16%	1.06%	1.27%
			Fedorka et al. (2014) [23]	U.S.A.	5	Unknown	159,975	8319	1.04%	1.02%	1.06%
			Harris et al. (2013) [40]	Australia	8	2	121,115	9110	0.94%	0.92%	0.96%
				U.K 1993		Unknown	6158	985	3.20%	3.00%	3.40%
			Hawker et al. (2008)[a] [24]	UK 1997	5		9048	1728	3.82%	3.64%	4.00%
				Canada 1993			3803	745	3.92%	3.65%	4.20%
				Canada 1997			3425	712	4.16%	3.86%	4.47%
			Zikria et al. (2016) [41]	U.S.A.	7	Unknown	842	131	2.22%	1.86%	2.63%

[a]Studies contain multiple unique study arms, which were separated for our analysis; Jackson rows: Severity stages I, II, III, IV

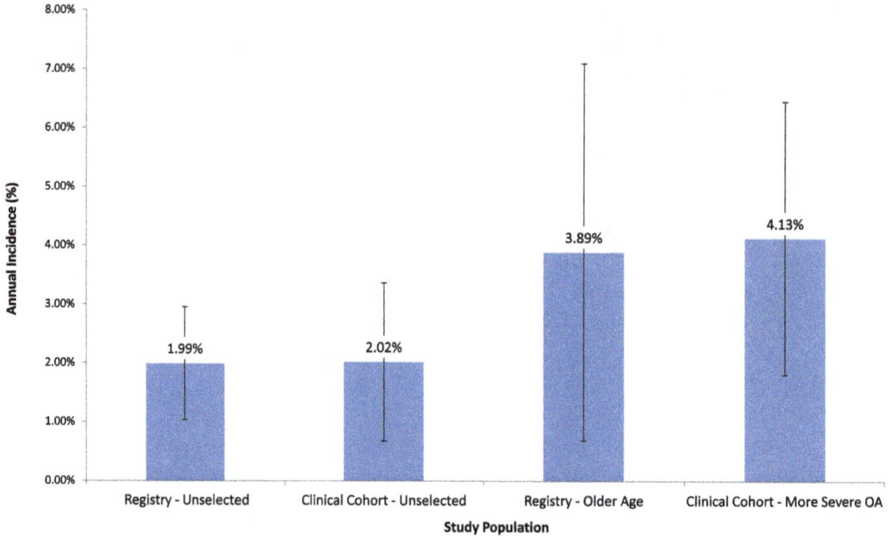

Fig. 2 Mean Annual Incidence of Registry – Unselected, Clinical Cohort – Unselected, Registry – Older Age, and Clinical Cohort – More Severe OA. Each bar represents the estimated yearly incidence of TKA from the logisitc random effects model. The vertical lines represent the 95% confidence intervals

whereas registry data included age but no information on OA severity nor on the details of surgery. The component studies did not perform analyses of subgroups that might be prognostically distinct, such as athletes and non-athletes, or males and females. Similarly, over half of the countries contributed just one cohort. This precludes meaningful analysis of between-country differences. While we performed replicate abstractions of all papers we did not repeat the screening of titles and abstracts in duplicate, creating the theoretical risk of our missing an eligible paper. As reflected in our quality assessment, the studies consistently defined the exposure and outcome explicitly. Since most of the larger studies used administrative data, the follow-up rates were generally 100%. We note as well that some patients with a medical 'need' for TKA (symptomatic, advanced OA) may not have received the procedure because of their own preferences or the practice styles of their physicians or still other reasons. When TKA is used as a health outcome, the role of these patient, physician and health system factors may attenuate the risk associated with specific variables such as prior arthroscopic surgery.

To the best of our knowledge, this is the first systematic review to analyze the yearly TKA incidence rate for those having undergone arthroscopic surgery for knee OA. Quality assessment of the studies generally reflected consistent specification of exposures, outcomes, and study samples and high rates of participation and follow-up. The findings suggest that OA patients undergoing arthroscopy and their physicians should anticipate an annual rate of TKA on the order of 2%, with higher rates among older patients and those with more advanced OA. These findings should be shared with patients when clinicians discuss the advantages and drawbacks of arthroscopy.

Conclusion

Clinicians and patients considering knee arthroscopy should discuss the likelihood of subsequent TKA as they weigh risks and benefits of surgery. Patients who are older or have more severe OA are at particularly high risk of TKA.

Abbreviations

KL: Kellgren-Lawrence; MRI: Magnetic resonance imaging; MT: Meniscal tear; NSAIDs: Nonsteroidal anti-inflammatory drugs; OA: Osteoarthritis; tka: Total knee arthroplasty

Acknowledgements

Not applicable.

Funding

National Institute of Arthritis, Musculoskeletal and Skin Diseases (National Institutes of Health) R01 AR 055557.

Authors' contributions

ARW and JNK developed final question and design of systematic review. ARW searched for and analyzed the included manuscripts, and was a major contributor to writing the manuscript. JEC performed the analysis in SAS, discussed the interpretation with the other authors and critically reviewed the manuscript. JNK consulted on final included manuscripts. All authors read, edited, and approved the final manuscript.

Competing interests

The authors declare they have no competing interests.

Author details
[1]Orthopaedic and Arthritis Center for Outcomes Research (OrACORe), Department of Orthopedic Surgery, Boston, MA, USA. [2]Division of Rheumatology, Immunology and Allergy, Brigham and Women's Hospital, 60 Fenwood St, Suite 5016, Boston, MA 02115, USA. [3]Harvard Medical School, Boston, MA, USA. [4]Departments of Epidemiology and Environmental Health, Harvard T. H. Chan School of Public Health, Boston, MA, USA.

References

1. Choong PF, Dowsey MM. Update in surgery for osteoarthritis of the knee. *Int J Rheum Dis*. 2011;14(2):167–74.
2. Dunlop DD, Manheim LM, Yelin EH, Song J, Chang RW. The costs of arthritis. *Arthritis Rheum*. 2003;49(1):101–13.
3. Deshpande BR, Katz JN, Solomon DH, Yelin EH, Hunter DJ, Messier SP, Suter LG, Losina E. Number of persons with symptomatic knee osteoarthritis in the US: impact of race and ethnicity, age, sex, and obesity. *Arthritis Care Res*. 2016;68(12):1743–50.
4. Bhattacharyya T, Gale D, Dewire P, Totterman S, Gale ME, McLaughlin S, Einhorn TA, Felson DT. The clinical importance of meniscal tears demonstrated by magnetic resonance imaging in osteoarthritis of the knee. *J Bone Joint Surg Am*. 2003;85-A(1):4–9.
5. Cullen KA, Hall MJ, Golosinskiy A. Ambulatory surgery in the United States. *Natl Health Stat Rep*. 2006;2009(11):1–25.
6. Kim S, Bosque J, Meehan JP, Jamali A, Marder R. Increase in outpatient knee arthroscopy in the United States: a comparison of National Surveys of Ambulatory Surgery, 1996 and 2006. *J Bone Joint Surg Am*. 2011;93(11):994–1000.
7. Moseley JB, O'Malley K, Petersen NJ, Menke TJ, Brody BA, Kuykendall DH, Hollingsworth JC, Ashton CM, Wray NP. A controlled trial of arthroscopic surgery for osteoarthritis of the knee. *N Engl J Med*. 2002;347(2):81–8.
8. Kirkley A, Birmingham TB, Litchfield RB, Giffin JR, Willits KR, Wong CJ, Feagan BG, Donner A, Griffin SH, D'Ascanio LM, et al. A randomized trial of arthroscopic surgery for osteoarthritis of the knee. *N Engl J Med*. 2008; 359(11):1097–107.
9. Herrlin SV, Wange PO, Lapidus G, Hallander M, Werner S, Weidenhielm L. Is arthroscopic surgery beneficial in treating non-traumatic, degenerative medial meniscal tears? A five year follow-up. *Knee Surg Sports Traumatol Arthrosc*. 2013;21(2):358–64.
10. Katz JN, Brophy RH, Chaisson CE, de Chaves L, Cole BJ, Dahm DL, Donnell-Fink LA, Guermazi A, Haas AK, Jones MH, et al. Surgery versus physical therapy for a meniscal tear and osteoarthritis. *N Engl J Med*. 2013;368(18):1675–84.
11. Sihvonen R, Paavola M, Malmivaara A, Itala A, Joukainen A, Nurmi H, Kalske J, Jarvinen TL. Arthroscopic partial meniscectomy versus sham surgery for a degenerative meniscal tear. *N Engl J Med*. 2013;369(26):2515–24.
12. Yim JH, Seon JK, Song EK, Choi JI, Kim MC, Lee KB, Seo HY. A comparative study of meniscectomy and nonoperative treatment for degenerative horizontal tears of the medial meniscus. *Am J Sports Med*. 2013;41(7):1565–70.
13. Gauffin H, Tagesson S, Meunier A, Magnusson H, Kvist J. Knee arthroscopic surgery is beneficial to middle-aged patients with meniscal symptoms: a prospective, randomised, single-blinded study. *Osteoarthr Cartil*. 2014;22(11): 1808–16.
14. Katz JN, Jones MH. Treatment of Meniscal Tear: the more we learn, the less we knowtreatment of meniscal tear: the more we learn, the less we know. *Ann Intern Med*. 2016,164(7):503–4.
15. Dervin GF, Stiell IG, Rody K, Grabowski J. Effect of arthroscopic debridement for osteoarthritis of the knee on health-related quality of life. *J Bone Joint Surg Am*. 2003;85-A(1):10–9.
16. Koyonos L, Yanke AB, McNickle AG, Kirk SS, Kang RW, Lewis PB, Cole BJ. A randomized, prospective, double-blind study to investigate the effectiveness of adding DepoMedrol to a local anesthetic injection in postmeniscectomy patients with osteoarthritis of the knee. *Am J Sports Med*. 2009;37(6):1077–82.
17. Losina E, Dervan EE, Paltiel AD, Dong Y, Wright RJ, Spindler KP, Mandl LA, Jones MH, Marx RG, Safran-Norton CE, et al. Defining the value of future research to identify the preferred treatment of meniscal tear in the presence of knee osteoarthritis. *PLoS One*. 2015;10(6):e0130256.
18. Healthcare Cost and Utilization Project. Nationwide Inpatient Sample. Rockville: Agency for Healthcare Research and Quality; 2014.
19. Quality Assessment Tool for Observational Cohort and Cross-Sectional Studies. [https://www.nhlbi.nih.gov/health-pro/guidelines/in-develop/cardiovascular-risk-reduction/tools/cohort]
20. Hamza TH, van Houwelingen HC, Stijnen T. The binomial distribution of meta-analysis was preferred to model within-study variability. *J Clin Epidemiol*. 2008;61(1):41–51.
21. Hunter DJ. Risk stratification for knee osteoarthritis progression: a narrative review. *Osteoarthr Cartil*. 2009;17(11):1402–7.
22. Bernard J, Lemon M, Patterson MH. Arthroscopic washout of the knee–a 5-year survival analysis. *Knee*. 2004;11(3):233–5.
23. Fedorka CJ, Cerynik DL, Tauberg B, Toossi N, Johanson NA. The relationship between knee arthroscopy and arthroplasty in patients under 65 years of age. *J Arthroplast*. 2014;29(2):335–8.
24. Hawker G, Guan J, Judge A, Dieppe P. Knee arthroscopy in England and Ontario: patterns of use, changes over time, and relationship to total knee replacement. *J Bone Joint Surg Am*. 2008;90(11):2337–45.
25. Jackson RW, Dieterichs C. The results of arthroscopic lavage and debridement of osteoarthritic knees based on the severity of degeneration: a 4- to 6-year symptomatic follow-up. *Arthroscopy*. 2003;19(1):13–20.
26. Johanson NA, Kleinbart FA, Cerynik DL, Brey JM, Ong KL, Kurtz SM. Temporal relationship between knee arthroscopy and arthroplasty. a quality measure for joint care? *J Arthroplast*. 2011;26(2):187–91.
27. McGinley BJ, Cushner FD, Scott WN: Debridement arthroscopy. 10-year followup. *Clin Orthop Relat Res* 1999(367):190-194.
28. Raaijmaakers M, Vanlauwe J, Vandenneucker H, Dujardin J, Bellemans J. Arthroscopy of the knee in elderly patients: cartilage lesions and their influence on short term outcome. A retrospective follow-up of 183 patients. *Acta Orthop Belg*. 2010;76(1):79–85.
29. Sansone V, de Girolamo L, Pascale W, Melato M, Pascale V. Long-term results of abrasion arthroplasty for full-thickness cartilage lesions of the medial femoral condyle. *Arthroscopy*. 2015;31(3):396–403.
30. Skedros JG, Knight AN, Thomas SC, Paluso AM, Bertin KC. Dilemma of high rate of conversion from knee arthroscopy to total knee arthroplasty. *Am J Orthop (Belle Mead NJ)*. 2014;43(7):E153–8.
31. Steadman JR, Briggs KK, Matheny LM, Ellis HB. Ten-year survivorship after knee arthroscopy in patients with Kellgren-Lawrence grade 3 and grade 4 osteoarthritis of the knee. *Arthroscopy*. 2013;29(2):220–5.
32. Wai EK, Kreder HJ, Williams JI. Arthroscopic débridement of the knee for osteoarthritis in patients fifty years of age or older: Utilization and outcomes in the province of Ontario. *Journal of Bone and Joint Surgery - Series A*. 2002; 84(1):17–22+Adv26.
33. Total Knee Replacement. American Academy of Orthopaedic Surgeons. 2015. http://orthoinfo.aaos.org/topic.cfm?topic=a00389. Accessed 4 April 2017.
34. Bin SI, Lee SH, Kim CW, Kim TH, Lee DH. Results of arthroscopic medial meniscectomy in patients with grade IV osteoarthritis of the medial compartment. *Arthroscopy*. 2008;24(3):264–8.
35. Lyu SR. Knee health promotion option for knee osteoarthritis: A preliminary report of a concept of multidisciplinary management. *Healthy Aging Research*. 2015;4
36. Pearse EO, Craig DM. Partial meniscectomy in the presence of severe osteoarthritis does not hasten the symptomatic progression of osteoarthritis. *Arthroscopy*. 2003;19(9):963–8.
37. Rand JA. Arthroscopic management of degenerative meniscus tears in patients with degenerative arthritis. *Arthroscopy*. 1985;1(4):253–8.
38. Dearing J, Brenkel IJ. Incidence of knee arthroscopy in patients over 60 years of age in Scotland. *The surgeon : journal of the Royal Colleges of Surgeons of Edinburgh and Ireland*. 2010;8(3):144–50.
39. Adelani MA, Harris AHS, Bowe TR, Giori NJ. Arthroscopy for Knee Osteoarthritis Has Not Decreased After a Clinical Trial. *Clin Orthop Relat Res*. 2016;474(2):489–94.
40. Harris IA, Madan NS, Naylor JM, Chong S, Mittal R, Jalaludin BB. Trends in knee arthroscopy and subsequent arthroplasty in an Australian population: a retrospective cohort study. *BMC Musculoskelet Disord*. 2013;14:143.
41. Zikria B, Hafezi-Nejad N, Wilckens J, Ficke JR, Demehri S. Determinants of knee replacement in subjects with a history of arthroscopy: data from the osteoarthritis initiative. *European journal of orthopaedic surgery & traumatology : orthopedie traumatologie*. 2016;26(6):665–70.

Permissions

All chapters in this book were first published in BMC MD, by BioMed Central; hereby published with permission under the Creative Commons Attribution License or equivalent. Every chapter published in this book has been scrutinized by our experts. Their significance has been extensively debated. The topics covered herein carry significant findings which will fuel the growth of the discipline. They may even be implemented as practical applications or may be referred to as a beginning point for another development.

The contributors of this book come from diverse backgrounds, making this book a truly international effort. This book will bring forth new frontiers with its revolutionizing research information and detailed analysis of the nascent developments around the world.

We would like to thank all the contributing authors for lending their expertise to make the book truly unique. They have played a crucial role in the development of this book. Without their invaluable contributions this book wouldn't have been possible. They have made vital efforts to compile up to date information on the varied aspects of this subject to make this book a valuable addition to the collection of many professionals and students.

This book was conceptualized with the vision of imparting up-to-date information and advanced data in this field. To ensure the same, a matchless editorial board was set up. Every individual on the board went through rigorous rounds of assessment to prove their worth. After which they invested a large part of their time researching and compiling the most relevant data for our readers.

The editorial board has been involved in producing this book since its inception. They have spent rigorous hours researching and exploring the diverse topics which have resulted in the successful publishing of this book. They have passed on their knowledge of decades through this book. To expedite this challenging task, the publisher supported the team at every step. A small team of assistant editors was also appointed to further simplify the editing procedure and attain best results for the readers.

Apart from the editorial board, the designing team has also invested a significant amount of their time in understanding the subject and creating the most relevant covers. They scrutinized every image to scout for the most suitable representation of the subject and create an appropriate cover for the book.

The publishing team has been an ardent support to the editorial, designing and production team. Their endless efforts to recruit the best for this project, has resulted in the accomplishment of this book. They are a veteran in the field of academics and their pool of knowledge is as vast as their experience in printing. Their expertise and guidance has proved useful at every step. Their uncompromising quality standards have made this book an exceptional effort. Their encouragement from time to time has been an inspiration for everyone.

The publisher and the editorial board hope that this book will prove to be a valuable piece of knowledge for researchers, students, practitioners and scholars across the globe.

List of Contributors

Ellen M. H. Selten, Johanna E. Vriezekolk and Cornelia H. M. van den Ende
Department of Rheumatology, Sint Maartenskliniek, Sint Maartenskliniek, GM, Nijmegen, The Netherlands

Henk J. Schers
Department of Primary and Community Care, Radboud University Nijmegen Medical Center, Nijmegen, The Netherlands

Marc W. Nijhof
Department of Orthopedics, Sint Maartenskliniek, Nijmegen, The Netherlands

Willemijn H. van der Laan
Department of Rheumatology, Sint Maartenskliniek, Woerden, The Netherlands

Roelien G. van der Meulen-Dilling
Physical Therapy and Manual Therapy Velperweg Partnership, Arnhem, The Netherlands

Rinie Geenen
Department of Psychology, Utrecht University, Utrecht, The Netherlands

Masayuki Miyagi, Gen Inoue, Kentaro Uchida and Masashi Takaso
Department of Orthopaedic Surgery, Kitasato University, School of Medicine, 1-15-1, Kitasato, Minami-ku, Sagamihara city, Kanagawa 252-0374, Japan

Tetsuhiro Ishikawa, Hiroto Kamoda, Miyako Suzuki, Yoshihiro Sakuma, Yasuhiro Oikawa, Sumihisa Orita, Kazuhisa Takahashi and Seiji Ohtori
Department of Orthopaedic Surgery, Graduate School of Medicine, Chiba University, Chiba, Japan

Chang Yong Suh, Yoon Jae Lee, Joon-Shik Shin, Jinho Lee, Wonil Koh and In-Hyuk Ha
Jaseng Spine and Joint Research Institute, Jaseng Medical Foundation, 858 Eonju-ro, Gangnam-gu, Seoul, Republic of Korea

Me-riong Kim
Department of Applied Korean Medicine, College of Korean Medicine, Graduate School, Kyung Hee University, Dongdaemun-gu, Seoul, Republic of Korea

Yun-Yeop Cha
Department of Rehabilitation Medicine of Korean Medicine, College of Korean Medicine, Sangji University, Wonju-si, Gangwon-do, Republic of Korea

Byung-Cheul Shin and Eui-Hyoung Hwang
Spine & Joint Center, Pusan National University Korean Medicine Hospital, Yangsan-si, Gyeongsangnam-do, Republic of Korea
Department of Korean Rehabilitation Medicine, School of Korean Medicine, Pusan National University, Yangsan-si, Gyeongsangnam-do, Republic of Korea

Kristin Suhr
Prevention Sciences, Rollins School of Public Health, Emory University, Atlanta, GA, USA

Mia Kim
Department of Cardiovascular and Neurological Diseases (Stroke Center), College of Korean Medicine, Kyung Hee University, Seoul, Republic of Korea

Zuogang Xiong, Jiulong Zhang, Yuyou Qiu, Ting Hua and Guangyu Tang
Department of Radiology, Shanghai Tenth People's Hospital, Tongji University School of Medicine, 301 Middle Yanchang Road, Shanghai 200072, China

Jingqi Zhu
Department of Radiology, Shanghai Tenth People's Hospital, Tongji University School of Medicine, 301 Middle Yanchang Road, Shanghai 200072, China
Department of Radiology, East Hospital, Tongji University School of Medicine, Shanghai 200120, China

Takahiro Makino, Yusuke Sakai, Masafumi Kashii, Shota Takenaka, Hideki Yoshikawa and Takashi Kaito
Department of Orthopaedic Surgery, Osaka University Graduate School of Medicine, 2-2, Yamadaoka, Suita, Osaka 565-0871, Japan

Kazuomi Sugamoto
Department of Orthopedic Biomaterial Science, Osaka University Graduate School of Medicine, 2-2, Yamadaoka, Suita, Osaka 565-0871, Japan

Shinji Tanishima and Hideki Nagashima
Department of Orthopedic Surgery, Faculty of Medicine, Tottori University, 36-1 Nishi-cho, Yonago, Tottori 683-8504, Japan

Chika Tanimura
School of Health Science, Tottori University Faculty of Medicine, 86 Nishi-cho, Yonago, Tottori 683-8503, Japan

Hiroshi Hagino
School of Health Science, Tottori University Faculty of Medicine, 86 Nishi-cho, Yonago, Tottori 683-8503, Japan
Rehabilitation Division, Tottori University Hospital, 36-1 Nishi-cho, Yonago, Tottori 683-8504, Japan

Hiromi Matsumoto
Rehabilitation Division, Tottori University Hospital, 36-1 Nishi-cho, Yonago, Tottori 683-8504, Japan

Martin Berli, Lazaros Vlachopoulos, Sabra Leupi, Thomas Böni and Charlotte Baltin
Department of Orthopedics, Balgrist University Hospital, University of Zurich, Forchstrasse 340, -8008 Zurich, CH, Switzerland

Liang Chen and Jun Zhong
Department of Orthopedics, Renmin Hospital of Wuhan University, 9 Zhangzhidong Street, Wuhan, Hubei 430060, People's Republic of China

Xianglei Wu
Laboratory of Immunology, University of Lorraine, Avenue du Morvan, 54511 Vandoeuvre lès Nancy, Nancy, France

Dongqing Li
Department of Microbiology, School of Basic Medical Science, Wuhan University, 185 Donghu Road, Wuhan, Hubei 430071, People's Republic of China

Dawei Liang, Jian Sun and Pengcui Li
Department of Orthopaedics, The Second Hospital of Shanxi Medical University, Taiyuan, China

Lei Wei
Department of Orthopedics, Renmin Hospital of Wuhan University, 9 Zhangzhidong Street, Wuhan, Hubei 430060, People's Republic of China
Department of Orthopaedics, Warren Alpert Medical School of Brown University and Rhode Island Hospital, Providence, RI, USA

Fangyuan Wei and Jianzhong Zhang
Foot and Ankle Orthopaedic Surgery Center, Beijing Tongren Hospital, Beijing, China

Yingke Xu
School of Community Health Science, Nevada Institute of Personalized Medicine, University of Nevada, Las Vegas, Nevada, USA

Xianwen Shang and Jin Deng
Department of Orthopaedics, Affiliated Hospital of Guizhou Medical University, Guiyang, China

Ting Zhao
Department of Orthopaedics, Warren Alpert Medical School of Brown University and Rhode Island Hospital, Providence, RI, USA

Takako Momose, Yutaka Inaba, Hyonmin Choe, Naomi Kobayashi, Taro Tezuka and Tomoyuki Saito
Department of Orthopaedic Surgery, Yokohama City University, 3-9 Fukuura, Kanazawa-ku, Yokohama, Japan

A. Guermazi, M. D. Crema and F. W. Roemer
Department of Radiology, Quantitative Imaging Center, Boston University School of Medicine, 820 Harrison Avenue, FGH Building, 3rd Floor, Boston, MA, USA

G. Kalsi, R. O. Copeland, A. Orlando and M. J. Noh
TissueGene, Rockville, MD, USA

J. Niu
Baylor College of Medicine, Houston, TX, USA

David M. Spranz, Hendrik Bruttel, Sebastian I. Wolf, Felix Zeifang and Michael W. Maier
Clinic for Orthopedics and Trauma Surgery, Heidelberg University Hospital, Schlierbacher Landstraße 200a, D-69118 Heidelberg, Germany

Alison Porter-Armstrong, Brendan Bunting and Sarah Howes
Centre for Health and Rehabilitation Technologies, Institute of Nursing and Health, School of Health sciences, Ulster University, Shore Road, Newtownabbey, Co Antrim BT37 0QB, UK

Joanne Marley
Centre for Health and Rehabilitation Technologies, Institute of Nursing and Health, School of Health Belfast Health and Social Care Trust, Chronic Pain Service, Belfast City Hospital, 51 Lisburn Road, Belfast BT9 7AB, UK

Suzanne M. McDonough
Centre for Health and Rehabilitation Technologies, Institute of Nursing and Health, School of Health Sciences, Ulster University, Shore Road, Newtownabbey, Co Antrim BT37 0QB, UK
UKCRC Centre of Excellence for Public Health (Northern Ireland), Centre for Public Health, School of Medicine, Dentistry and Biomedical Sciences, Queens University Belfast Room 02020, Institute of Clinical Science B, Royal Victoria Hospital, Grosvenor Road, Belfast, BT 12 6BJ, UK
Honorary Research Professor, School of Physiotherapy, University of Otago, Dunedin, New Zealand

Mark A. Tully
Centre for Public Health, Queens University Belfast, Royal Victoria Hospital, Grosvenor Road, Belfast BT12 6BA, UK
UKCRC Centre of Excellence for Public Health (Northern Ireland), Centre for Public Health, School of Medicine, Dentistry and Biomedical Sciences, Queens University Belfast Room 02020, Institute of Clinical Science B, Royal Victoria Hospital, Grosvenor Road, Belfast, BT 12 6BJ, UK

John O'Hanlon
Belfast Health and Social Care Trust, Chronic Pain Service, Belfast City Hospital, 51 Lisburn Road, Belfast BT9 7AB, UK

Lou Atkins
Centre for Behaviour Change, University College London, 1-9 Torrington Place, London, UK

Gernot Lang, Kaywan Izadpanah, Eva Johanna Kubosch, Dirk Maier and Norbert Südkamp
Department of Orthopedics and Trauma Surgery, Medical Center - Albert-Ludwigs-University of Freiburg, Faculty of Medicine, Albert-Ludwigs-University of Freiburg, Hugstetter Strasse 55, 79106 Freiburg, Germany

Peter Ogon
Department of Orthopedics and Trauma Surgery, Medical Center - Albert-Ludwigs-University of Freiburg, Faculty of Medicine, Albert-Ludwigs-University of Freiburg, Hugstetter Strasse 55, 79106 Freiburg, Germany
Center of Orthopedic Sports Medicine Freiburg, Breisacher Strasse 84, 79110 Freiburg, Germany

Nicolo Martinelli, Alberto Bianchi, Gloria Casaroli and Fabio Galbusera
IRCCS Istituto Ortopedico Galeazzi, Milan, Italy

Silvia Baretta, Jenny Pagano and Tomaso Villa
IRCCS Istituto Ortopedico Galeazzi, Milan, Italy
Laboratory of Biological Structure Mechanics (LaBS), Department of Chemistry, Materials and Chemical Engineering "Giulio Natta, Politecnico di Milano, 20133 Milan, Italy

Stephen Kelly
Barts Health NHS Trust, London, UK

Brian Davidson and Stephan Gadola
University Hospital Southampton NHS Foundation Trust, Southampton, UK

Sarah Keidel
Abbvie Limited, Maidenhead, UK

Claire Gorman and Piero Reynolds
Homerton University Hospital NHS Foundation Trust, London, UK

Gary Meenagh
Antrim Area Hospital, Antrim, Northern Ireland, UK

Ann Kristin Hansen
Department of Orthopaedic Surgery, University Hospital of North Norway, Tromsø, Norway
Bone and joint research group, Institute of Clinical Medicine, Faculty of Health Sciences, University of Tromsø, Tromsø, Norway

Inigo Zubiaurre-Martinez
Bone and joint research group, Institute of Clinical Medicine, Faculty of Health Sciences, University of Tromsø, Tromsø, Norway

Yngve Figenschau
Department of Laboratory Medicine, University Hospital of North Norway, Tromsø, Norway
Endocrinology Research Group, Institute of Clinical Medicine, Faculty of Health Sciences, University of Tromsø, Tromsø, Norway
Department of Medical Biology, Faculty of Health Sciences, University of Tromsø, Tromsø, Norway

Chenglei Liu, Liping Si and Weiwu Yao
Department of Radiology, Shanghai Jiao Tong University Affiliated Sixth People's Hospital, Shanghai, China

Chang Liu, Xvhua Ren and Qian Wang
Med-X Research Institute, School of Biomedical Engineering, Shanghai Jiao Tong University, Shanghai, China

Hao Shen
Department of Joint Surgery, Shanghai Jiao Tong University Affiliated Sixth People's Hospital, Shanghai, China

Index

www.ingramcontent.com/pod-product-compliance
Lightning Source LLC
Chambersburg PA
CBHW082021190326
41458CB00010B/3235
* 9 7 8 1 6 3 2 4 1 5 3 9 4 *